Concepts of Artificial Intelligence and Its Application in Modern Healthcare Systems

This reference text presents the usage of artificial intelligence in healthcare and discusses the challenges and solutions of using advanced techniques like wearable technologies and image processing in the sector.

Features:

- Focuses on the use of artificial intelligence (AI) in healthcare with issues, applications, and prospects
- Presents the application of artificial intelligence in medical imaging, fractionalization of early lung tumour detection using a low intricacy approach, etc.
- Discusses an artificial intelligence perspective on wearable technology
- Analyses cardiac dynamics and assessment of arrhythmia by classifying heartbeat using electrocardiogram (ECG)
- Elaborates machine learning models for early diagnosis of depressive mental affliction

This book serves as a reference for students and researchers analyzing healthcare data. It can also be used by graduate and post-graduate students as an elective course.

Concepts of Artificial Intelligence and Its Application in Modern Healthcare Systems

Edited by
Deepshikha Agarwal
Khushboo Tripathi
Kumar Krishen

CRC Press
Taylor & Francis Group
Boca Raton London New York

CRC Press is an imprint of the
Taylor & Francis Group, an **informa** business

Front cover image: Have a nice day Photo/Shutterstock

First edition published 2024
by CRC Press
6000 Broken Sound Parkway NW, Suite 300, Boca Raton, FL 33487-2742

and by CRC Press
4 Park Square, Milton Park, Abingdon, Oxon, OX14 4RN

CRC Press is an imprint of Taylor & Francis Group, LLC

© 2024 selection and editorial matter, Deepshikha Agarwal, Khushboo Tripathi and Kumar Krishen; individual chapters, the contributors

Library of Congress Cataloging-in-Publication Data
Names: Agarwal, Deepshikha, editor. | Tripathi, Khushboo, editor. | Krishen, Kumar, editor.
Title: Concepts of artificial intelligence and its application in modern healthcare systems / edited by Deepshikha Agarwal, Khushboo Tripathi, Kumar Krishen.
Description: First edition. | Boca Raton : Chapman & Hall/CRC Press, 2024. | Includes bibliographical references. |
Identifiers: LCCN 2023000905 (print) | LCCN 2023000906 (ebook) | ISBN 9781032361550 (hardback) | ISBN 9781032366456 (paperback) | ISBN 9781003333081 (ebook)
Subjects: LCSH: Artificial intelligence--Medical applications. | Medical care--Technological innovations.
Classification: LCC R859.7.A78 C655 2023 (print) | LCC R859.7.A78 (ebook) |
DDC 362.10285--dc23/eng/20230419
LC record available at https://lccn.loc.gov/2023000905
LC ebook record available at https://lccn.loc.gov/2023000906

ISBN: 978-1-032-36155-0 (hbk)
ISBN: 978-1-032-36645-6 (pbk)
ISBN: 978-1-003-33308-1 (ebk)

DOI: 10.1201/9781003333081

Typeset in Times
by MPS Limited, Dehradun

Contents

Preface

This book on Concepts of Artificial Intelligence and Its Application in Modern Healthcare Systems captures the use of AI in today's healthcare scenario. The book's material focuses on applications and challenges in relevant areas. The work is the result of our effort to put together a representative collection of chapters covering most advanced techniques and development in the healthcare domain. The chapter contents are listed according to the book's theme. The contents are explained in the application area where AI is applicable in medical and different technologies. This approach also helps readers to find the advances in healthcare areas together with technologies. The chapters include introductory contents in addition to the chapter introduction. The history and evolution of healthcare technology states that healthcare is in demand and a top priority today. Hence, the chapters have been collected and presented in the book. A more efficient and practical aspect of implementation of AI techniques should be further enhanced and applied in the healthcare area.

The book is intended for, and inclined to, researchers, students, and academicians, as well as developers and industry parties in multidisciplinary areas. The editors of the book envision the numerous problems and their solutions in the healthcare area and believe that this book provides ample references for improving the quality in a course of healthcare technology.

The editors sincerely thank all contributors who have agreed to present their work in our book. They are also grateful to the reviewers whose helpful remarks ensured the quality of the authors' presented work. Special thanks to Ms. Jubi and Ms. Isha for their invaluable collaborations in making this book a reality.

About the Authors

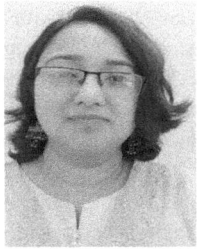

Dr. Deepshikha Agarwal, is currently working as Head of Department and Assistant Professor at the Indian Institute of Information Technology, Lucknow. She has more than 17 years of teaching and research experience. She published more than 40 research papers and guided projects in the fields of mobile and adhoc communications, optimization algorithms, wireless sensor networks, IOT & Machine Learning and Blockchain. She achieved a Ph.D from MNNIT Allahabad in 2015 and an M.Tech degree from IIIT Allahabad in 2004, with research work on wireless sensor networks. She is also guiding projects and Ph.D candidates.

She achieved membership in various professional bodies, including IEEE, IET, PcPro, and Oxford Journals. She is an active reviewer for reputed conferences and journals such as IEEE Sensors, IEEE Access, Science Direct, and Elsevier. She is an invited Speaker for International Conferences held in China and Japan, editor of CRC published book and chairman of sessions in international conferences. She is registered as an accomplished international author in the Scholar's book of world records. She has published several book chapters and books in international publishing houses like John Wiley and CRC. She received the University Grant from Amity University for presenting a research paper in IEEE at a Conference at Indonesia. She has recently been granted two innovation patents by the Australian government. She is also the receipient of several prestigious awards, including Swami Vivekanand changemaker award & Rise & Shine Women Eduvisionary Award by MentorX and International Academic Achievers Award (Excellent in Professional Achievement), JYD International School of Higher Education, Zurich, Switzerland in 2021.

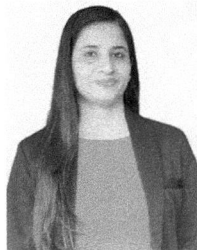

Dr. Khushboo Tripathi received a Ph.D in computer science from the University of Allahabad, Prayagraj, India in 2012. She received a Master of Science in Computer Science & Engineering from KNIT Sultanpur, M. Sc. (Mathematics) and B.Sc. from University of Allahabad, Prayagraj. She has more than 15 years of experience in teaching and research. Dr. Tripathi's interests include research and implementation aspects of wireless ad-hoc networks, MANET and SENSOR networks, secure routing protocols, SDN, advanced networking, security, and data interpretation. Dr. Tripathi has authored more than 30 papers and published in peer-reviewed international journals and conferences proceedings. Dr. Tripathi has authored various book chapters in scopus and science journals. She has supervised many Ph.D., M. Tech., MCA and B. Tech students in their thesis and other projects. She has served as session chair and organiser for IEEE, Springer conferences. Currently, she is serving as Assistant Professor in Department of Computer Science & Engineering at Amity University Haryana Gurgaon. Dr. Tripathi has been a reviewer for several international journals. She has earned many awards in her credits as a young researcher, including an award by InSc Bengaluru, India, Swami Vivekanand changemaker award by MENTORx Globally, and best paper presentation awards at AUH. Dr. Tripathi is a member of ACM, IEEE, IET U.K. and computer societies.

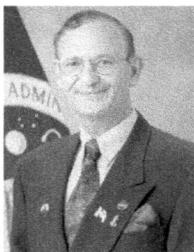

Dr. Kumar Krishen is the Chief Technologist at The Krishen Foundation, USA; Adjunct Professor, University of Houston, USA; Honorary Professor, Delhi Technological University, India; Adjunct Faculty, Indian Institute of Information Technology, Lucknow, India; and Honorary Distinguished Professor, Amity University, Haryana, India. Dr. Kumar Krishen has supported space exploration since January 1965 and was with NASA in various capacities from February 1976 to September 2018. Dr. Krishen has served as an Innovation Champion and ST/Chief Technologist for NASA Johnson Space Center (JSC) and represented JSC as the Principal Technologist on the NASA Council on Science and Technology. Dr. Krishen served at Virginia Tech as a University Fellow for Technology Transfer, Office of Special Initiatives, and Visiting Professor on a special NASA assignment. He has also served as an Adjunct Professor at Rice University. Authoring more than 170 technical papers/reports/proceedings, Dr. Krishen is a Fellow of the Society for Design and Process Science (SDPS), a Fellow and Distinguished Speaker of the Institution of Electronics and Telecommunication Engineers (IETE), and an Associate Fellow of the American Institute of Aeronautics and Astronautics (AIAA). Dr. Krishen's academic degrees are from Kansas State University (Ph.D. and M.S. – Phi Kappa Phi, Eta Kappa Nu & Sigma Xi honors), Calcutta University (M. Tech and B. Tech – Gold & Silver Medals), and Jammu and Kashmir University (B.A. – Highest University Merit) in electronics, electrical engineering, radio physics, physics, and mathematics. Dr. Krishen received the NASA Exceptional Service Medal in September 2018, recognizing his exceptional and sustained service to NASA and the United States in the realm of technological advancements in support of Human Spaceflight.

Contributors

Ayad Alkaim
Department of Computer Science Faculty
of Science for Women (SCIW)
University of Babylon
Babylon, Iraq

Pallavi Asthana
Amity University
Uttar Pradesh, India

Robin Kumar Attri
Department of Computer Science
School of Engineering and Technology
K.R. Mangalam University
Gurugram, India

B. Rajalingam
Department of Computer Science and
Engineering
St. Martin's Engineering College
Secunderabad, Telangana, India

N. Boroday
Institute for Problems of Cryobiology and
Cryomedicine of the National Academy of
Sciences of Ukraine
Ukraine

Vijayaraghavan M. Chariar
CRDT, IIT Delhi
New Delhi, India

Sarika Chaudhary
DPGITM Gurgaon
India

Rekha Devi
Chandigarh University
Mohali

Cheekireddy Dhamini
Sri Ramachandra Institute of Higher Education
and Research
Chennai, India

Vandana Dubey
Ashoka Institute of Technology and
Management
Varanasi, Uttar Pradesh, India

Juhi Dwivedi
Amity University
Uttar Pradesh, India

Jayanthi Ganapathy
Sri Ramachandra Institute of Higher Education
and Research
Chennai, India

K. Golubeva
Taras Shevchenko National University of Kyiv
Ukraine

Kartikey Gupta
Banaras Hindu University
Varanasi, Uttar Pradesh, India

Swati Gupta
Associate Professor
Centre of Excellence
Department of Computer Science
School of Engineering and Technology
K.R. Mangalam University
Gurugram, India

Bramah Hazela
Amity University
Uttar Pradesh, India

Jaiswal Dhirendra
Department of Nuclear Medicine
All India Institute of Medical Sciences
Raipur, Chhattisgarh, India

Samaher Al-Janabi
Department of Computer Science Faculty
of Science for Women (SCIW)
University of Babylon
Babylon, Iraq

Hemalatha Karnan
School of Chemical and Biotechnology
SASTRA
Thanjavur

Jyoti Singh Kirar
Banaras Hindu University
Varanasi, Uttar Pradesh, India

D. Klyushin
Taras Shevchenko National University of Kyiv
Ukraine

O. Kravets
Taras Shevchenko National University of Kyiv
Ukraine

Rahul Ramanathan Krishnamoorthy
University of Illinois Urbana
Champaign, IL, USA

Priti Kumari
Ashoka Institute of Technology and
    Management
Varanasi, Uttar Pradesh, India

Thanushree Latha A. S.
School of Chemical and
    Biotechnology
SASTRA
Thanjavur

Ameer M
Department of Computer Science
Faculty of Science for Women (SCIW)
University of Babylon
Babylon, Iraq

Pranav M.
School of Chemical and Biotechnology
SASTRA
Thanjavur

G. R. Mishra
Dr. Ram Manohar Lohia Avadh University
Faizabad, Uttar Pradesh, India

Shweta Mongia
MRIIRS Faridabad

Prince Nagpal
Banaras Hindu University
Varanasi, Uttar Pradesh, India

P. Deepan
Department of Computer Science
    and Engineering
St. Peter's Engineering College
Hyderabad, Telangana, India

P. Santosh Kumar Patra
Department of Computer Science
    and Engineering
St. Martin's Engineering College
Secunderabad, Telangana, India

Nisarg C. Patel
APMC College of Pharmaceutical Education &
    Research
College Campus, Motipura, Himatnagar
Gujarat Technological University
Gujarat, India

Beenkumar R. Prajapati
L.M. College of Pharmacy
Gujarat University
Gujarat, India

Bhupendra G. Prajapati
Shree S.K. Patel College of Pharmaceutical
    Education & Research
Ganpat University
Gujarat, India

Jigna B. Prajapati
Acharya Motibhai Institute of Computer
    Application
Ganpat University
Ganpat, Gujarat, India

Medha Raghavendra Prasad
Sri Ramachandra Institute of Higher Education
    and Research
Chennai, India

R. Santhoshkumar
Department of Computer Science and
    Engineering
St. Martin's Engineering College
Secunderabad, Telangana, India

Unnati Rastogi
Banaras Hindu University
Varanasi, Uttar Pradesh, India

Sapna M. Rathod
APMC College of Pharmaceutical Education &
    Research
College Campus, Motipura, Himatnagar
Gujarat Technological University
Gujarat, India

Sehrawat Abhishek
Chitkara School of Health Sciences
Chitkara University
Rajpura, Punjab, India

and

Department of Radiodiagnosis and Imaging
All India Institute of Medical Sciences
Bhopal, Madhya Pradesh, India

Nayankumar C. Ratnakar
L.M. College of Pharmacy
Gujarat University
Gujarat, India

Chandra Mani Sharma
CRDT, IIT Delhi
New Delhi, India

Sugandha Sharma
UPES Dehradun

Utpal Shrivastava
Chitkara University School of Engineering and
    Technology
Badi, Solan, Himachal Pradesh, India

Balwinder Singh
Centre for Development of Advanced
    Computing
Mohali

Mandeep Singh
Centre for Development of Advanced
    Computing
Mohali

O. P. Singh
Amity School of Engineering & Technology
Amity University
Lucknow, Uttar Pradesh, India

Pawan Singh
Department of Computer Science &
    Engineering
Amity School of Engineering and
    Technology
Amity University
Lucknow, Uttar Pradesh, India

Shikha Singh
Department of Computer Science &
    Engineering
Amity School of Engineering &
    Technology
Lucknow Amity University
Uttar Pradesh, India

Sudarshan Singh
Department of Chemistry
Faculty of Science
Chulalongkorn University
Bangkok, Thailand

Vineet Singh
Amity University
Uttar Pradesh, India

Aunu Singhal
SRM Institute of Science and Technology
Delhi NCR Campus
Ghaziabad, Uttar Pradesh, India

Shweta Sinha
Department of CSE
Amity University
Gurgaon, Haryana, India

Prateek Singhal
Department of Computer Science &
    Engineering
Sagar Institute of Research
    Technology-Excellence
Bhopal, Madhya Pradesh, India

Garima Srivastava
Department of Computer Science &
  Engineering
Amity School of Engineering & Technology
Lucknow Amity University
Uttar Pradesh, India

Prabhat Kumar Srivastava
Department of Computer Science &
  Engineering
IMS Ghaziabad
Uttar Pradesh, India

Rishikesh Swaminathan
Sri Ramachandra Institute of Higher Education
  and Research
Chennai, India

Vikas Thada
Department of CSE
Poornima University Jaipur
Rajasthan, India

Khushboo Tripathi
Department of Computer Science &
  Engineering
Amity University
Haryana, India

Milind Udbhav
Department of Computer Science
School of Engineering and Technology
K.R. Mangalam University
Gurugram, India

Meenu Vijarania
Centre of Excellence
Department of Computer Science
School of Engineering and Technology
K.R. Mangalam University
Gurugram, India

Animesh Singh Yadav
Department of Computer Science &
  Engineering
Amity School of Engineering & Technology
Lucknow Amity University
Uttar Pradesh, India

1 Artificial Intelligence (AI) in Healthcare
Issues, Applications, and Future

Sarika Chaudhary
DPGITM Gurgaon

Sugandha Sharma
UPES Dehradun

Shweta Mongia
MRIIRS Faridabad

Khushboo Tripathi
Amity University Haryana

CONTENTS

DOI: 10.1201/9781003333081-1

1.1 INTRODUCTION

In artificial intelligence (AI), "artificial" refers to objects that are made or produced by humans rather than occurring naturally, and "intelligence" refers to the ability to form tactics to achieve goals by interacting with an information-rich environment. In other words, AI is a broad term that refers to any technique that allows computers to simulate human intelligence through the use of logic [1]. In the twenty-first century, AI has gotten a lot of attention and applications, although its origins are far older. Since the stone era, humanity has progressed at an exponential rate. Because of the massive growth in the population, difficulties caused by such pressure have also increased. People today are dying at a far higher rate from cancer, mental problems, and depression, or as a result of modernised warfare. Humanity underwent many biological alterations over time to become what it is now. Such alterations, as well as the expanding human chain, have resulted in significant variances in specific human genes, resulting in a variety of physiological, psychological, and biological differences. In addition, as population clusters with various races of people develop, space accommodation has resulted in a vast junction of animal and human territory, which has led to many outbreaks and pandemics. Humans have been known to turn to prayers in the past, but this has changed as people have discovered medical characteristics in natural substances, and now modern technology, designed medications, and new procedures have replaced them [2]. The quantity of exposure of live beings to invisible rays that cannot be felt but can travel through our bodies varies depending on geography and technological support. Some of them have the power to wreak havoc on our DNA, resulting in genetic abnormalities that can spread to future generations or simply harm our health.

Even though we have the resources for treatment, we can't always fight nature, which is why so many people die every day. But, instead of relying on traditional ways, what if we focused on individualised or automated therapies, assisted surgeries, personalised lifestyle recommendations, and, most importantly, preventing such diseases in individuals? We don't need any psychic abilities to accomplish this goal, thanks to technological advancements. Imagine people predicting ailments your unborn child would acquire in the future by merely looking at your genes, allowing you enough time to consider methods, treatments, or even having a child when adoption seems more compassionate. Genetic profiling may be the solution. All of these new technologies go under the umbrella of artificial intelligence, a notion that was first envisioned in the mid-1990s and is still transforming the world every day, with a slew of new capabilities awaiting release until hardware issues are resolved [3].

AI simply refers to a machine's ability to think and act rationally and practically like a person. It is now aimed at automating basic tasks that need basic human intellect, such as computing, analysing, and predicting or recommending actions, among other things. AI could help doctors better manage patient pathways or treatment strategies, as well as provide them with practically all the information they need to make outstanding healthcare and medical decisions [4]. AI has already established itself in several fields of healthcare, and it is only beginning to change things radically, starting with the creation of treatment strategies and progressing through the automation of repetitive tasks through medication administration and drug research. Since the world has gone digital, mountains of data are awaiting analysis. Every day, a large amount of data is generated in healthcare as well. Patients' medical histories, eating habits, geographic location, and other factors can all be examined using modern algorithms. Various authorities and institutes are using large datasets containing medical records to anticipate probable diseases that may be on the rise in a specific area. Animal populations and their environs can be studied to forecast epidemics, and outbreaks can be tracked to determine their origin, clusters, routes, and mutations. People might be immediately reminded of their upcoming check-ups and appointments. Individuals can be advised to take a vaccination course based on their area and other factors. A genetic test can aid in the identification of defective/abnormal genes that can be used to forecast genetic disorders, as well as susceptibility to a specific disease or strain. Lifestyles can also be examined to determine if any issues could lead to the development of other diseases.

Doctors don't have to memorize nearly as much information as they did 50 years ago. AI is prepared to take this reality to the next level. The time spent on "thinking" is getting into a position to consider, make a choice, or research something. Much more time was spent finding or obtaining information than processing it. To get the data into a comparable format, it took more than a few hours of calculation. When they were in comparable form, it took only a few seconds to decide. As AI advances, it will be able to increase the energy of a person's thinking in three key areas: advanced computation, statistical analysis, and hypothesis development [5]. These three areas correspond to three distinct AI waves. Specialists typically monitor more than 50 patients each day, which can be a great degree of debilitating thinking when considering the amount of notice and information required for each individual. Unlike a doctor, AI is unaffected by the number of patients, the length of the workday, or task redundancy. AI assists doctors in assessing a patient's health risk and then applying intelligence to not only improve the quality of care but also to monitor and advise patients on the adverse effects of specific medications.

The influence of AI across the globe is troubling, with technologically advanced tools providing enhanced decision-making, disease discovery, and management of chronic and acute illnesses. Doctors and other medical professionals use AI to diagnose patients more accurately and quickly. In medicine, AI employs arithmetical algorithms as well as data science from the human body to create diagnoses that are superior to those made by doctors. This allows professionals to take immediate action in the case of disorders that could otherwise develop seriously. Healthcare systems must be viewed as a collection of heterogeneous, distributed, and omnipresent systems that speak different languages, integrate medical devices, and are personalized by different entities, which were set by people living in different situations and pursuing different aims. As a result, architecture has been designed to support medical uses in the form of an organization for the integration, dispersal, and archiving of medical data and the electronic medical record, in the shape of a web spider of the intelligent information-processing system, its main subsystems, their functional roles, and the flow of information and control among them, with modifiable autonomy. The quality of service will be improved with such web-based simulated systems. In the field of healthcare, artificial intelligence is being used in a variety of ways. Keeping track of medical records and data management is the most visible application of artificial intelligence in healthcare. This tracking involves getting it together, storing it, standardizing it, and tracking its lineage. It is the first step toward transforming the available healthcare systems. Recently, Google's AI research arm, Google DeepMind Health, launched its Google DeepMind Health project, which mines medical statistics to provide incredibly good and timely health services [6].

Data management is the most widely used application of artificial intelligence and digital automation in healthcare since accumulating and evaluating data is a necessary step. To provide faster, more consistent access, robots collect, store, re-layout, and trace data. The amount of health data that is currently available has increased over the last decade. Every day, large amounts of data (patient information, diagnosis information, new research discoveries, and so on) are generated in the healthcare industry. The use of big data and analytical tools has helped organizations gain the insights needed to collaborate more efficiently with patients and make better decisions; from cutting costs to streamlining hospital staff schedules, enabling remote patient monitoring to anticipate epidemics, and this reliance on big data and storing it has been growing noticeably [7]. AI is an area of computer science and technology that deals with the modelling of intelligent behaviour in computer systems. Combining the power of AI with the experience, information, and human interaction of clinicians will improve the high quality of patient care while simultaneously lowering its cost. AI can be used to examine data from entire patient populations to find new evidence and select high-quality healthcare practices. Performing routine tasks analysing tests, x-rays, CT scans, data entry, and other routine tasks are all part of the job.

1.2 REVOLUTIONS OF ARTIFICIAL INTELLIGENCE (AI) IN MEDICAL FIELD

AI improves the quality of care while simultaneously increasing the productivity and efficiency of care. In the sphere of healthcare, artificial intelligence is anticipated to rise from $2.1 billion to $36.1 billion by 2025, with a CAGR of 50.2 percent. Machine learning (ML) plays an important role in the development of innovative medical treatments for treatment. ML is also used to keep track of the patient's data and to administer treatment. Hospitals in the medical field have acknowledged the need to be digitalised and are integrating into administrative processes as time passes and the construction of digital India takes place. Finland, Germany, the United Kingdom, Israel, China, and the United States are some of the countries that are heavily investing in AI research [5].

Medical advancements are now being driven by ML in domains such as pharmaceuticals and vaccines, medical devices, medical imaging, and radio genomics. This process can result in a healthcare system that is both cost-effective and patient-centered. The main hurdle for AI is ensuring their use in regular clinical practise. On a large scale, AI will not replace human clinicians; rather, it will supplement their efforts to care for patients.

- **Inventions of AI**
  - In 2017, an artificial intelligence-assisted surgery was performed to suture constricted blood arteries. This research was carried out at the Maastricht University Medical Centre in the Netherlands.
  - A report published by Stanford University in 2017 described the successful application of AL algorithms to detect skin cancer [7].
  - In China, a robot passed the medical licensing exam in 2017, and this robot takes and analyses patient data autonomously. The robot gathers basic information and directs you to an actual doctor who is ready to begin therapy right away. This direction means that the robot does not replace doctors, but rather assists doctors and patients in providing faster and more precise care.
  - Robot doctors (dentists) are considerably superior to human dentists since they can work independently and more efficiently. A dental implant can be performed by the robot without any errors. In 2018, this transition occurred in China. The staff was just in charge of supervising the implant robot.
  - Leonardo da Vinci Si is a surgical robot that performs operations. It improves its technology in the future by using knowledge from previous procedures. It includes 3D cameras and surgical equipment that mimic the movements of the operating surgeon.
  - Deep-learning algorithms identified 23 patients who were at a higher risk of cardiovascular disease. Intel worked on this with the Scripps Research Institute in California [5].
  - According to a study, AI using deep learning was able to diagnose breast cancer at a higher rate than medical personnel. With the use of machine-learning technology, Path AI is assisting pathologists in making more accurate diagnoses. This system has also worked with pharmaceutical companies.
  - Atomize employs artificial intelligence to combat major diseases such as Ebola and multiple sclerosis. This use aids in the prediction of bioactivity and the identification of patient features for clinical studies [5].
- **Advantages of Artificial Intelligence (AI) in Field of Healthcare**
  - Increase productivity: the treatment and check-up procedure is rapidly accelerating. In a recent interview, Dr. Kevin Sandeman stated that AI systems can diagnose at a faster rate than humans.
  - Improved diagnosis accuracy: AI improves analytical accuracy and reduces bias.
  - Improve patient outcomes: AI benefits patients by improving treatment efficacy, reducing the number of needless surgeries, and improving the quality of services provided to them [8].

- According to Dr. Tuomas Mirtti, AI can make quick decisions and solve issues more precisely and quickly than humans.

1.3 APPLICATION AREAS OF AI IN HEALTHCARE

AI has incredibly expanded the healthcare sector in past decades. AI applications have been applied to unveil information and assist healthcare providers in a wide range of clinical tasks, like assistance with case triage, enhanced image scanning and segmentation, supported decision making, integration and improvement of workflow, disease risk prediction, patient appointment scheduling, and treatment tracking. However, the applications of AI technology to disease detection, cancer patient screening, therapy selection, reducing medication errors and productivity improvement is now creating its way [8].

Furthermore, COVID-19 has created tremendous chaos around the world, affecting people's lives and causing a large number of deaths. In such a situation, AI application to COVID- 19 has increased, especially to the medical-imaging data, screening positive cases, predictive and analytical model in decision making, treatment planning, prediction of future cases, and vaccine development. AI technology has already shown its potential to track the spread of COVID- 19, as well as satisfy high-risk patients. It has also shown vast effectiveness in predicting real-time infection rates by adequately analysing the previous data [8]. It is noticeable that AI platforms such as Bluedot Global have predicted the COVID- 19 cases before the cases started from China.

There are different ways to build AI systems for healthcare, i.e., find healthcare problems to apply AI solutions without due consideration to the local context. Hence, when establishing an AI system in healthcare, it is important not to replace the principal elements of human interaction in medicine but to focus on those interactions and improve their efficiency and effectiveness. Moreover, AI innovation in healthcare will come through in-depth, human-centered understanding of the complexity of patient journey and care pathway [8]. Figure 1.1 illustrates application area of AI in healthcare and medicines.

1.3.1 PATIENT CARE

One of the biggest benefits of AI is to help people stay fit and healthy so they don't need a doctor, or not at least as often. AI has increased the ability for healthcare professionals to clearly understand day-to-day patient needs, and with that understanding, they are able to judge, provide feedback, and support for staying healthy. Babylon Health provides relevant information on health and triage based on symptoms explained by the patient [10].

- **Jvion:** Identifying hidden patient risk across various diseases and if the risk trajectory can be changed to a positive outcome [11].
- **Wellframe:** Wellframe delivers interactive-care programs directly to patients on mobile devices. Clinical portfolio based on evidence-based care enables the care team to provide a personalized experience for any patient [12].
- **GNS Healthcare:** The company uses machine learning to reveal the driver of disease progression and how patients respond to drugs [13].
- **Zakipoint Healthcare:** The company displays all relevant health-related data at the member level on the dashboard to understand healthcare expenses and population risk and how to mitigate these risks [14].

For pregnant women, early identification and management of risk are essential to provide them with early treatments. 'SAFER' is a risk assessment and risk management approach that has been developed to assess antenatal risk and develop a comprehensive clinical management plan.

- Assisted or automated diagnosis & prescription
- Real time case prioritization and triage
- Personalized medications and care
- Patient data analytics
- Pregnancy Management

Diagnostic error prevention •
Medical imaging insights •
Early diagnosis •

PATIENT CARE

MEDICAL IMAGING AND DIAGNOSTIC

(Ai) **IN** HEALTHCARE

RESEARCH & DEVELOPMENT

MANAGEMENT

- Drug discovery
- Gene analytics and editing
- Device and drug comparative effectiveness

Market research •
Pricing and risk •
Brand management and marketing •

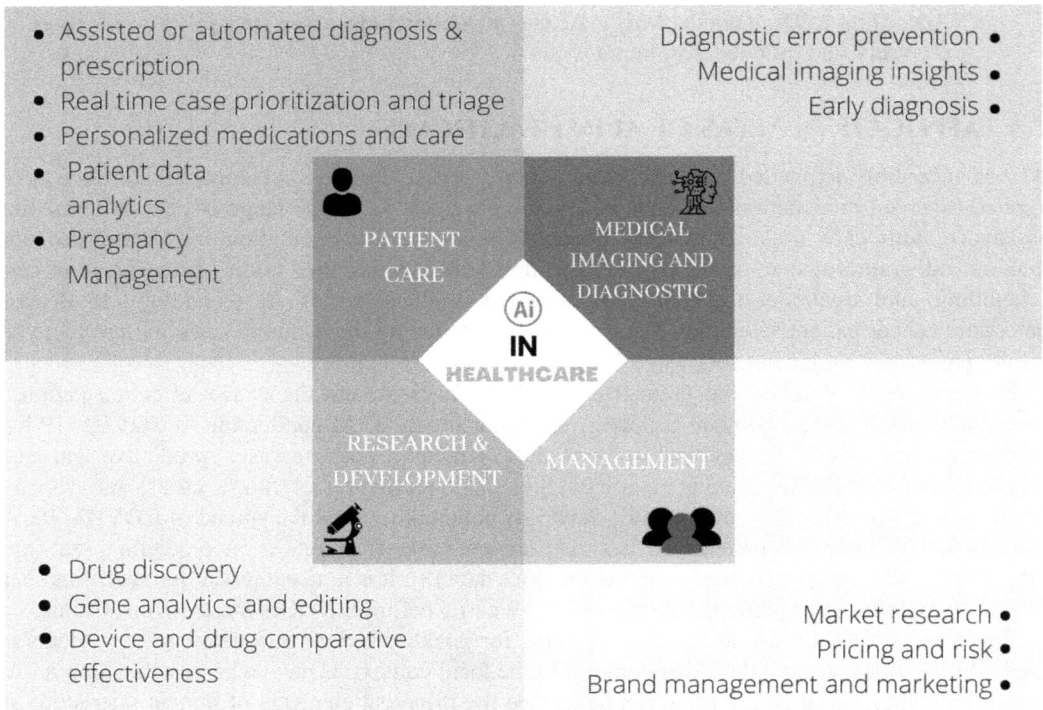

FIGURE 1.1   Areas where AI is used in healthcare and medicine [9].

1.3.2 Medical Imaging and Diagnostic

The bulk of medical data that is associated with each patient in today's healthcare system is staggering and increasing every day. Though the doctors and medical personnel are extremely knowledgeable and well trained, they are like other human beings who can make mistakes in absence of adequate data. So AI is helping to make more accurate diagnoses at a faster rate while reducing cost. Advanced medical imaging helps precisely analyse and transform images and model possible situations [10].

- **SkinVision:** SkinVision enables to the assessment of skin spots and common skin cancer by taking photos of skin from phones and sending risk indications by the clinical validation technology within 30 seconds.
- **MammoScreen:** MammoScreen with mammography to aid breast cancer detection. The system is designed to identify the suspicious spots for breast cancer on 2D digital mammograms and assess their likelihood of malignancy.

In recent years, AI is widely used in diagnosing COVID-19 cases and identifying patients with ventilator support. Huiying Medical, a company in China, has developed an AI-based medical-imaging system solution with 96% accuracy.

1.3.3 Research and Development

Drug research and development is one of the recent applications of AI in healthcare. New drugs are discovered based on previous data and medical intelligence [15].

- **NuMedii:** NuMedii is a biopharma company that discovers de-risk effective new drugs by translating life science big data and AI into therapies. The company has built a technology AIDD (Artificial Intelligence of Drug Discovery) that uses big data and AI to discover connections between drugs and diseases.

Genome editing in AI is very powerful. AI in genetics is used to identify harmful genes and treatment of diseases. Gene editing has the ability to cut out disease-causing genes. CRISPR (clustered regularly interspaced short palindromic repeat) can edit deoxyribonucleic acid with remarkable precision.

- **4Quant:** The company utilizes big data and deep-learning technology to extract meaningful, actionable information from images and videos for experiment design to help pick and choose which components make the most sense for the needs.

1.3.4 Healthcare Management

Healthcare management is creating an optimal market strategy for a brand based on market perception and target segment.

- **Healing:** The company's Migraine Buddy is an advanced migraine reporting and tracking application. The application has recorded terabytes of data that help patients, doctors, and researchers better understand the cause and effect of neurological disorders.

Process automation technologies such as intelligent automation and RPA helps hospitals automate routine reporting. Customer service chatbots help patients' clear queries regarding bill payments, appointments, and medication refill. Patients may make false claims leveraging AI-powered fraud-detection tools that can help hospital managers to identify fraudsters. There are too many possible AI use cases in healthcare to be listed here, and they can be identified by the practitioners. A machine-learning-based solution can be built in areas where significant training data is available, and the problem statement can be formulated in a clear way [16].

1.3.5 Artificial Intelligence in Statistical Analysis

AI has exploded in popularity in a variety of fields and regions during the previous decade. Unsurprisingly, healthcare is one of the industries that has been transformed by artificial intelligence. While companies have broadened their applications of artificial intelligence, the fundamental application of AI remains in high demand: data analysis and prediction. With so many technical breakthroughs, storage and processing technologies have grown in their own right, allowing infrastructures to keep a digital footprint or record of everything they've done in the past. Logs aren't the only thing that's being saved now that storage isn't an issue. People's responses and medical histories, as well as test results, symptoms, medication, medication response, genetical constitution, and other information, are collected anonymously or not, freely or not, to keep track of everything related to healthcare. People have created numerous innovative methods to analyse this massive mountain of data and draw meaningful conclusions as technology has progressed. To maintain a deployable dataset, private organisations or the government may record all data from hospitals or clinics [16].

1.3.5.1 Pharmaceutical Use

Response to drugs is one example of where statistical analysis has been shown to be beneficial. People willingly participate in surveys in which their medical records, including tests and progress, are kept to determine the efficacy of a treatment or procedure against a specific medical problem.

The public can learn about any recurring pattern of symptoms, depending on location, gender, food habits, culture, and other factors, as well as the effectiveness of a particular prescription in people classified into various groups and their treatment progress. Once completed, it is easy to determine if a certain population is segregated on any possible criteria for the majority of the population, which improves treatment efficiency. Studies can be carried out to see if there is a link between symptoms and lifestyle, culture, or geography, and this information can then be utilised to map the condition accordingly.

1.3.5.2   Outbreak Prevention and Tracking

Data capturing a strange or novel symptom in a region progressively moving across the vicinities can be used to detect illness outbreaks, their origins, symptoms, impacts, and, most crucially, the pattern and pace with which they travel. This detection can save a lot of lives since it enables governments, healthcare organisations, and pharmaceutical companies, both worldwide and locally, to be prepared for a potential epidemic and begin working on determining the reason and root of the problem to create a defence. This ability was demonstrated in the last pandemic, where scientists and health organisations predicted the speed and scope of infection, the appearance of new variations due to mutation, their origin, symptoms, and path every day. This ability has saved lives since people were aware of the scope of the harm and were prepared for it. The same method was utilised to discover patterns, which aided in the discovery of any potential medicine or vaccination adverse effects that may or may not affect people depending on their lifestyles, age, or geographic region. This made it possible to build a working vaccination with minimal side effects in a short amount of time, which would not have been conceivable in the past [16]. This enabled super-quick vaccine development and manufacture, which would not have been possible without statistical analysis of volunteer responses to prototypes.

1.3.5.3   Genetics

It's also employed in the field of analysing the recurrence/susceptibility of a given disease in persons who share specific genes. Genetic illnesses can be inherited through a lengthy family history, and blood tests are often ineffective in detecting them. People rely on symptoms to determine whether they have a genetic disease that is incurable. People can now use artificial intelligence to discover defective genes even before a child is born by looking at the genetic makeup of the child's parents, and so prevent a child's quality of life from deteriorating. Identification of specific genes among millions of genes necessitates extensive investigation. People can also use AI to map probable genetic diseases or abnormalities in people all over the world based on their geographical birthplace, ancestry, race, and other factors.

It is fair to conclude that all of these, as well as a slew of additional AI benefits, have aided in improving the quality of life through greater preparedness and responsiveness. So much data and data analysis tools have aided individuals and organisations in doing research, seeing trends, learning and understanding the causes, and inventing treatments and techniques. As a result of these capabilities, our healthcare business is making rapid progress and assisting people in surviving ailments that were once thought to be fatal.

1.4   USE IN THE DEVELOPMENT OF MEDICINE AND VACCINES

The drug development process begins with existing data gathered from a variety of sources, including high-throughput compound and fragment screening, computer modelling, and publicly available information. AI is employed in many areas of the pharmaceutical business, including medication development and discovery. It decreases human workload and allows for the achievement of goals in a short time. AI can also help with decision-making and determining the best treatment for a patient.

It will provide the healthcare business a huge boost because they can now produce more and more efficiently in less time, and vaccines can be manufactured in less time with fewer drawbacks. Machine-learning models learn to discover patterns from a large number of training instances that would be impossible for a human to remember. However, using AIML technology is a difficult task because, first and foremost, we must feed and save all data to the machine, and then train it according to that data, which can be difficult at times, and we must conduct numerous trials to ensure that it is remembered. Additionally, its maintenance costs are high and take a long time. However, in the end, it greatly aided us and saved us time. This method enabled the rapid development of the COVID-19 vaccine, which benefited the entire country.

1.4.1   CHALLENGES FACED IN DRUG DEVELOPMENT

Vaccine and medicine development can be a lengthy and laborious process due to the large amount of data available and the inability to recognise all previous trials, primarily due to the complexity of different people's immune systems and the various tasks involving fragment screening, computational modelling, and information from the literature. Another issue in drug research is increasing R&D efficiency, which is defined as the number of medications authorised by the FDA per billion dollars spent on R&D alone. That is why AI is the technology that can save all of the data and trials while also making them less expensive and more successful.

1.4.2   AI IN DRUG DEVELOPMENT

By reducing the number of produced compounds that are then tested in either an in vitro or in vivo system, AI systems can lower attrition rates and R&D costs. Validated artificial intelligence approaches can be utilised to improve drug development success rates; however, the AI techniques that are used in the development process must be validated before being applied to the drug development process.

The first step in the retrosynthesis process is to recursively and sequentially analyse the target compounds, breaking them down into small fragments or building blocks that can be easily purchased and prepared. The second stage is to figure out how these fragments will be converted into target molecules. Some technologies, such as SPiDER, which is based on AI and is used to forecast the molecular target of B-lapachone or other compounds, save development time. The process of drug repurposing becomes more appealing and practical using AI. The idea of adapting an existing therapeutic for a new disease has advantages because the new drug is qualified and can proceed directly to phase II trials for a different indication without having to go through phase I clinical trials and toxicology testing.

1.4.3   AI IN PATTERN RECOGNITION

Artificial intelligence aids in the development of vaccines that contain highly immunogenic viral components. Artificial intelligence can identify hit and lead compounds, allowing for faster validation of the vaccine target and therapeutic structure design optimization. AI can also forecast prospective toxicity risks, as well as possible synthetic routes for drug-like molecules, pharmalogical properties, protein characteristics, efficacy, drug combination and drug target connection.

The binding affinity of a medicine is measured using AI-based methods that conssider either the features or similarities of the drug and its target. Machine-learning algorithms were taught by the researchers to anticipate the intensity of viral fragments displayed on the human cell interface. Machine-learning techniques and predictive model software also aid in the discovery of target-specific virtual molecules and their connection with their particular targets, all while maximising safety and efficacy [17].

1.5 LIMITATION OF ARTIFICIAL INTELLIGENCE IN HEALTHCARE

AI depends on digital data, so inconsistencies in the availability and quality of data restrict the potential of AI. Also, significant computing power is required for the analysis of large and complex data sets. While many are enthusiastic about the possible uses of AI in the NHS, others point to the practical challenges, such as the fact that medical records are not consistently digitized across the NHS, and the lack of interoperability and standardization in NHS IT systems, digital recordkeeping, and data labelling [18]. There are questions about the extent to which patients and doctors are comfortable with digital sharing of personal health data [19]. Humans have attributes that AI systems might not be able to authentically possess, such as compassion [20]. Clinical practice often involves complex judgments and abilities that AI currently is unable to replicate, such as contextual knowledge and the ability to read social cues [21]. There is also debate about whether some human knowledge is tacit and cannot be taught [22]. Claims that AI will be able to display autonomy have been questioned on grounds that this is a property essential to being human and by definition cannot be held by a machine [9].

While AI offers a number of possible benefits, there also are several risks:

1.5.1 SECURITY CONCERNS

The prerequisite of enormous datasets means designers are motivated to gather such information from numerous patients. A few patients might be worried that this assortment might disregard their security, and claims have been documented dependent on information dividing among enormous wellbeing frameworks and AI developers [11]. AI could embroil protection in another manner: AI can foresee private data about patients despite the fact that the calculation never got that data. (To be sure, this is regularly the objective of medical services AI.) For example, an AI framework could possibly distinguish that an individual has Parkinson's infection dependent on the shaking of a PC mouse, regardless of whether the individual had never revealed that data to any other person (or didn't have a clue). Patients should seriously think about this as an infringement of their protection, particularly if the AI framework's surmising were accessible to outsiders, for example, banks or extra security organizations.

1.5.2 INFORMATION ACCESSIBILITY TRAINING

AI frameworks require a lot of information from sources, for example, electronic well-being records, drug store records, protection claims records, or purchaser-created data like wellness trackers or buying history. In any case, well-being information is regularly hazardous. Information is ordinarily divided across a wide range of frameworks. Indeed, even besides the assortment recently referenced, patients ordinarily see various suppliers and switch insurance agencies, prompting information split in different frameworks and numerous configurations. This discontinuity builds the danger of blunder, diminishes the breadth of datasets, and expands the cost of get-together information—which likewise restricts the sorts of elements that can foster successful medical care AI.

1.5.3 PREDISPOSITION AND IMBALANCE

There are risks, including inclination and disparity in medical care AI. Computer-based intelligence frameworks gain from the information on which they are prepared, and they can join predispositions from that information. For example, if the information accessible for AI is mainly accumulated in scholastic clinical focuses, the subsequent AI frameworks will think less about—and, along these lines, will treat less adequately—patients from populaces that don't normally visit scholarly clinical focuses. Essentially, if discourse acknowledgment AI frameworks are utilized to interpret experience notes, such AI might perform more regrettable when the supplier is of a race or sexual orientation underrepresented in preparing data.

1.5.4 WOUNDS AND BLUNDERS

The clearest danger is that AI frameworks will at times be off-base, and that patient injury or other medical care issues might result. On the off chance that an AI framework suggests some unacceptable medication for a patient, neglects to see cancer on a radiological sweep, or designates a clinic bed to one patient over another in light of the fact that it anticipated wrongly which patient would help more, the patient could be harmed. Obviously, numerous wounds happen because of clinical blunders in the medical care framework today, even without the association of AI. Simulated intelligence blunders are possibly unique for no less than two reasons. To begin with, patients and suppliers might respond contrastingly to wounds coming about because of programming than from human blunders. Second, if AI frameworks become broad, a basic issue in one AI framework may harm many patients—as opposed to the set number of patients harmed by any single supplier's mistake.

Most AI-based clinical gadgets exist as programming, and they are by and large new gadgets unique in relation to the conventional gadgets as far as administrative issues. Thus, new approaches should be set up to support and direct such gadgets. The International Medical Device Regulators Forum has sorted these AI programming planned to be utilized for clinical purposes as "Programming as a Medical Device (SaMD)" [13]. In the U.S., the Digital Health Unit was set up by the FDA's Center for Devices and Radiological Health in May 2017 to advance the skill in computerized medical services gadget endorsements and guidelines, and the FDA has reported the rules for SaMD in December 2017 [14]. The FDA recognizes that the current guidelines for conventional clinical gadgets are not reasonable for SaMDs that are quickly being developed and modified [23]. FDA has as of late fostered a Software Precertification Program, which empowers quicker advertising of SaMD through an engineer-focused affirmation pathway, not at all like the current pathway fixated on individual items. Makers who accomplished 'authoritative greatness' in this pathway can get an exclusion from premarket audits for generally safe items. Japan, as per the AI clinical improvement plans reported in 2018, is intending to make thorough principles overseeing the utilization of AI in clinical gadgets to limit the current AI clinical gadget-related debates and forestall the subsequent R&D hindrances [24]. Lastly, in Korea, the "Endorsement and Review Guidelines for Big Data and AI-based Medical Devices" and "Audit Guidelines for Clinical Effectiveness of AI-based Medical Devices" were declared in 2017, making them a portion of the primary AI-related endorsement rules in the world [25] However, the normalized survey file for the security and viability of AI-based clinical gadgets is as yet missing worldwide [26].

1.6 PREDICTIONS OF FUTURE ARTIFICIAL INTELLIGENCE (AI) IN HEALTHCARE

When we talk about artificial intelligence, we can't just treat it as one technology, but a collection of them. Most of these technologies are relevantly connected to the healthcare field, but the processes and the tasks they do vary widely. Looking at our current progress in AI, we can see that AI will play a very important role in the healthcare offerings of the future.

So, let's talk about some particular AI technologies of high importance to healthcare.

As we can see that the form of machine learning is the primary capability behind the development of precision medicine, agreed worldwide to be a sorely needed advance in healthcare. Although the current AI technology can't provide diagnosis and treatment recommendations to all the diseases, with the early efforts we can make great progress. Even though it may prove challenging, we expect that AI will ultimately master this domain as well. Given the significant advancements in AI for imaging analysis, most radiology and pathology images are expected to be reviewed by AI at some time. Speech and text recognition are already being used for tasks like patient communication and clinical note capture, and this trend will continue.

The most difficult hurdle for AI in many healthcare fields is assuring its acceptance in daily clinical practice, not whether the technologies are capable enough to be useful. AI systems must be approved by regulators, integrated with EHR systems, standardized to the point that similar products work in a similar way, taught to physicians, paid for by public or private payer organizations, and updated over time in the field for widespread adoption to occur. These obstacles will be overcome in the end, but they will take considerably longer than the maturation of the technologies themselves. As a result, we predict AI will be used in therapeutic settings only to a limited extent.

It's also becoming clear that AI systems will not replace human clinicians on a large scale, but rather will enhance their efforts to care for patients. Human physicians may progress toward activities and job designs that rely on essentially human skills like empathy, persuasion, and big-picture integration in the future. Those that refuse to work with artificial intelligence may be the only ones who lose their careers in the long run.

The most common application of classical machine learning in healthcare is precision medicine, which involves predicting which treatment techniques are most likely to succeed on a patient based on a variety of patient characteristics and the treatment context. The great majority of machine-learning and precision medicine applications require supervised learning, which requires a training dataset with the end variable (e.g., illness onset) known.

If we talk about the most complex forms of machine learning, we'll learn that it involves deep learning or neural network models with many levels of features or variables that are meant to predict outcomes. There could be thousands of hidden elements in such models, which are revealed by today's graphics processing units and cloud architectures' speedier processing. Recognizing possibly malignant tumors in radiography pictures is a common application of deep learning in healthcare. Deep learning is increasingly being used in radionics, which is the discovery of clinically significant patterns in imaging data that are beyond what the human eye can see. In oncology-focused image analysis, both radionics and deep learning are routinely used. Their combination appears to promise improved diagnostic accuracy than the previous generation of computer-aided detection (CAD) techniques for image analysis.

Patient participation and adherence have long been seen as the 'last mile' challenge in healthcare, the final barrier between ineffective and good health results. The more patients actively participate in their own well-being and treatment, the better the outcomes—utilization, financial outcomes, and member experience. To overcome these difficulties, big data and artificial intelligence are increasingly being deployed.

Clinical experience is frequently used by providers and hospitals to establish a plan of care that they know will improve the health of a chronic or acute patient. That doesn't matter if the patient doesn't make the necessary behavioural changes, such as losing weight, arranging a follow-up visit, filling medicines, or adhering to a treatment plan. Noncompliance, or when a patient fails to follow a treatment plan or take prescription medications as directed, is a big issue. In a survey of more than 300 clinical leaders and healthcare executives, more than 70% of respondents claimed that less than half of their patients were highly involved, and 42% said that less than a quarter of their patients were extremely engaged.

In healthcare, there are numerous administrative applications.

First and foremost, radiologists do more than simply read and analyse pictures. Radiology AI systems, like other AI systems, accomplish a single task. Deep-learning models are trained for specific image-identification tasks in labs and start-ups (such as nodule detection on chest computed tomography or haemorrhage on brain magnetic resonance imaging). To properly identify all potential findings in medical imaging, many of such limited detection jobs are required, and only a few of these can currently be done by AI.

In addition, radiologists consult with other physicians on diagnosis and treatment, treat diseases (for example, by providing local ablative therapies), and perform image-guided medical interventions such as cancer biopsies and vascular stents (interventional radiology), define the technical parameters of imaging examinations to be performed (tailored to the patient's condition), relate findings from images to other medical records and test results, and discuss procedures and results with patients.

Second, clinical techniques for using AI-based image work are still in the early stages of development. The probability of a lesion, the probability of cancer, the characteristic or location of a nodule is all different foci for different imaging technology providers and deep learning algorithms. Deep-learning systems would be challenging to integrate into existing clinical practice because of these unique foci.

Third, deep-learning image identification algorithms require 'labeled data,' which consists of millions of photographs from patients who have been diagnosed with cancer, a broken bone, or another pathology. However, there is no centralized archive of tagged or unlabeled radiological images.

Finally, for automated image analysis to take off, significant changes in medical legislation and health insurance will be required.

Artificial intelligence (AI) has far-reaching ramifications in the medical field. The current global COVID-19 pandemic, which has overburdened hospitals, stretched resources, and infected millions of individuals before testing and therapy were available, has brought this to light. The model was only trained on data on healthcare costs, not on data about healthcare that was sought or provided. Because the payment data showed that black patients in this scenario spent less money on healthcare, the algorithm thought they didn't require it. After the bias was eliminated from the AI model, the results revealed that this group had a 28.8% higher need for healthcare services. There are currently no established frameworks for analysing models for bias. This incident was only discovered because the data was considerably distorted.

Despite the hurdles that AI faces in healthcare, scientists expect that AI will continue to make significant advances in the medical industry in the years to come. Udacity recently organized a virtual conference on the future of AI in healthcare, where leading experts in technology and medicine discussed their predictions on anything from future pandemics to disease diagnosis [17]. What they foresee as being on the cutting edge of AI in healthcare is as follows.

- **Future challenges in artificial intelligence (AI)**

When it comes to implementing AI in the healthcare and medical fields, there are numerous obstacles to overcome. Because of the privacy and secrecy of the huge amount of data obtained from hospitals, AI had trouble acquiring access to those resources. Clinically proven diagnosis is less available and credible, which reduces the chances of an accurate diagnosis. Due to the export of imaging and medical record data, the work burden has increased. The clinical decision-making capabilities of AI is limited to solving one problem at a time, but patients in life-threatening situations may have a complex set of problems that require full examination from several angles. Hospitals must collaborate with software companies to construct a robust AI platform based on diagnosis and treatment data, which is a time-consuming and error-prone procedure. The proper labelling, annotations, segmentation, and quality verification of imaging (CT/MRI) data necessitate highly qualified specialists, which raises the entire cost and time. For the appropriate development of an AI system to diagnose disease, imaging data is insufficient. All of the aforementioned factors act as roadblocks to AI implementation in the healthcare and medical fields.

With the advancement of AI and software that can be used to analyse imaging data, diseases like cancer may now be predicted with high accuracy and precision. Work guidelines for future clinical practises will be aided by a wide range of study and analysis of imaging data. After integrating AI, rehabilitation exercises could be modified to accomplish tailored evaluation and rehabilitation training that improves desired neurological function in the context of various neurological dysfunctions. New technologies with strong learning ability and generalisation capacity are predicted to acquire human-like intelligence in the future, which will improve diagnostic approaches and decision-making systems, allowing for the provision of higher-quality and more inexpensive medical services. AI will help primary hospitals improve their medical services, as well as construct a black box model predictor to tackle black box problems and develop 5G technologies. The high-speed transmission capabilities of the 5G network will improve real-time remote technical guidelines for safe, dependable, and stable remote collaborative surgeries, lowering surgical risks.

- **AI could make medical professionals better**

There's no substitute for a human touch or years of medical experience, but that doesn't rule out AI as a useful tool for medical professionals. AI has been used to help detect high-risk patients during distinct peaks of the pandemic, for example; screening and diagnostic analysis is another interesting area where AI could supplement professional skills.

This capability isn't restricted to COVID-19 or even hospitals. Kendra Gaunt of The Trevor Project, an organisation dedicated to preventing suicide among LGBTQIA+ adolescents, was recently interviewed on our company's podcast to explore the role AI plays in their goal. Trevor has lately used AI to help educate counsellors by providing realistic scenarios that let them to practise before taking live calls, making them more successful in crisis situations, according to Kendra.

In the end, AI does not need to take centre stage to assist medical professionals, whether they be doctors, nurses, or therapists. It can still assist healthcare in making significant progress.

In a nutshell, the healthcare business has experienced remarkable growth in the recent year. But, in the midst of the chaos, we've seen some amazing technological developments that, in my opinion, could pave the way for a new, better healthcare system fuelled in part by AI. Furthermore, the healthcare industry's experience has revealed valuable lessons for business executives in general, not only in medicine. Specifically, now that we've all seen the power of AI, it's almost certain to stick around; however, to maximise its effectiveness, we must prioritise comfort, maintain a human touch, and, perhaps most importantly, ensure that we're using AI to make our daily lives better and easier as we move toward a new normal.

1.7   CONCLUSION AND FUTURE WORK

AI is now allowing the healthcare industry to get better results. It has increased its productivity and care efficiency. Doctors' and patients' roles have shifted as a result. The goal of AI is to expand and grow in the medical industry. It will transform how diseases are diagnosed, treated, and detected.

It has the potential to aid in the treatment of serious health problems. Its purpose is to leverage data and healthcare technologies to address ethical and social issues. The key difficulty for AI is to ensure that it is transparent and compatible with the public's interests.

AI has made significant progress in the health field, but it still has to evolve. And AI isn't a science that aims to replace human doctors with robots; rather, it aims to assist and support both doctors and patients.

Artificial intelligence (AI) has exploded in popularity in a variety of fields and regions during the previous decade. Unsurprisingly, health care is one of the industries that has been transformed by artificial intelligence. While companies have broadened their applications of artificial intelligence, the fundamental application of AI remains in high demand: data analysis and prediction. With so many technical breakthroughs, storage and processing technologies have grown in their own right, allowing infrastructures to keep a digital footprint or record of everything they've done in the past. Logs aren't the only thing that's being saved now that storage isn't an issue. People's responses and medical histories, as well as test results, symptoms, medication, medication response, genetical constitution, and other information, are collected anonymously or not, freely or not, in order to keep track of everything related to healthcare. People have created numerous innovative methods to examine this massive mountain of data and draw meaningful conclusions as technology has progressed. To maintain a deployable dataset, private organisations or the government may record all data from hospitals or clinics.

Response to drugs is one example of where statistical analysis has been shown to be beneficial. People willingly participate in surveys in which their records, including tests and progress, are kept to determine the efficacy of a treatment or procedure against a certain medical problem. Public findings of any repeating pattern of symptoms depending on location, gender, food habits, culture, etc., effectiveness of a particular drug in persons grouped by numerous groups, and treatment progress are all possible thanks to research in these records. Once completed, it is easy to determine if a certain population is segregated on any possible criteria for the majority of the population, which improves treatment efficiency. Studies can be carried out to see if there is a link between symptoms and lifestyle, culture, or geography, and this information can then be utilised to map the condition accordingly.

Data capturing a strange or novel symptom in a region progressively moving across the vicinities can be used to detect illness outbreaks, their origins, symptoms, impacts, and, most crucially, the pattern and pace with which they travel. This detection could save a lot of lives since it enables governments, healthcare organisations, and pharmaceutical companies, both worldwide and locally, to be prepared for a potential epidemic and begin working on determining the reason and root of the problem to create a defence. This ability was demonstrated in the last pandemic, where scientists and health organisations predicted the speed and scope of infection, the appearance of new variations due to mutation, their origin, symptoms, and path on a daily basis. This ability has saved lives since people were aware of the scope of the harm and were prepared for it. The same method was utilised to discover patterns, which aided in the discovery of any potential medicine or vaccination adverse effects that may or may not affect people depending on their lifestyles, age, or geographic region. This made it possible to build a working vaccination with minimal side effects in a short time, which would not have been conceivable in the past. This enabled super-quick vaccine development and manufacture, which would not have been possible without statistical analysis of volunteer responses to prototypes.

It's also employed in the field of studying the recurrence/susceptibility of a given disease in persons who share specific genes. Genetic illnesses can be inherited through a lengthy family history, and blood tests are often ineffective in detecting them. People rely on symptoms to determine whether they have a genetic disease that is incurable. People can now use artificial intelligence to discover defective genes even before a child is born by looking at the genetic makeup of the child's parents, and so prevent their quality of life from deteriorating. Identification of specific genes among millions of genes necessitates extensive investigation. People can also use AI to map probable genetic diseases or abnormalities in people all over the world based on their geographical birthplace, ancestry, race, and other factors.

It will improve the medicine's efficiency and make it more immunological, as well as reduce risk and select the best treatment for each patient. It aids researchers in developing vaccines that increase vaccine immunity levels, as well as providing speedy validation of vaccination targets and optimization results. To be effective in AI-assisted drug development, an individual must be able to train algorithms, which necessitates domain expertise. It necessitates a lot of upkeep and effort to rebuild and learn. This provides an appropriate venue for AI and medicinal chemists to collaborate and produce some output with correct analysis and efficiency.

It is fair to conclude that all of these, as well as a slew of additional AI benefits, have aided in improving the quality of life through greater preparedness and responsiveness. So much data and data analysis tools have aided individuals and organisations in doing research, seeing trends, learning and understanding the causes, and inventing treatments and techniques. As a result of these capabilities, our healthcare business is making rapid progress and assisting people in surviving ailments that were once thought to be fatal.

Because the AIML is based on previous results and trials, it will have a significant impact on the developing medical sector. It will take less time to provide proper and accurate results.

Its cost is very low, allowing industry to produce more for the general public.

Deep-learning technologies have also transformed cancer vaccine development by improvising neoantigen prediction in collaboration with AI businesses and other medical sectors. "It won't be long until these are exposed for what they are; the hoopla can't last very long because the truth will come out in the data over the next five years ago or so, if by then we are generating better pharmaceuticals, and doing it faster and cheaper, then AI will really take off," Narain previously stated.

By employing this technology in the future, we will be able to get more out of our lives and achieve our goals, and the medical business will benefit more. It is only the beginning of a healthcare revolution, and progress is being made and will continue to be made at an exponential rate.

- Future scope of artificial intelligence (AI)
  - To lower the death rate, AI will prioritise those who are in greater need. It can also assist the patient's blood pressure and anxiety, as well as increase social contact. The use of social assistive robot technology improves the quality of life for senior citizens.
  - AI is used to find and create new drugs in the fields of immune-oncology and neuroscience.
  - AI has also given hope for the detection of melanoma, which is extremely difficult to detect with the naked eye. It's a sort of skin cancer that arises from the pigment-producing cells called melanocytes.
  - Since tissue-based genomics can't sample other regions of the tumour, image-omics will be used in the future.

REFERENCES

[1] Fast, E. & Chen, B., "Can artificial intelligence help us design vaccines?". brookings.edu, (2020).

[2] Panch, T., Mattie, H., & Celi, L. A., "The "inconvenient truth" about AI in healthcare". *npj Digital Medicine*, 2, 77 (2019).

[3] Reddy, S., Allan,S., Coghlan, S., & Cooper, P. A., "A governance model for the application of AI in health care". *Journal of the American Medical Informatics Association*, 27(3), 491–497 (2020).

[4] Mak, K. K. & Pichika, M. R., "Artificial intelligence in drug development: Present status and future prospects". *Drug Discovery Today*, 24(3), 773–780 (2019).

[5] Salathé, M., Wiegand, T., & Wenzel, M., *Focus Group on Artificial Intelligence for Health*. Geneva, Switzerland: World Health Organization, (2018).

[6] Coeckelbergh, M., "Health Care, Capabilities, and AI Assistive Technologies". *Ethical Theory and Moral Practice*, 13, 181–190 (2010). 10.1007/s10677-009-9186-2.

[7] Weissman, I., "AI is the new reality: The 4th healthcare revolution in medicine". *Health Management*, 19(2), (2019).

[8] Davenport, T. & Kalakota, R., "The potential for artificial intelligence in healthcare". *Future Healthcare Journal*, 6(2), 94–98 (2019).

[9] Dilmegani, C., "Top 18 AI Use cases in Healthcare Industry". *research.aimultiple.com*, (April 2022).

[10] Jiang, F., Jiang, Y., Zhi, H., Dong, Y., Li, H., Ma, S., Wang, Y., Dong, Q., Shen, H., & Wang, Y., "Artificial intelligence in healthcare: Past, present and future". *Stroke and Vascular Neurology*, 2(4), 230–243 (2017).

[11] Jvion, "Healthcare & Clinical AI Platform | Jvion". *jvion.com*.

[12] Imran, T. F., Wang, N., Zombeck, S., & Balady, G. J., "Mobile Technology Improves Adherence to Cardiac Rehabilitation: A Propensity Score-Matched Study". *Journal of the American Heart Association*, 10(15), e020482 (2021).

[13] Reddy, S., Fox, J., & Purohit, M. P., "Artificial intelligence-enabled healthcare delivery". *Journal of the Royal Society of Medicine*, 112(1), 22–28 (2019).

[14] Cath, C., "Governing artificial intelligence: Ethical, legal and technical opportunities and challenges". *Philosophical Transactions of the Royal Society A: Mathematical, Physical and Engineering Sciences*, 376(2133), (2018).

[15] Chifley, L., "10 Powerful Examples of AI used in Healthcare Industry". *Referral md*, (2019).

[16] Agarwal, Y., Jain, M., Sinha, S., & Dhir, S., "Delivering high-tech, AI-based health care at Apollo Hospitals". *Global Business and Organizational Excellence*, 39(8), (2019).

[17] Shalamanov, J., "The Future of AI in Healthcare". *udacity.com*, (2020).

[18] Yin, J., Ngiam, K. Y., & Teo, H. H., "Role of Artificial Intelligence Applications in Real-Life Clinical Practice: Systematic Review", 23(4), (2021).

[19] Islam, M. M., Poly, T. N., Alsinglawi, B., Lin, L.-F., Chien, S.-C., Liu, J.-C., & Jian, W., "Artificial Intelligence in COVID-19 Pandemic: Bibliometric Analysis". *Healthcare*, 9, 441 (2021).

[20] Ellahham, S., "Artificial intelligence in the diagnosis and management of COVID-19: A narrative review". *Journal of Medical Artificial Intelligence*, 4(4), (2021).

[21] Bajwa, J., Munir, U., Nori, A., & Williams, B., "Artificial intelligence in healthcare: transforming the practice of medicine". *Future Healthcare Journal*, 8(2), e188–e194 (2021).

[22] Eszter, N., "AI and robotics are transforming healthcare: Why AI and robotics will define New Health: Publications: Healthcare: Industries: PwC". (2021).

[23] He, J., Baxter, S. L., Xu, J., Xu, J., Zhou, X., & Zhang, K., "The practical implementation of artificial intelligence technologies in medicine". *Nature Medicine*, 25(1), 30–36 (2019).

[24] Char, D. S., Shah, N. H., & Magnus, D., "Implementing machine learning in health care – addressing ethical challenges". *The New England Journal of Medicine*, 378, 981–983 (2018).

[25] Shah, P., Kendall, F., Khozin, S. et al. "Artificial intelligence and machine learning in clinical development: A translational perspective". *npj Digital Medicine*, 2, 69 (2019).

[26] Pacilè, S., "AI tool improves breast cancer detection on mammography". *Radiological Society of North America*, 4, (2020).

2 Artificial Intelligence in Medical Imaging for Developing Countries
Challenges and Opportunities

Balwinder Singh and Mandeep Singh
Centre for Development of Advanced Computing, Mohali

Rekha Devi
Chandigarh University, Mohali

CONTENTS

2.1 INTRODUCTION

As an increasingly emerging technology, artificial intelligence (AI) has arisen and gained broad acceptance in many areas. Healthcare is one of the fields where the introduction of AI is extremely promising. Currently, using AI in healthcare in India involves opportunities, various challenges, possible solutions, and the a future with this emerging technology. New startups and major companies provide AI solutions for healthcare problems in India, which are increasingly using AI. Such

DOI: 10.1201/9781003333081-2

issues and solutions include resolving the uneven ratio between qualified doctors and patients; making doctors more effective at their work; personalizing healthcare, delivering good healthcare in rural areas, and educating physicians and nurses in complex procedures. Companies provide several solutions, including medical diagnosis automation, automated medical test review, disease detection and tracking systems, wearable detection-based medical tools, patient engagement systems, predictive diagnostics of healthcare, and disease prevention. The lack of accurate, usable, interoperable, and clean data is a common problem in implementing such solutions; that problem is to be tackled through the Electronic Health Records Standards established by Health and Family Welfare Ministry in 2016. Specific challenges include access to open data sets and the practitioners' acceptance. This study aims to chart the existing state of AI in Indian healthcare. It explores the actual healthcare use of AI; India's AI-healthcare story; a key player in designing, implementing, and controlling AI in the health sector; possible and actual health effects of AI; and the problems in AI policymaking in the health sector. In every region, the health industry is facing unique challenges. The developed economies fail to build an effective system to efficiently combine various roles when it comes to the last miles of healthcare. If you look at the wide-area and number of potential recipients, problems are different in a country like India. There are other issues, such as demographic growth, unique regional problems, and digital literacy. To achieve the state-of-the-art research results, as well as facilities, the increasing application of artificial intelligence (AI) in healthcare is crucial for the scientific community. AI could significantly boost outcomes in reliable healthcare and the quality in facilities as it is used in healthcare. India is well-positioned to build solutions that tackle robustness and efficiency issues with its immense wealth of unstructured medical data and population diversity combined with its large pool of human talent. This report will address some of the problems that the Indian healthcare system is facing. Some cases studies have provide promising pathways for AI [1–3].

Artificial intelligence (AI) is a technology that accentuates the formation of smart and intelligent machines that work and respond like individuals [1,2]. The machines or smart computers with the capability to accomplish intellectual roles, such as observing, learning, decision making, reasoning, and problem solving, are called artificial intelligence computers or machines, as shown in Figure 2.1. According to the panel of Forbes technology council members, 13 different sectors, including the healthcare sector, will be revolutionized by artificial intelligence. This sector is progressing toward a modern epoch, where plentiful medical data are performing an incredibly

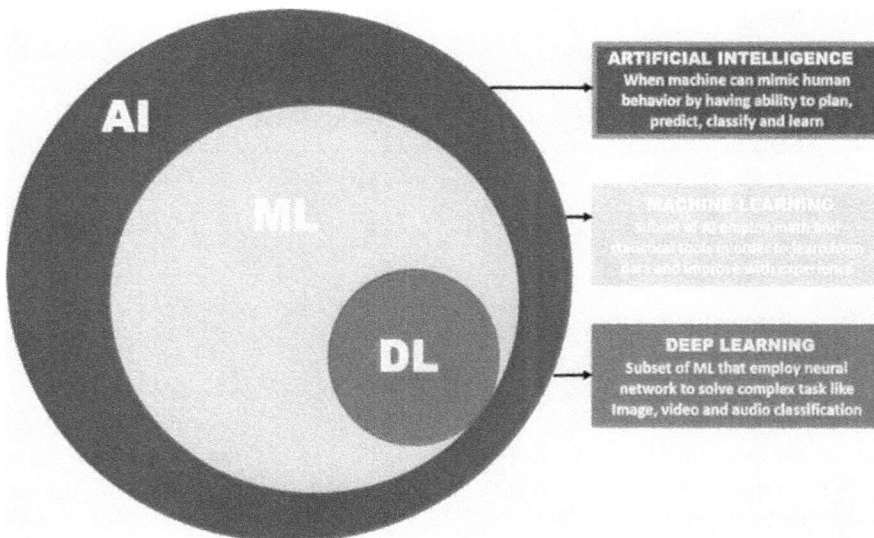

ARTIFICIAL INTELLIGENCE
When machine can mimic human behavior by having ability to plan, predict, classify and learn

MACHINE LEARNING
Subset of AI employ math and statistical tools in order to learn from data and improve with experience

DEEP LEARNING
Subset of ML that employ neural network to solve complex task like Image, video and audio classification

FIGURE 2.1 Differentiation of AI, ML, and DL.

significant role. In modern healthcare technologies, the primary objective is 'assurance of the affordable treatment is given to the needy patient within a short period deprived of complex documentation in Indian scenario' by using AI in healthcare [3].

Deep learning aims to transform the way medical tests are assessed and diagnosed by physicians, allowing them to recognize illnesses and begin care sooner. The immense accessibility of medical data creates incredible prospects and tasks for healthcare examination [4].

2.2 MACHINE LEARNING AND DEEP LEARNING

Machine learning is the ability of machines or computers to learn without being programmed. It uses numerous algorithms to analyze and evaluate data, and, after analyzing the data, learn from it, and then make judgments or deliver an output. In the field of medical imaging, conventional machine-learning methods have been applied more recently. With rapidly enhancing computational capacity, along with the readiness of massive volumes of clinical data, traditional machine learning (statistical tools based) has been replaced by the neural network-based deep learning. Too many complex patterns can be trained, learned, and acquired by deep learning compared to traditional machine-learning systems. Therefore, machine-learning algorithms permit systems to execute a task by training the machines by applying accessible data to inputs [5–8]. On the other hand, deep learning is a subset of machine learning, which is based on biological neural network-learning representations for solving complex problems as humans do, as shown in Figure 2.1.

Deep-learning approaches, unlike traditional machine-learning techniques, significantly simplify the process of feature engineering by applying directly to unstructured data, such as audio, video, and images, as shown in Figure 2.2. Alternatively, the machine learning in the featured area scales inadequately and loses the opportunities to find new patterns from unstructured data. As a replacement, the representation learning helps systematically find the representations required for extrapolation from unprocessed data. So, this makes it easier and faster for researchers to develop

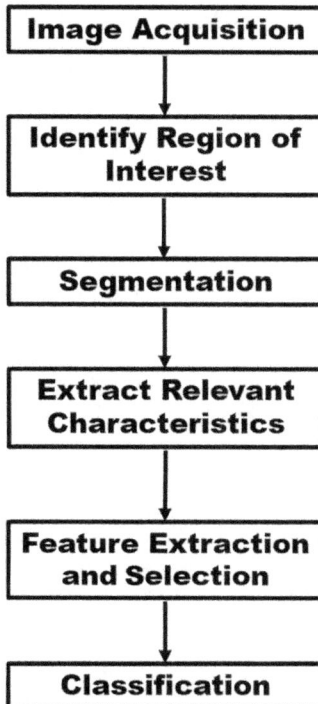

FIGURE 2.2 Deep-learning steps for the classification process.

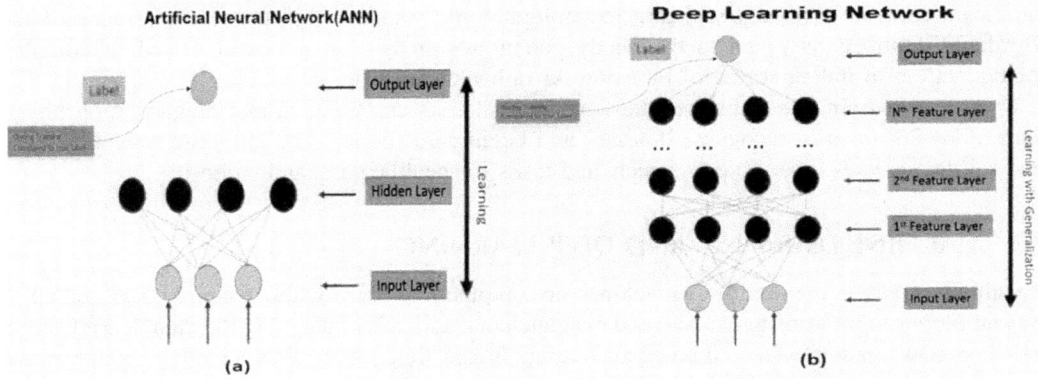

FIGURE 2.3 Deep-learning steps for the classification process.

the newest concepts [9]. Deep learning-based CNNs algorithm is of special importance in the field of medical imaging among all deep-learning methods. There are, of course, several recent works that aim to apply CNN to medical image analysis. The deep-learning techniques are also a part of representation learning with many stages of illustration, accomplished by comprising nonlinear data that separately changes the depiction at a single point (beginning with the input data), switching to a subsequent representation at an advanced level with the help of multiple hidden layers, a somewhat abstract level. Deep learning takes things a step further by imitating the layered or "deep" structure of the human brain, called an artificial neural network (Figure 2.3(a)). It emulates this layered structure by creating a similar artificial neural network with the potential to be even more powerful than state-of-the-art machine-learning software (Figure 2.3(b)).

Deep-learning algorithms exhibited wonderful performance in the early detection, diagnosis, and precautionary measures in biomedical healthcare through hidden layers, as explained in Figure 2.3. Moreover, it has exceptionally good potential in other related technologies, such as speech recognition, natural language-processing tasks, and computer vision. As per the implementation of deep learning in various areas and the quick advances of methodological enhancements, AI models, especially subset deep-learning algorithms with framework, present an energizing new open door for medical healthcare worldwide [7–10].

The most recent innovations in artificial intelligence technologies offer successful models to obtain supervised, reinforcement, semi-supervised, or unsupervised learning models from such complex data. For the medical research industry, this kind of active learning is important. That is because computers can learn to improve the quality and accuracy of diagnoses from new medical research and past performance data. By incorporating more advanced data processing into research efforts and removing the need for a human expert with years of training, deep learning would change the medical research field. This cutting-edge technology is also expected to reduce the time it takes for a diagnosis to be made. Instead of moving from doctor to specialist for several months or longer, patients would quickly work with their physician to type their symptoms and test results into a device [4]. The deep-learning program uses data from millions of other patients to make appropriate assessments months or years before a doctor could. This helps to reduce patient anxiety and improve early therapy health outcomes. Deep-learning techniques are being applied to human services, especially in the healthcare sector, and are now coordinated or some modules are in progress. For instance, Google DeepMind has declared blueprints to employ its research team and expertise in the health sector. and Enlitic business is also developing new deep-learning models to point health issues from X-rays as well as computed tomography scans. Yet, deep-learning methodologies have not been broadly examined practically in diverse health applications that might gain from its facilities [6–10]. Hence, various characteristics of representation learning (deep learning) frameworks can be beneficial in the medical field because of its exceptional performance, overall learning structure along with unified feature learning, the ability to manage complicated data, and on and on. To quicken the endeavors, the AI technology subset, i.e. deep learning, have to tackle numerous challenges concerning the in-depth characteristics such as noisy, heterogeneous, sparse, and time dependency of raw data for enhanced techniques and frameworks that permit artificial intelligence subfields such as deep learning to help in healthcare data workflows, along with medical decision support systems. Newly upcoming methods, such as the deep belief network, rectified linear unit, recurrent neural network, RBM, and deep residual learning, mitigate problems like the disappearing gradient; hence, it is possible to train deeper models with much more ability and thus transform the deep learning technology in medical imaging to next level. Nonetheless, some remaining issues continue to be resolved, for example, data format inconsistencies and the lack of reliable training data [11,12].

2.3 AI HEALTHCARE IN INDIA

Indian countries that use AI in healthcare also become part of a growing list. New start-ups and major core companies occur through AI adoption in India with practical solutions for healthcare problems in the region. These include resolving the unequal relationship between trained physicians and patients and enhancing their performance at work, delivering customized healthcare and first-class healthcare in far-flung areas, and educating physicians and nursing staff in clinical practices. Industries provide a variety of solutions, including medical diagnostic automation, digital processing of medical tests, advanced disease detection with screening, and real-time monitoring equipment using automated software [13]. A common problem in the implementation of these solutions has been setting up the electronic hygiene standards established by India's health department for detailed, accurate, interoperable, and clean data. Specific challenges include access to and acceptance by clinicians of the online medical data. A CIS India report published in 2018 estimates that AI will allow the Indian economy to add US$ 957 billion by 2035. Microsoft, together with Apollo and other hospitals, has taken a major effort to increase its usage to explore the diverse uses of AI in the healthcare sector. Microsoft has announced that it will create an AI-centric cardiology network in collaboration with Apollo hospitals. In the analysis of cardiovascular risks in patients, the organization will use AI models and assist doctors with tailored treatments. Siemens researchers and its engineers' team have developed an AI system to create a digital double heart, which imitates real cardiac cell electrical and physical characteristics, which allow surgeons to perform simulations of the patient before surgery. Philips offers AI-based cardiac frameworks that help doctors to diagnose conditions automatically using these models, to support surgeons for their next step treatments or further processes. Google has designed a suite of AI-based frameworks that include deep-learning algorithms for the analysis of medical images to diagnose eye disease. Max Healthcare, one of Northern Indian's largest hospital chains, uses AI for critical-care monitoring [13,14].

2.3.1 GOVERNMENT INITIATIVES

AI integration in India's healthcare has been considered an important technology to improve the efficiency, quality, costs, and scope of healthcare. In India, helping AI has the greatest growth potential, whereas innovations that can replace doctors have the least chance of success; one explanation is a medical institution's conflict of interest. Many AI health programs concentrate on escalating healthcare services to poor populations that lack the necessary infrastructure or adequate primary doctors. Therefore, the use of AI technology in healthcare appears to be addressing the subject of monetary difference in India instead of increasing present gaps [8–13]. NITI Aayog focuses on early diagnosis and identification, based on AI models of diabetic retinopathy and cardiac risk. These interventions would, in the long term, benefit patients in the early stages of preventive treatment rather than reactive healthcare, reducing healthcare costs and increasing recovery chances. NITI Aayog and Google join forces to collaborate on several plans to develop India's AI-enabled clinical care system. The collaboration between Google and NITI Aayog will develop major educational initiatives, fund start-ups, and promote AI work through Ph.D. grants, which will contribute to the broader concept of the latest state-of-the-art technology in India. Google will organize hands-on workshops and development programs through NITI Aayog to raise awareness among policymakers and government technical experts of specific AI technologies and how they can be used for streamlining governance. A nationwide platform for innovation in cross-border technologies, including clinical practices using AI, has been funded by NITI Aayog [14]. As part of this mandate, NITI Aayog, together with its national data and analysis platform, has established India's national AI strategy for the large implementation and use of AI. India is currently witnessing major health developments, a growing prevalence, for example, of non-communicable diseases and marked demographic changes. For most families, it is incredibly difficult to manage out-of-pocket costs. To simplify medical information and promote efficient execution, the National Help Stack (NHS) provides comprehensive central health records to all citizens in the country. The new NHS is a challenging strategy that aims to use the latest technology to create a unified citizen health identity—while navigating services at various levels. The Ministry of Health is also establishing a National Digital Health Authority, a statutory authority that establishes interoperability frameworks, regulations, guidelines, and digital information exchanges. It would also entail cooperation if the government plans to use AI and mechanical technology for healthcare workers in hospitals or community settings. State governments fund AI start-ups as well. The Karnataka government, for example, mobilizes Rs 2000 core to fund them by 2020. Karnataka also has a start-up strategy and a fund that can support AI start-ups. Karnataka Information Technology Venturing Capital Fund. Besides, an MoU with the government of Telangana to establish a data science & artificial intelligence center of excellence was signed in Feb 2018 by the National Association of Software & Services Companies (NASSCOM). The government also partners with other nations on AI technology to boost the healthcare sector [15]. In April 2018, Theresa had addressed strategic partnerships and increasing convergence in regional and international matters underneath the UTP collaboration. All sides will strengthen collaboration on future technology to solve global challenges; realize AI's potential, the digital economy, health innovation, and cybersecurity; and foster sustainable growth, clever urban development, and economic mobility while improving our young people's future skills and abilities. As a portion of the rising joint technology partnership in India, the Indian government applauded the initiative of the UK to set up the UK-India tech center in India [13,14].

2.3.2 THE STARTUPS IN INDIA

The technology hub will bring high-tech companies together to build investments and exports, as well as offer a new forum for exchanging the best technologies and advancing policy collaboration, advanced development, and health AIs under India's district ambition program. A host of start-ups have taken onboard technologies like AI-enabled healthcare, mHealth, telemedicine, patient data management, and remote diagnostics, which have developed in the health industry in India. Companies are providing technology-based services in the Indian public health sector for positive changes. The government's policy to promote start-ups has further reinforced this service growth. The Indian health sector has seen an explosion of innovation in AI application. Such companies are providing customer service from cancer detections to the search for a new healthcare provider, although its implementation tends to slowly be gaining momentum in rural towns, primarily in urban areas. Tricog Health, a start-up targeted for its cloud-based cardiac-monitoring software by the GE healthcare accelerator program. Tricog provides access to heart care in 340 cities in 23 countries, as well as in some of India's most remote areas. The company's app gathers clinical data along with ECGs from field devices and applies the best deep-learning algorithms in real-time and diagnoses the diseases. A second company, Aindra Systems from Bengaluru, uses AI as its second most common cancer in Indian women ages 15 to 60 to cope with cervical cancer. The AI-enabled software solution of Aindra can observe cervical cancer in the initial phases and escalate the probability of life [11–14]. This firm improves the effectiveness of cervical cancer research pathologists, who usually need to analyze each sample and mark the case manually, with a high probability of cancer getting further analysis by an oncologist. HealthifyMe focuses on lifestyles, such as obesity, high blood pressure, and diabetes. HealthifyMe brings the best elite fitness experience in the world with its AI-enabled wellness coach Ria. The healthcare AI revolution is just starting, and the future players' list is never-ending. Early breast cancer screening is underway at Niramai. Ten3 T provides RDM services through algorithms to sense irregularities and warn the doctor about the patient's condition. Advancells offers stem cell therapy that has great potential for an organ transplant, also known as regenerative medicine. Doctors and healthcare professionals may help patients who are unable to access hospitals with remote diagnostics and monitoring devices. SigTuple decreases pathologist pressure with smart automated blood sample analysis. AI diagnoses start-up SigTuple. The Supercraft 3D printing company is designing and developing imagining tools based on artificial intelligence that allows physicians, nursing staff, and medical researchers to gain a deeper understanding of human structure. In the end, AI can become a force that improves precautionary healthcare for all rather than only those in urban or wealthy societies. In other words, simpler algae only must have a larger training dataset, as AI experts frequently claim. This produces accurate, useful results for payers as well as providers. With a population in the billions, a country like India can deliver a massive amount of health data to solve global health problems [13,14].

Furthermore, we review the opportunities, applications, and challenges related to these artificial intelligence techniques, while implementing in precision diagnosis, early detection, treatment, medicine, and next-generation healthcare in India.

2.4 BACKGROUND AND RELATED WORK

Extensive worldwide research is moving toward the implementation of artificial intelligence in the healthcare sector. We will review the existing literature on the subject to get preliminary knowledge and the scope of investigations. A detailed literature survey is conducted in the domain of healthcare technologies using artificial intelligence, and their applications. Some research gaps have been identified based on the literature review. In the paper, numerous machine-learning and deep-learning algorithms are studied in-depth for improving effective decision support systems for healthcare applications. AI algorithms are applied to find different patterns from medical data sets and deliver an outstanding capability to guide patients and to predict most of the diseases. The use of this technology is predominant and is used in numerous medical applications. In this section, we have reviewed the leading contemporary literature of deep-learning models for medical imaging. More than 50 articles published were reviewed to explore applications of artificial intelligence, traditional machine learning, and deep learning in medical diagnosis. Table 2.1 encapsulates all the research papers stated in the literature survey, in specific emphasizing the diseases addressed, algorithms/models used, and the data source incorporated. The intense architectures employed in the healthcare domain have been mainly centered on neural network algorithms such as convolutional neural networks (CNNs), Restricted Boltzmann Machines (RBMs), recurrent neural networks (RNNs), and Autoencoders (AEs). The algorithms and techniques, and the key concepts behind their models, are demonstrated in Table 2.2. There are two main approaches when it comes to the application of medical diagnoses. A first approach is to identify the outcome by linking data to specific results (diagnostic results). The second approach is the detection and diagnosis of tumors or other diseases using physiological data. Deep learning applies to medical diagnosis in various ways. Table 2.1 presents brief analyses of individual research papers in the fields of deep learning and medical diagnosis.

TABLE 2.1

Summary of the Recent Research Papers Listed with Medical Diagnosis, Algorithms, and Performance Using AI in Medical Imaging

Subspecialty	Author	Model	Conclusion/Remarks	Ref.
Brain	J.Dolz et al.(2020)	3D-CNN	Precise 3D segmentation of infant brain tissues, the method shows very competitive results among 21 teams, ranking 1st or 2nd in most metrics on segmentation of the 6-month infant brain MRI.	[16]
Skin	J. Czajkowska et al.(2020)	HBSA	The Hypoechoic band segmentation algorithm contains three parts which result in epidermis layer detection, segmentation of the epidermis layer and delineation of the SLEB region. The accuracy of the proposed system has been checked by 2 independent experts on 45 clinical images	[17]
Fetal echocardiography	L. Xu et al.(2020)	DW-Net	The CNN centered deep learning method is used in the segmentation of several anatomical structures for A4C views of early fetal echocardiography (FE).	[18]
Brain Tumor	M.I. Sharif et al.(2020)	CNN	The dice score achieved for the core tumor is 83.73%, for the whole tumor 93.7% and for the enhanced tumor 79.94%. Complete findings demonstrate that the method submitted outstrips both for classification as well as brain tumor segmentation.	[19]
Liver and Heart	Q. Dou et al. (2017)	CNN	Automated segmentation; segmentation of the liver, heart, and great vessels; this technique has great clinical potential.	[20]
Brain tumour	Y. Pan et al. (2015)	CNN	Tumor classification of the brain; 3-layered CNN has an increase of 18 percent relative to the baseline neural network.	[21]
Alzheimer	A.Payan et al.(2015)	AE& 3D CNN	Prediction of Alzheimer's disease based on the MRI scan of the patient. 3D CNN is better than other classifiers reported previously.	[22]
Brain tumour	M.Havaei et al.(2017)	DNN	Segmentation of the brain tumors; this procedure makes the entire brain a broad tool of segmentation within 25 seconds to 3 minutes.	[23]
Brain lesion	K.Kamnitsas et al.(2017)	CNN	Segmentation of brain lesions, which resulted in great results	[24]
Brain tumor	F. isensee et al.(2017)	U-Net	Segmentation of Glioblastoma; this method has allowed a broad U-Net training without substantial overfitting with small data sets. Given that patients are moving during the segmentation process, the move to 3D convolutions that improve efficiency.	[25]
Alzheimer	T.Brosch et al. (2013)	Multiple RBM	Multiple brain MRI's to spot types of changes in Alzheimer disease	[26]
Skin cancer	A.Esteva et al. (2017)	CNN	Categorization of skin cancer using a lone convolution neural network, focused end-to-end from images precisely, using only pixels and disease labels as inputs.	[27]
Diabetes	V. Gulshan et al. (2016)	CNN	Finding of diabetic retinopathy by deep-learning algorithm training using images of retinal fundus	[28]
Lung cancer	JL. Causey(2018)	CNN	Lung cancer nodule malignancy classification made with 0.99 AUC. Accuracy equal to that of an experienced radiologist	[29]

Topic	Author (year)	Method	Description	Ref.
Pancreas segmentation	HR. Roth et al.(2015)	(SLIC) & CNN	Precise segmentation of the pancreas, using a convolution network technique and compared favorably with state-of-the-art approaches. Using ConvNets average Dice scores of 68%±10% (range, 43–80%) in testing is achieved.	[30]
Osteoarthritis	Prasoon et al.(2013)	T-CNN	Applied voxel classification integrating three 2D CNNs technique and predicted the risk of osteoarthritis using automatic segmentation of knee cartilage	[31]
Alzheimer	S. Liu et al.(2014)	Stacked AE with S-Layer	Detection of Alzheimer's disease at an early stage from brain MRI	[32]
Sclerosis lesion	y. yoo et al.(2014)	DL&RF	Deep learning and the random forest is used for multiple sclerosis (MS) lesion segmentation into the multiple-channel 3D MRI.	[33]
Breast lesions and lung nodules	J-Z.Cheng et al.(2016)	SDAE-based CADx	Detection and diagnosis of the pulmonary nodule; the results indicated significant performance improvements. However, it was observed that deep-learning systems can modify the traditional CAD systems effortlessly without structural reconstruction. The SDAE outperforms the two texture-based algorithms for classification of breast ultrasound lesion and lung CT nodules.	[34]
Heart diseases	B.D De Vos et al.(2016)	DCNN	Deep CNNs improve the process by retrieving feature representations, as well as to identify functional ROIs in 2D images to localize it in 3D.	[35]
Breast tissue classification	A.Dubrovina (2016)	CNN/CL	The supervised based new deep learning-based framework has been developed for tissue classification with convolution layers. The pectoral muscles & nipple muscle detected with 83 and 56% accuracy respectively.	[36]
Myocardial infarction	Ur. Acharya et al.(2017)	CNN	Accuracy of 93.53% and 95.22% achieved for automatic recognition of myocardial infarction with and without noise respectively	[37]
Brain-related diseases	R. Mehta et al.(2017)	CNN	Suggest a complementary methodology using a convolutional neural network that categorizes a voxel into one of many structures.	[38]
Breast cancer	A.M. Abdel Zaher & A.M. Eldeib(2016)	CAD based DBN	Automatic breast cancer diagnosis; the overall proposed method accuracy was 99.68% with 100% sensitivity; the 99.47% specificity.	[39]
Drug-induced liver injury prediction	Y. xu et al.(2015)	UGRNN	The model had 86.9% accuracy, 82.5% sensitivity, and 92.9% specificity. Overall, deep learning in contrast to other DILI prediction models gave significantly better results.	[40]
Breast cancer	B.Ehteshami et al.(2018)	DCNN	An algorithm is trained to distinguish between two different types of cancer, such as stroma encircling invasive cancer and benign biopsies. AUC achieved with the trained algorithm is 0.962.	[41]
Metastatic spinal lesions	J.Chmelik et al.(2018)	DCNN	The results obtained were compared quantitatively to other approaches, and it was finally decided that even for minor lesions, this method can provide better accuracy.	[42]
Breast cancer	J. xu et al(2016)	SSAE	Breast cancer nuclei detection; the stacked sparse autoencoder (SSAE) method will outperform nuclear detection strategies of state-of-the-art requirements.	[43]
Pulmonary disease & mortality in smokers	G. Gonzalez et al.(2018)	CNN	A deep-learning methodology that employs only CT imaging data to classify and predict those smokers with COPD and highly expected to have ARD instances along with the highest mortality.	[44]

(Continued)

TABLE 2.1 (Continued)

Summary of the Recent Research Papers Listed with Medical Diagnosis, Algorithms, and Performance Using AI in Medical Imaging

Subspecialty	Author	Model	Conclusion/Remarks	Ref.
Brain structure	H. Choi et al.(2016)	CNN	Created a rapid and accurate striatum segmentation system for application in neuroscience by using two serial CNN, global, and local algorithms.	[45]
Eye diseases	X. Gao et al.	CRNN	This approach has enhanced this cataract disease's clinical management and can diagnose other eye diseases.	[46]
Skin cancer	A.Masood et al.	SA-SVM	Diagnosis of malignant melanoma; the results have been encouraging, and there is a chance of using this type of method in incidents where inadequate labeled data are available.	[47]
Breast cancer	Z. Han et al.	CSDCNN	The research on a large-scale dataset has achieved an overall accuracy of 93.2%, a method is an efficient tool for multi-classification of breast cancer in clinical settings.	[48]
Urinary bladder segmentation	K.H.Cha et al.	DL-CNN	This technique can surmount robust boundaries between the two such regions which have great variations in gray levels.	[49]
Breast tumour	Q.Zhang et al.	RBM	Results suggested that the model attained a significant precision rate of 93.4%, with an overall sensitivity of 88.6% and a specificity of 97.1%.	[50]
Cancer	P.Danaee et al.	SDAE	The study succeeded in extracting genes that are useful in cancer prediction	[51]
Brain segmentation	J.Kleesie k et al.(2016)	3DCNN	Approach manages an arbitrary number of modalities, such as enhanced contrast scans with a mean 95.19 Dice score	[52]
Lung cancer	D.Kumar et al.(2015)	CAD+AE	This methodology ensued in 75.01% accuracy and 83.35% sensitivity; 0.39 per patient on the 10 crosses over validations.	[53]
Lung cancer	W.Sun et al.(2016)	CNN+DBN +SDAE	Highest accuracy of 81.19% was achieved with Deep belief network	[54]
Breast cancer	R. Rasti(2017)	CNN	The accuracy, sensitivity, and specificity obtained was 96.39%, 97.73%, and 94.87% reported respectively.	[55]
Lung cancer	R. Anirudh(2017)	3DCNN	To learn highly biased nodule detection features, the network equipped with these weak labels can generate relatively low false-positive levels with high sensitivity, even in the absence of specific 3D labels	[56]
Breast cancer	R.K. Samala et al.(2016)	DLCNN	The detection of microcalcifications in breast tomosynthesis and AUC achieved is 0.933.	[57]
Breast, fibroglandular tissue	M.U.Dalmis et al.(2017)	U-Net	Average Coefficients of Dice Similarity (DSC) for the proposed methods were 0.850, 0.811 and 0.671 respectively.	[58]

TABLE 2.2

Extensive Study of Artificial Neural Networks that form the Future Deep Learning Designs that Employed in the Latest Medical Diagnosis

Architecture	Description
CNN	CNN is a kind of deep-learning model for data processing that has images motivated by animal visual cortex organization. It depends upon the local contacts along with attached weights throughout the stable units pursued by feature sharing (sampling) to achieve unvarying descriptors for translation. It is programmed to learn function hierarchies, from low- to high-level patterns, automatically and adaptively. CNN is composed of a mathematical construct consisting of 3 types of layers such as convolution layer, pooling layer, and completely interconnected layers [45]. The feature extraction task was carried out by both layers such as convolution and pooling layers, whereas a completely interconnected layer carried out the classification task by mapping the extracted features for concluding output. The convolution layer performs a crucial part in CNN, comprises a stack of operations including convolution and specialized linear mathematical operation [55].
RBM	It is a two-layer neural network that makes up a whole deep-belief network. It comprises of the input or visible layer followed by the second layer or hidden layer. Node pairs from each of the two groups may have a symmetrical relation between them but within a group, there are no contacts between nodes. This constraint creates these algorithms more influential than the conventional Boltzmann machines, which enables links between the hidden layers. RBMs were effective in reduced dimensionality and joint filtering. Therefore, deep-learning systems built using stacking RBMs to form the Deep Belief Networks [50].
AE	AE is an unsupervised learning algorithm that uses the backpropagation method, where the target values equivalent to the inputs. i.e. $y(i)=x(i)$. Autoencoders are comprised of a digital decoder that converts all the input into a hidden representation, and again the decoder reconstructs that representation's inputs [34,43,51]. These are prepared to reduce reconstruction errors. To minimize dimensionality an auto-encoder uses a neural network. This is beneficial to reduce the size of the set function before it is transferred through another neural network [54].
RNN	RNN is a sort of neural network in which the prior phase output is given as feedback to input in the present step. The crucial role is the hidden state that retains information about every sequence. It is employed in dropping the complexity of growing parameters and for storing data streams [40]. Therefore, these alternates are effective in apprehending extensive tenure needs, which lead to an outstanding outcome in natural language processing (NLP) based applications [46].

2.4.1 Medical Imaging

For decades, ML algorithms have been used in medical-imaging equipment, beginning with approaches to evaluate or assist in taking radiographic pictures in the 1970s. In the mid-1980s, computer-aided diagnosis systems began to create automotive healthcare progress, leading with severe cancer identification and treatment, algorithms for chest X-rays, mammograms, and then widening to more advanced methods like scan, ultrasound, and other computed tomography (CT) methods. The CAD algorithms used a data-driven approach predominantly in the early days, as most deep-learning algorithms do today [15]. According to a new report by Signify Research, the healthcare market for artificial intelligence in medical imaging is prepared for robust growth and is expected to reach more than $2 billion by the end of 2023. The report states that AI will change the medical imaging industry, concerning increased productivity, enhanced diagnosis precision, additional personalized medication scheduling, and, eventually, better clinical results. AI will perform a crucial part in radiology to manage the continuously growing number of diagnostic-imaging procedures, even though shortages of a persistent radiologist in most of the countries [35]. Signify Research said the implementation of deep-learning technology and inexpensive cloud computing, graphics processing units, and storage is faster than ever before. This not only leads to increasing the availability of the product from a wider choice of vendors but with added functionalities. Gradually, AI-based tools become more precise and sophisticated. For predicting Alzheimer's disease and its variations, the primary application of medical imaging using deep learning is spitting image processing for brain MRI scans analysis [51,54]. CNNs have been employed in other medical fields to indicate a categorized description of knee MRI scans and along with cartilage segmentation for prediction of the threat of severe osteoarthritis problems [53]. Deep learning was also applied in the multi-channel 3D MRI segment of multiple sclerosis lesions and ultrasonic visual differential treatment of benign and malignant breast nodules [54,55]. More recently, Gulshan and research team [48] used CNNs in retinal fundus images to recognize diabetic retinopathy, achieving a high sensitivity as compared to certified annotations by ophthalmologists. CNN's algorithms have performed as good as certified dermatologists, in the classification of biopsy-verified medical photos of various forms based on skin cancers [49].

2.5 METHODOLOGY

The study would focus on these three aspects of artificial intelligence applicability in healthcare and bring out the technologies being developed by academic institutions and R&D labs. The outcome of the study would be useful for various R&D labs, industrial organizations including startups, that can adapt and build upon the identified technologies and roll out to the Indian populace. This would also eliminate the unnecessary cycle of reinventing the technology, and with a transfer of technology, the technologies could be adopted by industries/ SMEs/start-ups and made commercial.

This study project aims to provide a platform where researchers, start-ups, and doctors can discuss technologies designed using AI for improving healthcare services in the Indian context. C-DAC has also shared its findings understudy project with many start-ups, academics, medical practitioners, and thinkers to validate the study. This study aims to summarize what has been achieved so far in AI healthcare, identify challenges, use researcher tactics to tackle the present challenges, and recognize some of the promising applications and innovations for the future healthcare in India. Based on the recent examined review in healthcare, the report suggests that deep-learning (DL) methods can be the platform for transforming immense health data into better human health. The DL algorithms ranging from convolution neural networks (CNN), radial basis function (RBF) to variable auto-encoders have applied in countless applications in the field of medical image analysis in recent medical research in detection, evaluation, facilitation, treatment, and prediction of various critical diseases.

2.6 ISSUES AND CHALLENGES IN INDIAN HEALTHCARE SECTOR

The health condition of the people in India has greatly improved after Independence. Nevertheless, the condition is less than in the case of the WHO report. Among 191 countries in the world, it placed India in 112th place.

While the economy is rising rapidly, India spends little on its healthcare needs. Nevertheless, over the period, India's total public-health investment has decreased; India spends only around 1% of its GDP on public health. Experts think that India needs to invest a significant amount of money to meet appropriate global rates of child and mother mortality. The government can raise resources in various ways from subsidies to welfare budgets optimization, especially by working closely with state governments. The government, as per the 2002 National Health Policy. The health sector contribution constitutes just 0.9% of GDP. It is not enough. Public health spending is 17.3 percent of the overall health expenditure in India, while 24.9 percent in China, and 45.4 and 44.1 in Sri Lanka and the USA, respectively. This is the key explanation for the country's low health standards. In the health sector, India also spends approximately 1.2% of its GDP, considerably less than some of the world's poorest countries. There are not enough facilities, appropriate management, committed personnel, and many other things required to ensure fair and effective healthcare. The density of physicians per 1000 people of various countries is not sufficient. The report illustrates that India ranks the worst compared to other countries in terms of medical personnel [14].

2.7 CHALLENGES OF AI IN HEALTHCARE

It is challenging to secure private data of patients and timely practical validation of AI research based on machine-learning and deep-learning algorithms by medical practitioners at clinics. Figure 2.4 shows the key challenges for integrating AI technology into healthcare, including those intrinsic to deep-learning and machine-learning technology, technical implementation difficulties, and recognition of the hurdles to adoption, along with the requisite sociocultural or pathway changes. Acquiring knowledge and perceptions from complicated, highly feature and diverse medical datasets continues a major task in transforming healthcare using artificial intelligence in the Indian context. Although existing studies involved very large numbers of patients with comprehensive benchmarking against expert results, most studies were retrospective, indicating that traditionally branded data were used to train and evaluate algorithms. We will only begin to understand the true usefulness of AI systems through prospective studies, as performance is likely to be worse when meeting real-world data that vary from that encountered during algorithm training. The limited number of prospective studies to date contains gradations of diabetic retinopathy. Detection of metastases of the breast cancer in sentinel lymph node biopsies, detection of wrist fractures, detection of colonic polyps and detection of congenital cataracts. By using wearables, consumer technology allows for huge prospective studies concerning historical standards. Given the promising outcomes achieved after applying deep-learning patterns, the medical application of new deep-learning algorithms to medical care remains faced with several unanswered challenges. Once AI is included in their program, a common mistake health professionals make often focuses on the benefits while ignoring the risk posed by the same system. There can be various potential drawbacks of relying only on computers rather than on humans. Therefore, full knowledge of any AI system that a healthcare platform intends to use is necessary.

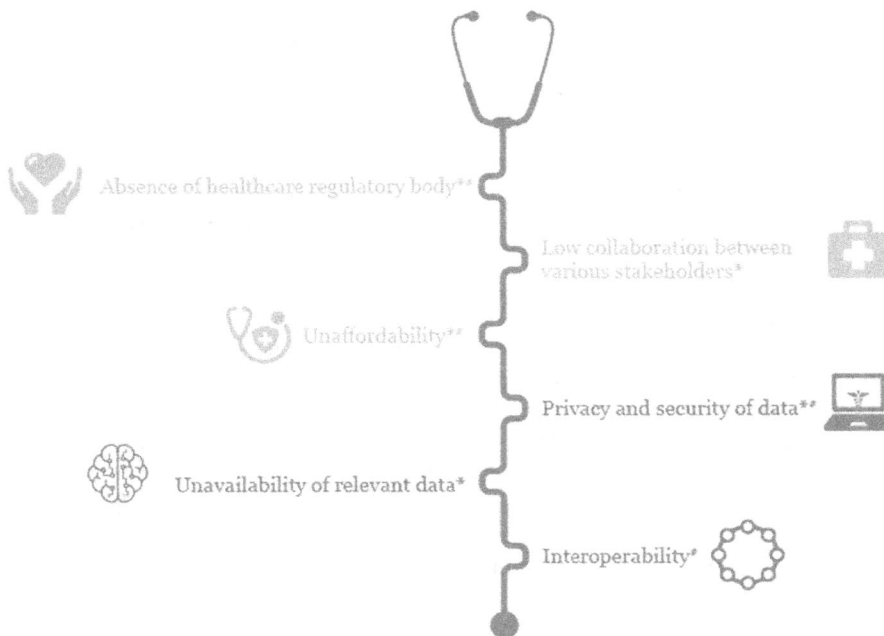

FIGURE 2.4 Challenges for AI implementation in healthcare.

AI itself has a long way to go before it can be integrated into any medical system without hesitation. Here are some of the obstacles for healthcare professionals in the AI industry and some things that can go wrong when health professionals rely only on AI instead of seeking ways to overcome the obstacles. This also helps in bridging the gap for developing an effective AI-based decision support mechanism for specific medical applications for healthcare in the Indian context. In particular, the following key challenges in Indian context are highlighted.

Government policies in healthcare: The firm's long-term business activities and traditions cannot be streamlined only by depending on an AI algorithm. Organizations need to consider strict and always changing government regulations. The data scientists are trained with the latest technologies because of the large volume of data available is primarily unstructured. This leads to a high demand in the healthcare sector for them.

Defective diagnosis: AI is based on a variety of data gathered from millions of patients who suffer from similar conditions to ensure the correct diagnosis for any specific disease. In addition, the data of patients belonging to a specific group should be appropriate for a fair comparison in AI databases. If patients with a particular background don't have sufficient data, AI will then make an inaccurate diagnosis and doctors will be mistaken to do this if they aren't sufficiently experienced to see it as being wrong.

Absence of compassion: AI-based computers lack compassion and an understanding of human existence and living circumstances. They often have economic and social implications after patients have been diagnosed. For example, an AI algorithm may indicate poor social support and recommend a nursing facility for patients from a community with low revenues. Because it is more expensive than home treatment, it may prevent the patient from continuing. Only a doctor will evaluate the family and home environment of patients to decide what kind of treatment plan they can afford, and which is most appropriate for their particular needs. Quartz, therefore, suggests that creators of AI apps get better textbooks to research the world, and everyone in it, without class, ethnic, or gender differences if they want AI to replace doctors.

Infringement of data privacy: Although important in all industries, privacy is usually particularly strongly enforced when it comes to medical data. The patient's data is usually not allowed to be disclosed, and hospitals and research institutions are vigilant about cloud platforms and servers. The start-up companies are unable to develop AI-based medical products due to difficulty in accessing patient personal data. Patients need to take care of data privacy and malfunctioning aspects while working with the AI systems. All patient information has been processed conveniently by AI applications. It covers everything from previous conditions, personal data, and blood test medical reports, etc. Although a person can ensure confidentiality for doctors and patients, machines do not make such promises. The loss of these data may result in a malfunction due to algorithmic bias or failure to maintain the program. Or even worse, the wrong people could use this information easily; that can occur if the network is not secured properly against hackers. Artificial intelligence developments pose a threat to health data, and therefore, appropriate steps must be established and taken to safeguard any AI machines in the medical sector.

Data quality and volume: Designing frameworks presently require huge data, and thus, the cutting-edge industry is a huge information environment. In any case, mechanical information, as a rule, is organized but may be of poor quality. The quality of the information may be poor and not at all like other consumer-faced applications; information from mechanical frameworks often have clear physical implications, which makes it harder to compensate for the quality with volume. Information collected for preparing machine-learning models, as a rule, is missing a comprehensive set of working conditions and well-being states/fault modes, which may cause untrue positives and untrue negatives in online usage of AI frameworks. Therefore, we cannot find the patients as required to teach a complete model of a machine or deep learning. Moreover, knowledge of diseases and their unpredictability is far more complex than other relevant tasks. Therefore, from a large data perspective, the amount of medical information necessary to train an accurate and reliable learning model would be considerably higher compared to other media.

Healthcare data are extremely unclear, chaotic, incomplete, and heterogeneous, unlike other environments in which information is smooth and well structured. It is challenging to form a decent learning model of diverse data sets to get rid of several problems, such as data sparseness, redundancy or lost values.

Domain complexity: Biomedicine and healthcare issues are more complex than in other fields (for example, image as well as speech analysis). The diseases are heterogeneously, and their causes and progress in most diseases are not yet fully known. Consequently, the sum of patients generally is constrained in a practical medical field, and we cannot apply to most of the patients as we would like too.

Incorporating expert knowledge: To healthcare problems, proven knowledge of medical problems is important. Because of the small amount and the various quality issues of medical data, expert expertise must be implemented for AI-based systems to monitor it in the appropriate path.

Temporal modeling: All healthcare problems have a time factor. Especially in the case of EHRs along with monitoring equipment. Therefore, time-vulnerable deep-learning model training is essential for awareness and timely clinical support for patients.

Feature enrichment: Due to the limited amount of data for patients suffering from specific diseases in the world, the challenge is to collect as many characteristics as feasible to identify and discover new aspects of treating every patient collectively.

Transparency: A physician must be able to understand why an algorithm has been approved for a certain treatment. This means the methods for prediction explaining are more intuitive and clearer. There is often a deal between projecting accuracy and transparency, particularly with the newest group of AI techniques embedded with artificial neural networks, which makes this problem even more crucial.

Sociocultural: Doctors, physicians or medical practitioners give treatments based upon their knowledge, experience, insight and problem-solving skills. It can be difficult for doctors to get suggestions from an AI-enabled automated system. Specific aspects likely to be assimilated into the medical programs to ensure that emerging technology is not seen as a threat to the medical doctor, but as medical assistance and updated knowledge for them. Indeed, if emerging technologies like AI are incorporated in such a manner that they empower doctors to treat more significantly and allows more people than to replace them.

Problem of infrastructure: In the last five to seven years, the latest deep-learning models have been used against traditional deep neural networks. However, the devices and infrastructure essential to support these algorithms are not accessible. Moreover, a small number of individuals acquire the required technical knowledge needed to deal with problems in data and software technology. AI solutions are often confronted with problems, particularly in medicine, with small amounts of data and variable data quality. Predictive models must be retrained as new information is provided so that improvements in data collection processes and other problems in the real world are closely monitored that can lead to a drift in data distribution over time.

All these problems present many opportunities for developing the sector and future research possibilities. Hence, we come across the resulting instructions with all of them in mind, encouraging the prospect of deep learning in medical care [59,60].

2.8 APPLICATIONS OF AI

AI plays a major role in various disciplines such as finance, marketing, banking, cybersecurity, and healthcare. There are important key points of AI-enabled healthcare applications such as:

Making healthcare accessible: In poor healthcare infrastructure nations, retrieving healthcare facilities is merely difficult, particularly for those residing in isolated areas. The integration of recent AI systems with healthcare in these isolated areas to establish an automated AI-enabled healthcare infrastructure in these rural areas. This provides a way to help patients understand their symptoms and find appropriate medications rather than full-service care. Health guidance for

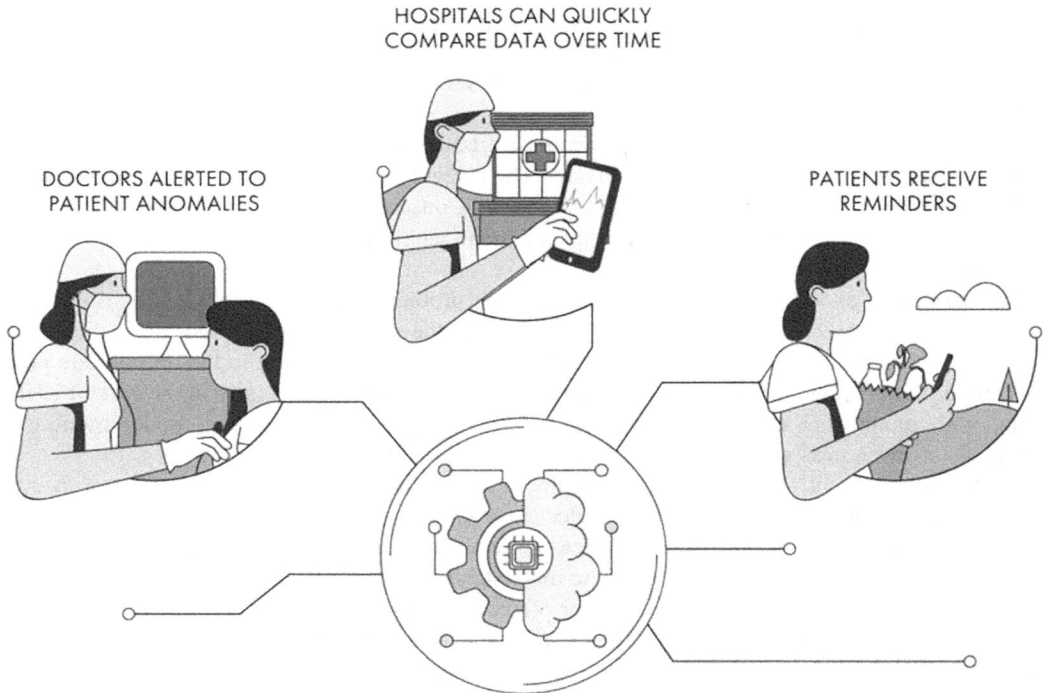

FIGURE 2.5   Healthcare accessible through AI technologies to patient.

underdeveloped populations is provided with applications such as Ada. Such solutions are easily accessible in the local languages of the areas where they are introduced (Figure 2.5).

Predicting diseases: Deep-learning algorithms of AI technology are capable of storing all records of people in one site and gaining access to this data for a more precise diagnosis of future illnesses in patients with current symptoms. Applications using algorithms predicted these diseases and have millions of the prior diagnoses stored; patients may consult these AI applications without taking any second opinion from any physician. However, AI can predict a person's health problems in the future by integrating and analyzing data from various sources. An application such as Verily by Google is predicting non-communicable diseases such as hereditary genetic illnesses, cancer, and heart attacks. The goal is to allow doctors to predict any potential problems so that they can establish plans for care to avoid or treat them promptly. Another method AI can assist with is diagnosis by detecting biomarkers. Biomarkers are unique particles that appear in biological fluids that can detect the existence of a specific illness in an individual's body. Emerging technology such as AI will automate manual work, saving a lot of time and energy in diagnosing a disease. These deep-learning algorithms can competently categorize molecules to recognize a specific state; they are also more cost-effective; if clinicians practice AI aid for diagnostic diseases, persons won't have to undertake costly laboratory tests.

Assisting in surgery: AI is now employed in surgical procedures as artificial intelligence-based applications have demonstrated to be exceptional support for the surgeons in the surgery. Robot surgery has currently opened the path for effective treatment of uncommon disorders in the healthcare industry. Complicated surgical procedures can now be conducted with accuracy, minimum side effects, and decreased pain along with a faster recovery. In addition to these, AI now has details for surgeons on existing patients under care in real-time. This includes scans showing the brain's different portions and MRI scans needed to assist in surgery. This is a security and relief for the subjects under anesthesia.

2.9 OPPORTUNITIES IN AI HEALTHCARE

India is one of the world's countries with the most scope to improve life-based advanced, safe, and scalable healthcare technologies due to its massive disparity in the delivery of healthcare, a strong shortage of qualified medical practitioners and facilities, and low government expenditures for healthcare. Nonetheless, it is still difficult to name more than a few digital technology deployment examples in the nation of one billion people, many of them now fitted with internet access and smartphones that have greatly influenced or commonly used health outcomes. This article discusses a variety of success stories and highlights some troubling developments surrounding artificial intelligence (AR) and Indian healthcare, as well as difficulties preventing smaller initiatives. Some of the opportunities in AI in Healthcare are shown in Figure 2.6.

2.9.1 MEDICAL IMAGING

The interpretation and comprehension of medical imaging are some of the biggest challenges for medical specialists. This is incredibly important because medical imaging, together with symptoms and blood tests, is a vital element for developing a medical diagnosis. For example, when viewing MRIs and CT scans, oncologists continue to strive to distinguish cancerous cells and noncancerous cells. They look unbelievably alike, and a misread picture with a corresponding somber overvivid rate can cause a late diagnosis. This is one reason why cell biopsies are still so relevant in this area. Medical research firms, however, change this model by machine learning. They teach these machine models on how to accurately read medical imaging by exposing machine-learning software to millions of stored images and the corresponding disease diagnosis. IBM Watson is a leader in the field of artificial intelligence education in the medical picture. The machine-learning software of the technology company is superior to many rivals because of the enormous amount of IBM data. The company has been buying medical companies like Merge over the last decade. As a result, more than 315 health data points are available today. Expect IBM in the next five years to obtain FDA approval for its AI technology. IBM public announcements indicate that the company expects permission to do more than basic medical imaging with deep-learning technology.

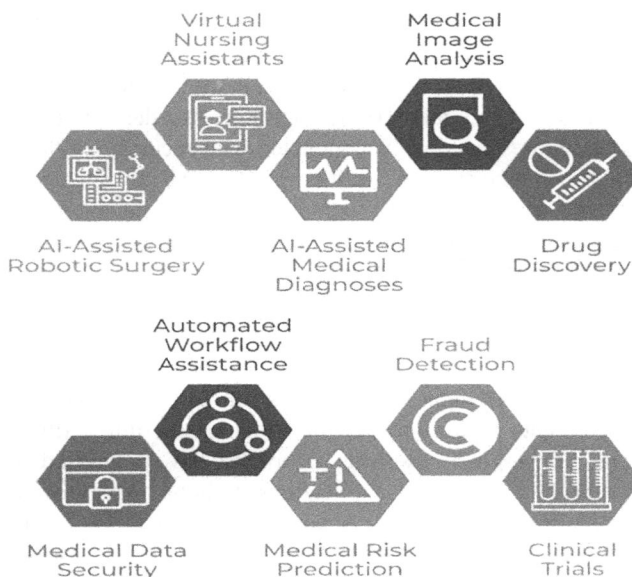

FIGURE 2.6 Opportunities in AI in healthcare.

2.9.2 PHARMACEUTICAL DISCOVERY

In deep learning, the pharmaceutical industry quickly becomes a leader. Major firms such as Amgen, AstraZeneca, Bayer, Eli Lilly, and others are expanding their internal research teams to increase the efficiency of their process of discovery. These organizations have a massive amount of data, including research information and patient outcomes to do research and development on deep-learning technology. The vast amount of information is important to the development of accurate predictions, the major reason for investing so much in deep learning by the pharmaceutical industry. A good example of this is the Benevolent AI. The company created a collection of custom algorithms to find clues about potential new medicines in current and past medical research. Different classes of drugs can be useful in the treatment of undesirable diseases by using software data. In particular, in comparison, organizations such as Sophia Genetics use deep learning, to inform patients about their hereditary disease vulnerability, using specific genetic markers linked to cancer, heart disease, diabetes, and more.

2.9.3 DISEASE IDENTIFICATION

Disease detection is one of the most important areas of machine and deep-learning science. Research showed that at least 5% of medical diagnoses were wrong in any given year. This has an annual effect of 12 million people, resulting in between 40,000 and 80,000 deaths. Deep knowledge and AI are used by medical research organizations to improve the accuracy of disease detection. A good example of the value of deep learning is the medical company's equity. To improve patient outcomes and disease identification, the company uses deep neural networks. It used its advanced AI technology recently to improve various diagnoses of sclerosis. This started by gathering millions of data points from insurance claims for multiple sclerosis in the state of New York. The comprehensive learning program finally was able to reliably "at least 8 months" identify the disease before doctors could carry out the test using standard medical technology. The deep-learning process is dedicated by helping medical professionals to treat diseases in advance of irreversible damage and to improve their longevity and quality of life.

2.9.4 AI-ENABLED SURGERY

AI is now employed in the surgical procedure as artificial intelligence-based applications have demonstrated to be exceptional support for the surgeons in the surgery. Robot surgery has currently opened the path for effective treatment of uncommon disorders in the healthcare industry. Complicated surgical procedures can now be conducted with accuracy, with minimum side effects, decreased pain, and a faster recovery. In addition to this, AI now has details for surgeons on existing patients under care in real-time. This includes scans showing the breakdown of the brain in its different portions and MRI scans that are needed to assist in the surgery. This is a security and relief for the subject while handing themselves to the doctors in anesthesia.

2.9.5 DISEASES PREDICTION

Deep-learning algorithms of AI technology are capable of storing all records of people in one site and gaining access to this data for a more precise diagnosis of future illnesses in patients with current symptoms. Prediction applications using algorithms have diagnosed and stored millions of results, with patients consulting these AI applications without taking second opinion from any physician. However, AI can predict a person's health problems in the future by integrating and analyzing data from various sources. An application such as Verily by Google is predicting non-communicable diseases, such as hereditary genetic illnesses, cancer, and heart attacks. The goal is to allow doctors to predict any potential problems so that they can establish care plans to avoid or treat them promptly. Another method AI can assist with is diagnosing by detecting biomarkers. Biomarkers are unique particles that appear in biological fluids that can detect the existence of a specific illness in an individual's body. The emerging technology such as AI will automate the manual work, saving a lot of time and energy in diagnosing a disease. These deep-learning algorithms can competently categorize molecules to recognize a specific state; they are also more cost-effective; if clinicians practice AI aid for diagnostic diseases, persons won't have to undertake costly laboratory tests [13,14].

2.10 STUDY FINDINGS

The major findings include deep-learning algorithms of AI technologies used in medical imaging, disease prediction, detection, and supervision for medical experts such as doctors and nurses, pharmaceutical discovery, and less invasive diagnostics. Numerous journals have been reviewed in the medical imaging for better findings in AI healthcare and the benefit of society. Internet of things of AI technology used in remote-monitoring solutions and digital platform integrations. Robotics is another field of AI technology used in remote-assisted surgery and ancillary services. Machine-learning is another artificial intelligence technology used in teleconsultation application, patient mobile interface, disease-detection prediction, and treatment. Software languages such as Java, php are used in healthcare for designing teleconsultation applications. C-DAC, Mohali has designed the teleconsultation application name esanjeevani to serve the nation during the COVID-19 pandemic in India. Most of the states have been utilizing the healthcare technologies for the benefits of patients and doctors in the pandemic situation currently. The study also identified list start-ups, academic institutes, government organizations such as IITs/IISC funded by various ministries working in the field of AI in healthcare. The study has also included case studies of AI-based technologies in healthcare. AI algorithm testing and validation methods are developed to assess algorithm output under conditions that vary from the training set. The development of AI systems can boost the efficiency of modern mobile surveillance tools and applications; build data infrastructure to collect and incorporate smart device-generated data to support AI applications; and identify and build methods for addressing critical health data gaps. Developing protocols and IT infrastructure to collect and incorporate different data. More significant steps need to implement such as a robust open data policy, comprehensive privacy policy, government funding on the healthcare sector, increased investment in R&D in AI, robust national infrastructure, providing staff with the necessary skills to implement AIs and be prepared for the changes that AI may bring. A regulatory framework ensuring transparency and accountability are some of the actions necessary to set up a functioning health environment for AI in India.

2.11 PRESENT AND FUTURE SCOPE

The article presented the latest literature survey on applying AI technologies, along with other allied fields to improve the healthcare domain in the Indian context. It will not be easy for AI to take control of the health sector and completely replace doctors. Next, we will find ways to address the above problems and solve them. Ultimately, we need to find ways to educate people and convince them of the different benefits that AI can offer in the healthcare industry to make them feel as safe as with doctors only. Consumers should be educated about not only AI; they should also be informed of the use of algorithms by healthcare professionals. They can only be convinced to use them in their facilities if they can trust these algorithms. Only a great number of clinical validations can build this trust, which can only be obtained through extensive studies and research on the ground. There is no question we still have a very long way to go before the healthcare sector can take on AI because in smaller facilities and developing countries, it still needs to prove value. This can not be denied, but there is a competitive advantage to those who have incorporated AI into their facility. However, AI makes it easier for doctors, not to completely replace them, even in such cases, we must bear in mind that AI is highly dependent on algorithms of machine learning; only a human, a specialist physician, can see a patient holistically and consider several other factors before creating a treatment plan. In fact, as Eliezer Yudkowsky, co-founder of the Institute for Machine Intelligence, warns: "The biggest risk of artificial intelligence is by far that people find it too early to understand." Professionals must have a clear understanding of the system they use and know how to protect it. Therefore, though AI has no doubt several advantages for the healthcare industry, HitConsultant argues that AI should help rather than replace healthcare professionals.

2.12 CONCLUSION

The studies demonstrate that emerging deep learning and its advanced algorithms in medical diagnosis are far superior to AI-enabled solutions in the healthcare field and various medical applications. India is currently in a unique position to push national and foreign companies in the field of AI and healthcare. Artificial intelligence is where it will reshape the healthcare industry in India. Nevertheless, AI-driven applications have many challenges: an efficient legal structure for privacy and data integrity is required, and we must address issues of cultural recognition, informed consent, and liability. The most important role played will be patients' data, which assists in integrating AI into clinical care in India. There is a need to standardize/centralize hospital management systems. It can assist in the creation of electronic health data repositories for AI applications. Furthermore, the live demonstration of AI-based products and specialist training to the doctors is the right approach for integrating AI into clinical care in developing countries like India. Precision treatment and early detection of diseases are the benefits of implementing AI-enabled solutions in healthcare in a country like India. India has the potential to tackle many health concerns using AI, with a wide range of knowledge and an increasing start-up community. The government has also taken a variety of steps to promote the adoption of AI across India, in its search for India to join the AI revolution. Still more significant steps need to implement such as a robust open data policy, comprehensive privacy policy, government funding on the healthcare sector, increased investment in R&D in AI, robust national infrastructure, providing staff with the necessary skills to implement AIs and be prepared for the changes that AI may bring, and a regulatory framework ensuring transparency and accountability are some of the actions necessary to set up a functioning health environment for AI in India.

ACKNOWLEDGMENTS

This study was supported by the following grants from the DSIR, New Delhi (A2K+ studies program). The authors would like to thank the Department of Scientific and Industrial Research, Ministry of Science and Technology for providing financial assistance and timely guidance to undertake this study.

REFERENCES

[1] Miotto, R., Wang, F., Wang, S., Jiang, X., Dudley, J. T. Deep learning for healthcare: Review, opportunities and challenges. *Briefings in Bioinformatics* 2017.

[2] Nature.com. A fairer way forward for AI in health care. 2020. [online] Available at: https://www.nature.com/articles/d41586-019-02872-2 [Accessed 2 Mar. 2020].

[3] Forbes.com. Council Post: 13 Industries Soon To Be Revolutionized By Artificial Intelligence. 2020. *[online]* Available at: https://www.forbes.com/sites/forbestechcouncil/2019/01/16/13-industries-soon-to-be-revolutionized-by-artificial-intelligence/#59f9f1f03dc1 [Accessed 2 Mar. 2020].

[4] Cichocki, Poggio, T., Osowski, S., Lempitsky, V. Deep Learning: Theory and Practice. *Bulletin of the Polish Academy of Sciences: Technical Sciences* 2018, (66), 757–759.

[5] Pourjavan, S. Definitions: Machine learning, deep leerning and AI understanding. *Acta Ophthalmologica* 2019, 97(S263).

[6] Stasiak, B., Tarasiuk, P., Michalska, I., Tomczyk, A. Application of convolutional neural networks with anatomical knowledge for brain MRI analysis in MS patients. *Bulletin of the Polish Academy of Sciences: Technical Sciences* 2018, (66), 857–868.

[7] Suzuki, K. Overview of deep learning in medical imaging. *Radiological Physics and Technology* 2017, 10, 257–273.

[8] Ravì, D., Wong, C., Deligianni, F., Berthelot, M., Andreu-Perez, J., Lo, B., Yang, G.-Z. Deep learning for health informatics. *IEEE Journal of Biomedical and Health Informatics* 2017, 21, 4–21.

[9] Lee, J. G., Jun, S., Cho, Y. W., Lee, H., Kim, G. B., Seo, J. B., Kim, N. Deep Learning in Medical Imaging: General Overview. *Korean Journal of Radiology* 2017, 18, 570–584.

[10] Mamoshina, P., Vieira, A., Putin, E., Zhavoronkov, A. Applications of Deep Learning in Biomedicine. *Molecular Pharmaceutics* 2016, 13, 1445–1454.

[11] Liu, J., Pan, Y., Li, M., Chen, Z., Tang, L., Lu, C., Wang, J. Applications of deep learning to MRI images: A survey. *Big Data Mining and Analytics* 2018, 1, 1–18.

[12] Bhargava, C., Aggarwal, J., Sharma, P. K. Residual life estimation of fabricated humidity sensors using different artificial intelligence techniques. *Bulletin of the Polish Academy of Sciences: Technical Sciences* 2019, (67), 147–154.

[13] Srivastava, S. Artificial Intelligence: Way Forward for India. *IAES International Journal of Artificial Intelligence (IJ-AI)* 2018, 7(1), 19.

[14] Anon, (2020). [online] Available at: https://cis-india.org/internet-governance/files/ai-and-healtchare-report [Accessed 2 Mar. 2020].

[15] Greenspan, H., Van Ginneken, B., Summers, R. M. Guest editorial deep learning in medical imaging: Overview and future promise of an exciting new technique. *IEEE Transactions on Medical Imaging* 2016, 35, 1153–1159.

[16] Dolz, J., Desrosiers, C., Wang, L., Yuan, J., Shen, D., Ben Ayed, I. Deep CNN ensembles and suggestive annotations for infant brain MRI segmentation. *Computerized Medical Imaging and Graphics* 2020, 79, 101660.

[17] Czajkowska, J., Korzekwa, S., Pietka, E. Computer Aided Diagnosis of Atopic Dermatitis. *Computerized Medical Imaging and Graphics* 2020, 79, 101676.

[18] Xu, L., Liu, M., Shen, Z., Wang, H., Liu, X., Wang, X., Wang, S., Li, T., Yu, S., Hou, M., Guo, J., Zhang, J., He, Y. DW-Net: A cascaded convolutional neural network for apical four-chamber view segmentation in fetal echocardiography. *Computerized Medical Imaging and Graphics* 2020, 80, 101690.

[19] Sharif, M., Li, J., Khan, M., Saleem, M. Active deep neural network features selection for segmentation and recognition of brain tumors using MRI images. *Pattern Recognition Letters* 2020, 129, 181–189.

[20] Dou, Q., Yu, L., Chen, H., Jin, Y., Yang, X., Qin, J., Heng, P. A. 3D deeply supervised network for automated segmentation of volumetric medical images. *Medical Image Analysis* 2017, 41, 40–54.

[21] Pan, Y., Huang, W., Lin, Z., Zhu, W., Zhou, J., Wong, J., Ding, Z. Brain tumor grading based on neural networks and convolutional neural networks. In Proceedings of the 2015 37th Annual International Conference of the IEEE Engineering in Medicine and Biology Society (EMBC), Milan, Italy, 25–29 August 2015, 699–702.

[22] Payan, A., Montana, G. Predicting Alzheimer's disease: A neuroimaging study with 3D convolutional neural networks. arXiv 2015, arXiv:1502.02506.

[23] Havaei, M., Davy, A., Warde-Farley, D., Biard, A., Courville, A., Bengio, Y., Larochelle, H. Brain tumor segmentation with Deep Neural Networks. *Medical Image Analysis* 2017, 35, 18–31.

[24] Kamnitsas, K., Ledig, C., Newcombe, V. F. J., Simpson, J. P., Kane, A. D., Menon, D. K., Glocker, B. Efficient multi-scale 3D CNN with fully connected CRF for accurate brain lesion segmentation. *Medical Image Analysis* 2017, 36, 61–78.

[25] Isensee, F., Kickingereder, P., Bonekamp, D., Bendszus, M., Wick, W., Schlemmer, H. P., Maier-Hein, K. Brain Tumor Segmentation Using Large Receptive Field Deep Convolutional Neural Networks. *Bildverarbeitung für die Medizin* 2017, 86–91.

[26] Brosch, T., Tam, R. Manifold learning of brain MRIs by deep learn- ing. *Medical Image Computing and Computer Assisted Intervention* 2013, 16, 633–640.

[27] Esteva, A., Kuprel, B., Novoa, R. A., Ko, J., Swetter, S. M., Blau, H. M., Thrun, S. Dermatologist-level classification of skin cancer with deep neural networks. *Nature* 2017, 542, 115–118.

[28] Gulshan, V., Peng, L., Coram, M., et al. Development and valida- tion of a deep learning algorithm for detection of diabetic retinopathy in retinal fundus photographs. *JAMA* 2016, 316, 2402–2410.

[29] Causey, J. L., Zhang, J., Ma, S., Jiang, B., Qualls, J. A., Politte, D. G., Prior, F., Zhang, S., Huang, X. Highly accurate model for prediction of lung nodule malignancy with CT scans. *Scientific Reports* 2018, 8, 9286.

[30] Roth, H. R., Farag, A., Lu, L., Turkbey, E. B., Summers, R. M. Deep convolutional networks for pancreas segmentation in CT imaging. *Medical Image Processing* 2015, 9413, 94131G.

[31] Prasoon, A., Petersen, K., Igel, C., et al. Deep feature learning for knee cartilage segmentation using a triplanar convolutional neural network. *Medical Image Computing and Computer Assisted Intervention* 2013, 16, 246–253.

[32] Liu, S., Liu, S., Cai, W., et al. Early diagnosis of Alzheimer's dis- ease with deep learning. In: International Symposium on Biomedical Imaging, Beijing, China 2014, 1015–1018.

[33] Yoo, Y., Brosch, T., Traboulsee, A., et al. Deep learning of image features from unlabeled data for multiple sclerosis lesion segmentation. In: International Workshop on Machine Learning in Medical Imaging, Boston, MA, USA, 2014, 117–124.

[34] Cheng, J-Z, Ni, D., Chou, Y-H, et al. Computer-aided diagnosis with deep learning architecture: applications to breast lesions in US images and pulmonary nodules in CT scans. *Scientific Reports* 2016, 6, 24454.

[35] Kurek, J., Świderski, B., Osowski, S., Kruk, M., Barhoumi, W. Deep learning versus classical neural approach to mammogram recognition. *Bulletin of the Polish Academy of Sciences: Technical Sciences* 2018(66), 831–840.

[36] Dubrovina, A., Kisilev, P., Ginsburg, B., Hashoul, S., Kimmel, R. Computational mammography using deep neural networks. *Computer Methods in Biomechanics and Biomedical Engineering: Imaging and Visualization* 2016, 6, 243–247.

[37] Acharya, U. R., Fujita, H., Oh, S. L., Hagiwara, Y., Tan, J. H., Adam, M. Application of deep convolutional neural network for automated detection of myocardial infarction using ECG signals. *Information Science* 2017, 415, 190–198.

[38] Mehta, R., Majumdar, A., Sivaswamy, J. BrainSegNet: A convolutional neural network architecture for automated segmentation of human brain structures. *J. Med. Imaging (Bellingham)* 2017, 4, 024003.

[39] Abdel-Zaher, A. M., Eldeib, A. M. Breast cancer classification using deep belief networks. *Expert Systems with Applications* 2016, 46, 139–144.

[40] Xu, Y., Dai, Z., Chen, F., Gao, S., Pei, J., Lai, L. Deep Learning for Drug-Induced Liver Injury. *Journal of Chemical Information and Modeling* 2015, 55, 2085–2093.

[41] Ehteshami Bejnordi, B., Veta, M., Johannes van Diest, P., van Ginneken, B., Arssemeijer, N., Litjens, G., Venancio, R. Diagnostic Assessment of Deep Learning Algorithms for Detection of Lymph Node Metastases in Women With Breast Cancer. *JAMA* 2017, 318, 2199–2210.

[42] Chmelik, J., Jakubicek, R., Walek, P., Jan, J., Ourednicek, P., Lambert, L., Amadori, E., Gavelli, G. Deep convolutional neural network-based segmentation and classification of difficult to define metastatic spinal lesions in 3D CT data. *Medical Image Analysis* 2018.

[43] Xu, J., Xiang, L., Liu, Q., Gilmore, H., Wu, J., Tang, J., Madabhushi, A. Stacked sparse autoencoder (SSAE) for nuclei detection on breast cancer histopathology images. *IEEE Transactions on Medical Imaging* 2016, 35, 119–130.

[44] González, G., Ash, S. Y., Vegas-Sánchez-Ferrero, G., Onieva Onieva, J., Rahaghi, F. N., Ross, J. C., Washko, G. R. Disease staging and prognosis in smokers using deep learning in chest computed tomography. *American Journal of Respiratory and Critical Care Medicine* 2018, 197, 193–203.

[45] Choi, H., Jin, K. H. Fast and robust segmentation of the striatum using deep convolutional neural networks. *Journal of Neuroscience Methods* 2016, 274, 146–153.

[46] Gao, X., Lin, S., Wong, T. Y. Automatic Feature Learning to Grade Nuclear Cataracts Based on Deep Learning. *IEEE Transactions on Biomedical Engineering* 2015, 62, 2693–2701.

[47] Masood, A., Al-Jumaily, A., Anam, K. Self-supervised learning model for skin cancer diagnosis. In Proceedings of the 2015 7th International IEEE/EMBS Conference Neural Engineering (NER), Montpellier, France, 22–24 April 2015, 1012–1015.

[48] Han, Z., Wei, B., Zheng, Y., Yin, Y., Li, K., Li, S. Breast Cancer Multi-classification from Histopathological Images with Structured Deep Learning Model. *Scientific Reports* 2017, 7, 4172.

[49] Cha, K. H., Hadjiiski, L., Samala, R. K., Chan, H. P., Caoili, E. M., Cohan, R. H. Urinary bladder segmentation in CT urography using deep-learning convolutional neural network and level sets. *Medical Physics* 2016, 43, 1882.

[50] Zhang, Q., Xiao, Y., Dai, W., Suo, J., Wang, C., Shi, J., Zheng, H. Deep learning based classification of breast tumors with shear-wave elastography. *Ultrasonics* 2016, 72, 150–157.

[51] Danaee, P., Ghaeini, R., Hendrix, D. A. A deep learning approach for cancer detection and relevant gene identification. *Pacific Symposium on Biocomputing* 2017, 2017, 219–229.

[52] Kleesiek, J., Urban, G., Hubert, A., Schwarz, D., Maier-Hein, K., Bendszus, M., Biller, A. Deep MRI brain extraction: A 3D convolutional neural network for skull stripping. *Neuroimage* 2016, 129, 460–469.

[53] Kumar, D., Wong, A., Clausi, D. A. Lung nodule classification using deep features in CT images. In Proceedings of the 2015 12th Conference on Robot VisionComputer and Robot Vision (CRV), Halifax, NS,Canada, 3–5 June 2015, 133–138.

[54] Sun, W., Zheng, B., Qian, W. Computer aided lung cancer diagnosis with deep learning algorithms. In Proceedings of the Medical Imaging 2016: Computer-Aided Diagnosis, San Diego, CA, USA, 27 February–3 March 2016; Volime 9785.

[55] Rasti, R., Teshnehlab, M., Phung, S. L. Breast cancer diagnosis in DCE-MRI using mixture ensemble of convolutional neural networks. *Pattern Recognition* 2017, 72, 381–390.

[56] Anirudh, R., Thiagarajan, J. J., Bremer, T., Kim, H. Lung nodule detection using 3D convolutional neural networks trained on weakly labeled data. In Proceedings of the Medical Imaging 2016: Computer-Aided Diagnosis, San Diego, CA, USA, 27 February–3 March 2016; Volume 9785.

[57] Samala, R. K., Chan, H. P., Hadjiiski, L. M., Cha, K., Helvie, M. A. Deep-learning convolution neural network for computer-aided detection of microcalcifications in digital breast tomosynthesis. In Proceedings of the Medical Imaging 2016: Computer-Aided Diagnosis, San Diego, CA, USA, 27 February–3 March 2016; Volume 9785.

[58] Dalmis, M. U., Litjens, G., Holland, K., Setio, A., Mann, R., Karssemeijer, N., Gubern-Merida, A. Using deep learning to segment breast and fibroglandular tissue in MRI volumes. *Medical Physics* 2017, 44, 533.

[59] (2020). Retrieved 15 April 2020, from https://cis-india.org/internet-governance/files/ai-and-healtchare-report

[60] Indian Healthcare Is All Set To Be Transformed By AI. 2020. Retrieved 15 April 2020, from https://www.medicalbuyer.co.in/indian-healthcare-is-all-set-to-be-transformed-by-ai/

3 Artificial Intelligence in Medical Imaging

Sehrawat Abhishek

Chitkara School of Health Sciences, Chitkara University, Rajpura, Punjab, India

Department of Radiodiagnosis and Imaging, All India Institute of Medical Sciences, Bhopal, Madhya Pradesh, India

Jaiswal Dhirendra

Department of Nuclear Medicine, All India Institute of Medical Sciences, Raipur, Chhattisgarh, India

CONTENTS

3.1 IMAGE SEGMENTATION

Image segmentation refers to the process of partitioning an image into multiple regions. These regions are a group of connected pixels with similar properties, such as gray level, color, texture, brightness, and contrast, etc. They also may correspond to a particular object or different parts of an object. The object/region of interest can be extracted manually on a good quality[18] F-FDGPET/CT fused image by simply selecting image intensity ranges; however, it is a time-consuming process and also subject to variation depending on the users. Segmentation carries a risk of generating incorrect object boundaries. Splitting the image into too many objects, called over-segmentation, may generate many small regions, which is problematic for good texture analysis and time-consuming to label when generating ground truth data. Under-segmentation is a much more serious problem; in that case, different objects can be merged into one cluster. We find that it is better to risk over-segmentation than under-segmentation because in the first case, all the pixels belonging to a region belong to the same class. On the other hand, in the case of under-segmentation, different regions are merged together; that means one region can contain pixels belonging to more than one class. Semi-automatic and fully automatic methods of segmentation are active areas of research in nuclear medicine ^{18}F-FDG PET/CT or SPECT/CT imaging. The simplest fully automatic method of segmentation is a thresholding-based segmentation method, which encompasses most of the voxel intensities of a particular tissue type. However, none of the segmentation methods are 100% successful for different types of images, whether using the automatic or semi-automatic method of segmentation [1–8].

It is very rare to achieve a useful segmentation using a single procedure, even under the most favorable conditions. Successful segmentation algorithms typically use a carefully constructed combination of procedures to achieve useful results. Some modern algorithms, especially the family of routines related to geodesic active contours, may seem to be an exception to this rule because they are often presented as achieving good segmentation results entirely on their own. However, close examination will show that a variety of preprocessing steps, in addition to careful parameter tuning, are necessary to achieve useful information.

3.2 WATERSHED ALGORITHM

The watershed transform was first proposed by Beucher and Lanteuejoul as a geophysical model of rain falling on a terrain. The idea is that a raindrop falling on a surface will trickle down the path of steepest descent to a minimum. The set of points on the surface that lead to the same minimum are known as a catchment basin, and borders between catchment basins are watershed lines. If an image is considered as a terrain and divided into catchment basins, then the hope is that each catchment basin would contain an object of interest [9].

Watershed Implementation Methods: These three are commonly used in conjunction with the watershed transform for segmentation.

- Distance transform approach
- Gradient method
- Marker-controlled approach

3.2.1 WATERSHED WITH DISTANCE TRANSFORM

Distance transform is a common tool used in watershed transform for image segmentation. The concept is the distance from every pixel to its nearest non-zero valued pixel. Every single valued pixel has a distance transform value of 0, as it is the closest non-zero valued pixel of itself [10].

3.2.2 GRADIENT-BASED METHOD

The principle of a gradient-based segmentation is to associate the boundaries of an object of interest with the gradient intensity crests observed in the image. To obtain meaningful image segmentation, several conditions must be satisfied. If the intrinsic resolution of the imaging device is low compared with the voxel size, transitions between regions of different activities in the images look blurred. As a consequence, the gradient-intensity peaks are not sharp and are thus more difficult to identify. Another caveat is related to the fact that noise gets amplified in the gradient-intensity image, compared with the initial image. As a first approximation, the effects of resolution and noise can be modeled as follows. First, the unknown 'ideal' image (i.e. with an infinitely large resolution and free of noise) is blurred by convolving it with the point spread function of the considered imaging device. Second, the blurred image is corrupted by statistical noise. Really acquired images can be assumed to result from this two-step model. This suggests that the ideal image could be recovered by reversing the above model, in the first approximation. For this purpose, the acquired image should be first denoised and then deblurred before segmentation [11].

3.2.3 MARKER-CONTROLLED METHODS

Direct application of watershed transform to a gradient image can result in over-segmentation due to noise. Over-segmentation means a large number of segmented regions. An approach used to control over-segmentation is based on the concept of markers. A marker is a connected component belonging to an image. Markers are used to modify the gradient image. Markers are of two types, internal and external, internal for object and external for boundary. The marker-controlled watershed segmentation has been shown to be a robust and flexible method for segmentation of objects with closed contours, where boundaries are expressed as ridges. Markers are placed inside an object of interest; internal markers associate with objects of interest, and external markers associate with the background. After segmentation, the boundaries of the watershed regions are arranged on the desired ridges, thus separating each object from its neighbours [12].

Image segmentation based on a watershed algorithm can be understood by visualizing a gray-scale image as a topographical surface, where the values of f(x, y) are implemented as heights. In geography, a watershed is the ridge that divides areas drained by different river systems. A catchment basin is the geographical area draining into a river or reservoir. The watershed transform finds the catchment basins and ridges lines in a gray-scale image. During the segmentation based on watershed transformation, the key concept is to change the starting image into another image whose catchment basins are the objects or regions we want to identify.

In image analysis, there are issues that need to be addressed, like development of a unified approach to the image-segmentation technique, which can be applied to all type of images, and selection of an appropriate technique for a specific type of image. In spite of profuseness in segmentation techniques, there is no universally accepted method for image segmentation; therefore, it remains a challenging problem. In this study, we studied the feasibility of using the gradient method of watershed algorithm of segmentation on ^{18}F-FDG PET/CT image of lung, liver, lymphoma, and breast tumors and tried to assess whether this method could provide appropriate segmentation.

Drever et al. (2007) [13] compared three image-segmentation techniques for target volume delineation in positron emission tomography. The authors compared thresholding, Sobel edge detection, and the watershed approach to yield accurate delineation of PET target cross-sections. A phantom study employing well-defined cylindrical and spherical volumes and activity distributions provided an opportunity to assess the relative efficacy with which the three approaches could yield accurate target delineation in PET. Results revealed that threshold segmentation can accurately delineate target cross-sections, but that the Sobel and watershed techniques both consistently fail to correctly identify the size of experimental volumes. The usefulness of threshold-based segmentation is limited, however, by the dependence of the correct threshold on target size.

Geets et al. (2007) [14] proposed a new gradient-based method and hierarchical cluster analysis for segmenting FDG-PET images. In this study, iteratively reconstructed images were first denoised and deblurred with an edge-preserving filter and a constrained iterative deconvolution algorithm. The authors first performed validation on computer-generated 3D phantoms containing spheres and then on a real cylindrical Lucite phantom containing spheres of different volumes ranging from 2.1 to 92.9 ml. Then, this validation segmentation on PET images was performed on preoperative laryngeal tumours from seven patients by the gradient-based method and the thresholding method based on the source-to-background ratio. For the spheres, the calculated volumes and radii were compared with the known values; for laryngeal tumours, the volumes were compared with the macroscopic specimens. Volume mismatches were also analysed. The authors concluded that gradient-based segmentation method applied on denoised and deblurred images proved to be more accurate than the source-to-background ratio method.

Ray et al. (2008) [15] compared two-dimensional and three-dimensional iterative watershed segmentation methods in hepatic tumor volumetrics. The authors compared the accuracy of two-dimensional (2D) and three-dimensional (3D) implementations of a computer-aided image segmentation method to that of physician observers (using manual outlining) for volume measurements of liver tumors visualized with diagnostic contrast-enhanced and PET/CT-based non-contrast-enhanced CT scans. The method assessed was a hybridization of the watershed method using observer-set markers with a gradient vector-flow approach. The authors called this method the iterative watershed segmentation (IWS) method. Initial assessments were performed using software phantoms that model a range of tumor shapes, noise levels, and noise qualities. IWS was then applied to CT image sets of patients with identified hepatic tumors and compared to the physician's manual outlines on the same tumors. IWS utilized multiple levels of segmentation performed with the use of fuzzy regions that could be considered part of a selected tumor. The results indicated that 2D-IWS is likely to be more accurate than 3D-IWS in relation to the observer volume estimate.

Wang et al. (2009) [16] studied the "automated liver segmentation" for whole-body low-contrast CT images from PET-CT scanners." The main objective of this study was to improve the identification and localization of hepatic tumor. The authors proposed a novel automated three-stage liver segmentation technique for PET-CT whole body studies, where: 1) the starting liver slice was automatically localized based on the liver-lung relations; 2) the "masking" slice containing the biggest liver section was localized using the ratio of liver ROI size to the right half of abdomen ROI size; 3) the liver segmented from the "masking" slice formed the initial estimation or mask for the automated liver segmentation. They concluded that this method can automatically segment the liver for a range of different patients, with consistent objective selection criteria and reproducible accurate results.

Campadelli et al. (2009) [17] in their study reviewed semi-automatic and automatic liver segmentation technique and compared their own fully automatized method. They used a gray-level based liver segmentation method and tested it on 40 patients with satisfactory results, which were comparable to the mean intra- and inter-observer variation. The authors concluded that their method outperformed the techniques in the literature.

Ballangan et al. (2011) [18] evaluated the impact of reconstruction algorithms on semi-automatic small lesion segmentation for PET in a phantom study. The aim of this study was to investigate the impact of different reconstruction methods on semi-automated small lesion segmentation for PET images. Four conventional segmentation methods were evaluated, including a region-growing technique based on maximum intensity (RGmax), mean intensity (RGmean) thresholds, fuzzy c-mean (FCM), and watershed (WS) technique. All these methods were evaluated on a physical phantom scan that was reconstructed with ordered subset expectation maximization (OSEM) with Gaussian post-smoothing and maximum a posteriori (MAP) with quadratic prior, respectively. The results demonstrated that: 1) the performance of all the segmentation methods were subject to the smoothness constraint applied on the reconstructed images; 2) FCM method applied on MAP-reconstructed images yielded overall superior performance than other evaluated combinations.

Zhang et al. (2011) [19] presented an interactive method for liver tumor segmentation from computed tomography (CT) scans. After some pre-processing operations, including liver parenchyma segmentation and liver contrast enhancement, the CT volume was partitioned into a large number of catchment basins under watershed transform. Then a support vector machines (SVM) classifier was trained on the user-selected seed points to extract tumors from liver parenchyma, while the corresponding feature vector for training and prediction was computed based upon each small region produced by watershed transform. Finally, some morphological operations were performed on the whole segmented binary volume to refine the rough segmentation result of SVM classification. The proposed method was tested and evaluated on MICCAI 2008 liver tumor segmentation challenge datasets. The experiment results demonstrated the accuracy and efficiency of the proposed method, which can be used routinely in clinical practice.

Christ et al. (2011) [20] **proposed** a methodology that integrates KMeans clustering with a marker-controlled watershed-segmentation algorithm and integrates fuzzy CMeans clustering with marker-controlled watershed-segmentation algorithm separately for medical image segmentation. The clustering algorithms are unsupervised learning algorithms, while the marker-controlled watershed-segmentation algorithm uses automated thresholding on the gradient magnitude map and post-segmentation merging on the initial partitions to reduce the number of false edges and over-segmentation. The authors concluded that integration of K-means clustering with a marker-controlled watershed algorithm gave better segmentation than integration of fuzzy C-means clustering with a marker-controlled watershed algorithm.

Ballangan et al. (2013) [21] assessed lung tumor segmentation in PET images using graph cuts. The aim of segmenting tumor regions in positron emission tomography (PET) was to provide more accurate measurements of tumor size and extension into adjacent structures than possible with visual assessment alone and hence improve patient management decisions. They proposed a segmentation energy function for the graph cuts technique to improve lung tumor segmentation with PET. Their segmentation energy was based on an analysis of the tumor voxels in PET images combined with a standardized uptake value (SUV) cost function and a monotonic downhill SUV feature. The monotonic downhill feature avoids segmentation leakage into surrounding tissues with similar or higher PET tracer uptake than the tumor, and the SUV cost function improves the boundary definition and also addresses situations where the lung tumor was heterogeneous. They evaluated the method in 42 clinical PET volumes from patients with non-small cell lung cancer (NSCLC). The authors concluded that their method improved segmentation and performed better than region-growing approaches, the watershed technique, fuzzy c-means, region-based active contour, and tumor customized downhill.

Bangara et al. (2014) [22] proposed a color-segmentation method for the detection of liver tumor in PET/CT scans. The authors attempted to segment the PET/CT images of liver using a binary tree quantization clustering method for the detection of a tumor. The problem of segmentation of gray scale is that intensity values between healthy tissue and tumor may be very close, but PET/CT provides more accurate measurements of tumor size than are possible with visual assessment alone. So they took 12 PET/CT images and processed them for segmentation of the liver tumor. The images are denoised using median filter, and a binary tree quantization clustering algorithm was used for segmentation. Finally, a region of interest (ROI) selection and shape-feature extraction was performed on the selected cluster to quantify the size of the tumor and the result compared to check the accuracy of the method with the original image and K-means clustering method. They concluded that this binary tree quantization clustering method is better than the k means clustering method in detecting tumors more accurately and precisely.

Altunbas et al. (2014) [23] evaluated the image-segmentation method to improve the accuracy of liver tumor contouring for treatment planning in stereotactic body radiation therapy (SBRT). They took pre-treatment PET-CT image sets for 26 patients who received SBRT to 28 liver lesions delineated using the following 3 methods: (1) percent threshold with respect to background-corrected maximum standard uptake values (SUV; threshold values varied from 10% to 50% with 10% increments); (2) threshold 3 standard deviations above mean background SUV (3σ); and (3) a gradient-based method that detects the edge of the FDG-PET avid lesion (edge). For each lesion, semi-automatically generated contours were evaluated with respect to reference contours manually drawn by 3 radiation oncologists. Two similarity metrics, dice coefficient and mean minimal distance (MMD), were employed to assess the volumetric overlap and the mean Euclidian distance between semi-automatically and observer-drawn contours. They found the mean dice and MMD values for 10%, 20%, 30% threshold, 3σ, and edge varied from 0.69 to 0.73, and from 3.44 mm to 3.94 mm, respectively (ideal dice and MMD values were 1 and 0 mm, respectively). A statistically significant difference was not observed among 10%, 20%, 30% threshold, 3σ, and edge methods, whereas 40% and 50% methods had inferior dice and MMD values. Finally, they concluded that the three PET segmentation methods are potential tools to accelerate liver-lesion delineation. The edge method appears to be the most practical for clinical implementation as it does not require calculation of SUV statistics. However, the performance of all segmentation methods showed large lesion-to-lesion fluctuations. Therefore, such methods may be suitable for generating initial estimates of FDG-PET avid volumes rather than being surrogates for manual volume delineation.

Arens et al. (2014) [24] studied the changes in tumour cell proliferation induced by radiotherapy for head and neck cancer, which can be depicted by the PET tracer ^{18}F-fluorothymidine (FLT). Three advanced semiautomatic PET segmentation methods for the delineation of the proliferative tumour volume (PV) before and during (chemo)radiotherapy were compared and related to clinical outcome in 46 patients with squamous cell carcinomas of the head and neck. The authors used background-subtracted relative-threshold level (PV RTL), a gradient-based method using the watershed-transform algorithm and hierarchical clustering analysis (PV W&C), and a fuzzy locally adaptive Bayesian algorithm (PV FLAB) applied to FLT PET/CT prior to treatment and in the 2nd and 4th week of therapy. Primary gross tumour volumes were visually delineated on CT images (GTV CT). PVs were visually determined on all PET scans. The authors concluded that in patients with head and neck cancer, FLAB proved to be the best performing method for segmentation of the PV on repeat FLT PET/CT scans during (chemo)radiotherapy. This may potentially facilitate radiation dose adaptation to changing PV.

Zhao et al. (2015) [25] proposed a new method of detecting pulmonary nodules with an improved watershed algorithm on (^{18}F-FDG PET/CT) PET/CT study. A dynamic threshold segmentation method was used to identify lung parenchyma in CT images and suspicious areas in PET images. Then, an improved watershed method was used to mark suspicious areas on the CT image. Next, the support vector machine (SVM) method was used to classify SPNs based on textural features of CT images and metabolic features of PET images to validate the proposed method. The proposed method in this process was more efficient than traditional methods and methods based on the CT or PET features alone (sensitivity 95.6%; average of 2.9 false positives per scan) [26,27].

The segmentation of tumor in PET/CT image is the pre-processing step of the image analysis. The segmented images are further analyzed for measurements of tumor size, tumor volume, or texture classification, etc. In texture classification, the basic issue is identifying the given textured region (tumor region) from a given set of texture classes (normal or other types of tumor). For example, a particular region in PET/CT image may belong to malignant tumor, benign tumor, or normal area. Each of these regions has unique texture characteristics. The texture analysis algorithms extract distinguishing features from each region to facilitate classification of such patterns. Implicit in this classification is the assumption that the boundaries between regions have already been determined for further analysis.

Therefore, a robust lesion-segmentation method is critical for the quantification of lesion activity in PET, especially for the cases where lesion boundary is not discernible in the corresponding computed tomography (CT). However, lesion delineation in PET is a challenging task, especially for small lesions, due to the low intrinsic resolution, image noise, and partial volume effect. The combinations of different reconstruction methods and post-reconstruction smoothing on PET images also affect the segmentation result significantly. Several authors have evaluated the watershed segmentation method on phantom studies, and limited studies have assessed its role in clinical scenarios. Watershed methods have been used in differentiating malignant and benign solitary pulmonary nodules, in segmentation of hepatic tumors for treatment planning in stereotactic body radiation therapy (SBRT), and to study changes in tumor cell proliferation induced by radiotherapy for head and neck cancer. However, different techniques of watershed algorithms have been used on different types of tumors with varying results, and the search for a more robust technique of this method continues. We have tried to address this issue by assessing watershed algorithm in segmentation of different types of solid tumors, including lung, liver, breast, and lymphoma. In this study, we performed tumor segmentation on FDG PET/CT images of these solid tumor malignancies using the watershed algorithm Figures 3.1–3.10.

Image segmentation is a process of partitioning a digital image into multiple segments. It describes the process through which an image is divided into constituent parts, regions, or objects to isolate and study separately areas of special interest. These regions are groups of connected pixels with similar properties, such as gray level, color, texture, brightness, and contrast, etc., and they may correspond to a particular object or different parts of an object.

The main goal of segmentation is to simplify and change the representation of an image into something that is more meaningful and simple to analyse. Image segmentation can be performed using automatic and semi-automatic methods. The simplest fully automatic method of segmentation is the thresholding-based segmentation method, which encompasses most of the voxel intensities of a particular tissue type; however, the automatic method may not be applicable to in all settings and provide desired results. The semi-automatic method gives an opportunity to the user to change the parameters as required to obtain good segmentation; however, it is a time-consuming process and also subject to variation depending on the users. Both semi-automatic and fully automatic methods of segmentation are the subject of intense research in imaging field and nuclear medicine F-18 FDG PET/CT or SPECT/CT imaging.

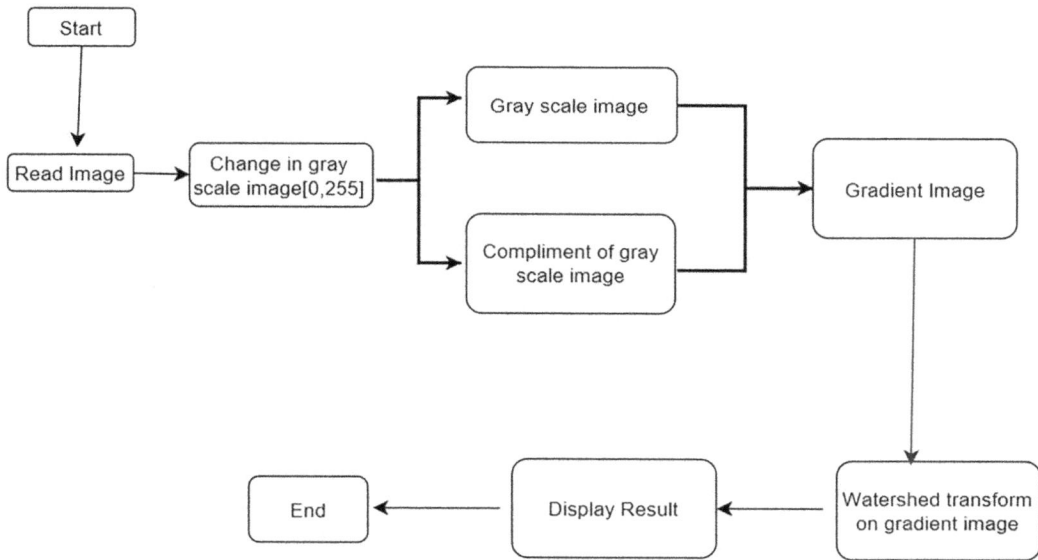

FIGURE 3.1   Watershed algorithm using gradient method.

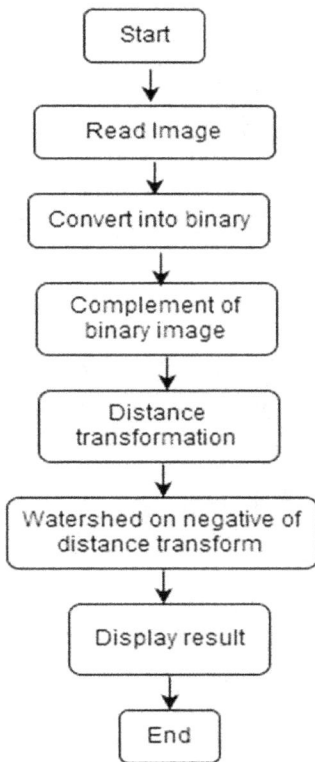

FIGURE 3.2   Watershed using distance transformation technique.

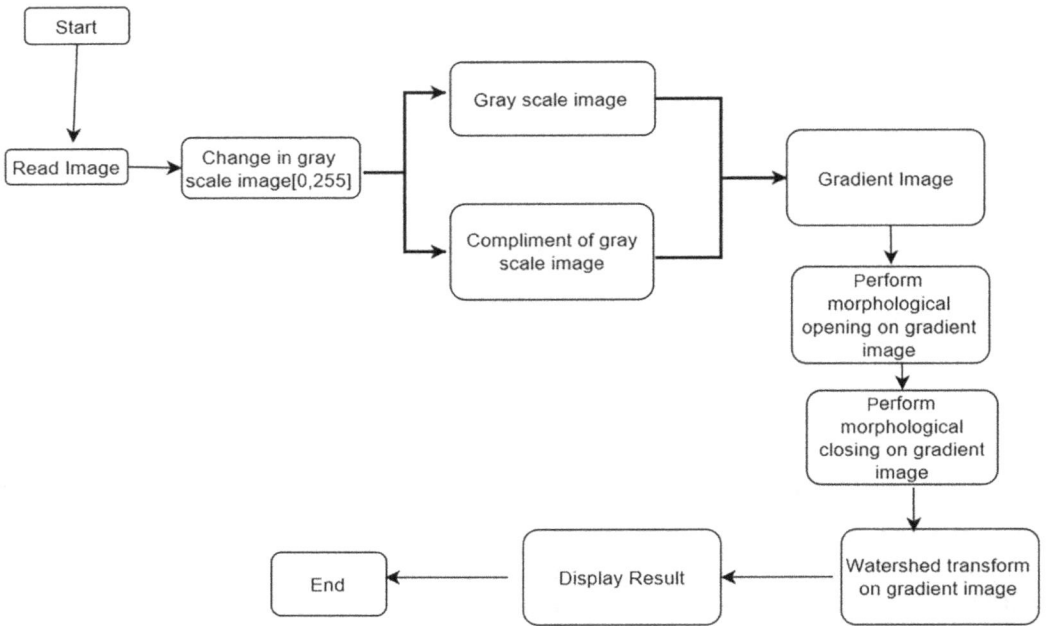

FIGURE 3.3   Watershed algorithm using gradient method with morphological operations.

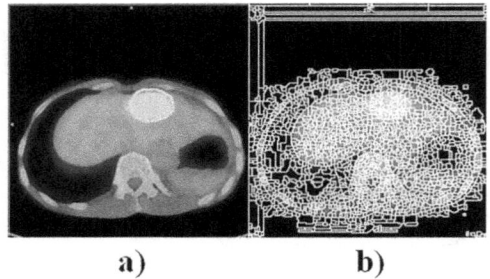

FIGURE 3.4   Shows a) Input image and b) Gradient image (transformed using watershed algorithm). Over-segmentation can be seen in the gradient image.

a)   b)

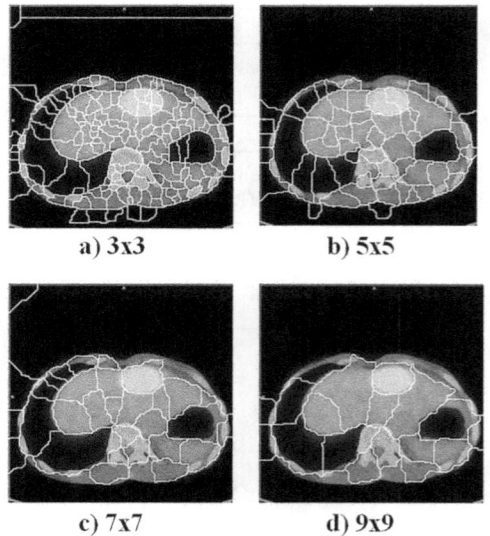

a) 3x3   b) 5x5

c) 7x7   d) 9x9

FIGURE 3.5   Shows morphological-operation gradient images with different parameters. The images show that over-segmentation still exists.

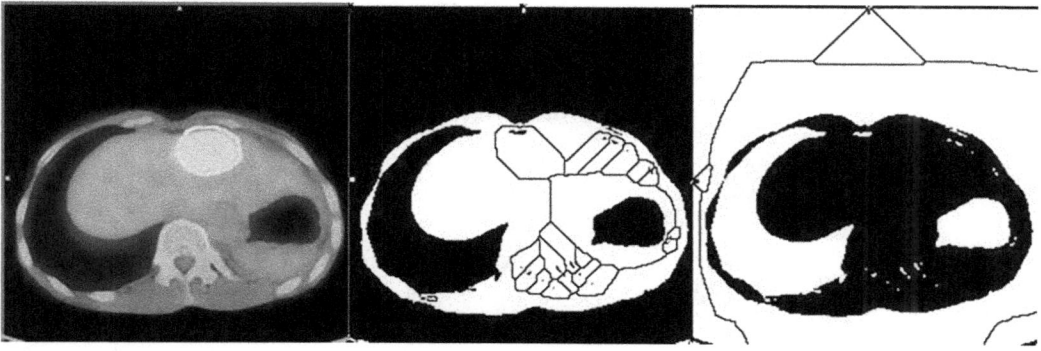

FIGURE 3.6 Shows image processed using watershed ridge lines of the negative of distance transformation and also with compliment distance transform, but over-segmentation still remains.

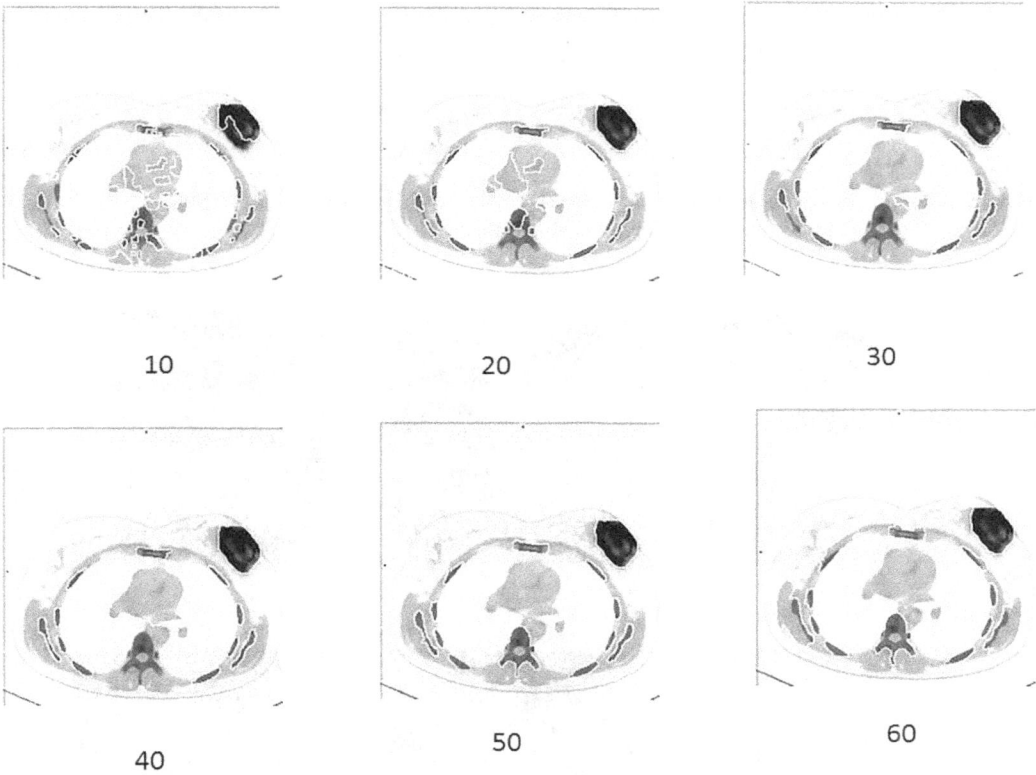

FIGURE 3.7 Shows over-segmentation resulting from applying the watershed transformation to the gradient magnitude image. Watershed ridge lines are superimposed in black over the original binary image; some over-segmentation is evident.

The first step of processing the input images was "segmenting grayscale images," which means dividing them into regions: generally, one of them stands for the background and each of the others corresponds to one of the objects or areas to be extracted. This segmentation comes down to the extraction of the contours of the desired objects. Now, the problem is to clearly define what a contour is and what is not. Edge detectors are commonly used to create contour of the objects in

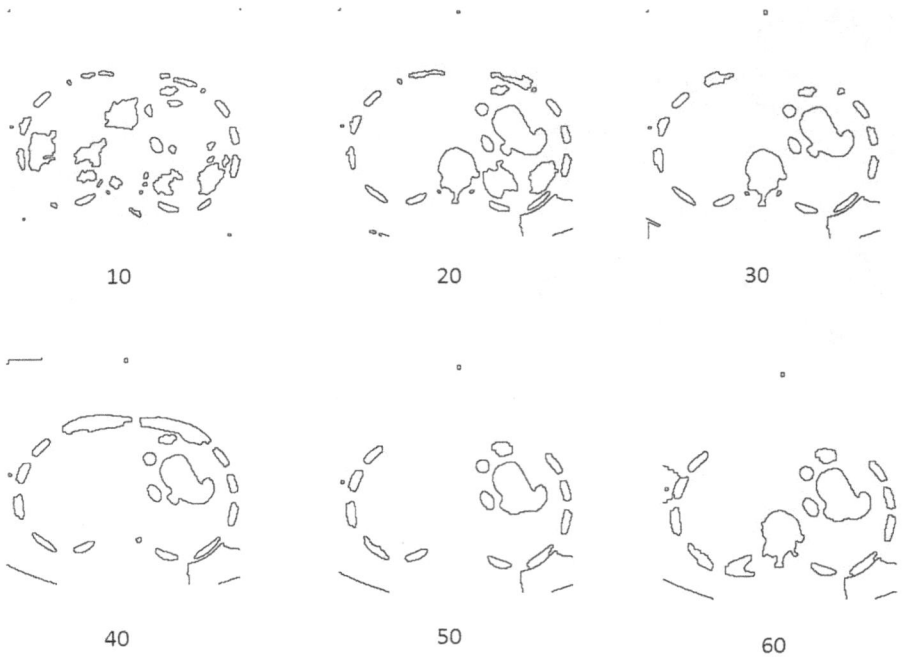

FIGURE 3.8 Shows watershed transform of the smoothed gradient image after applying several values of threshold (10 to 60); some over-segmentation is still evident.

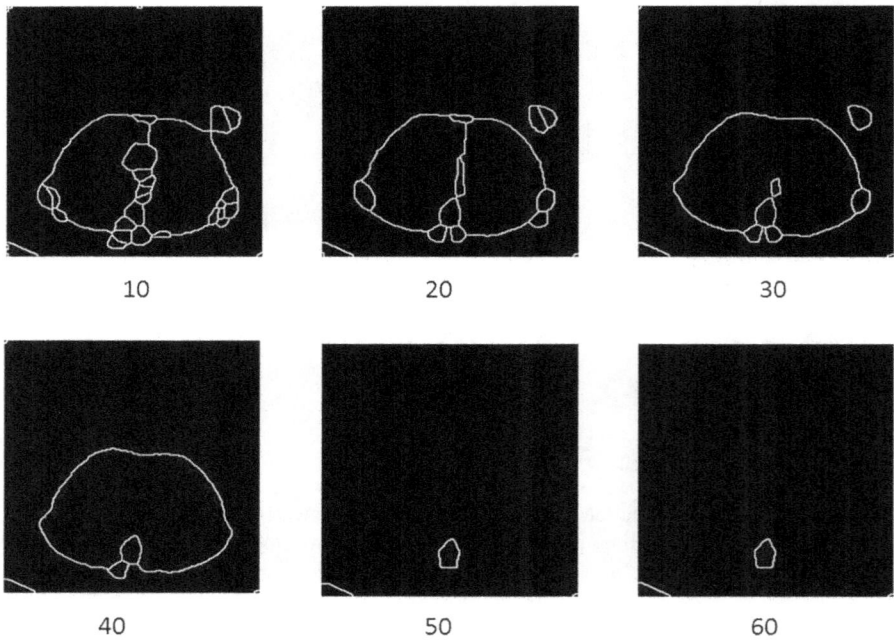

FIGURE 3.9 Shows external markers images with various threshold values.

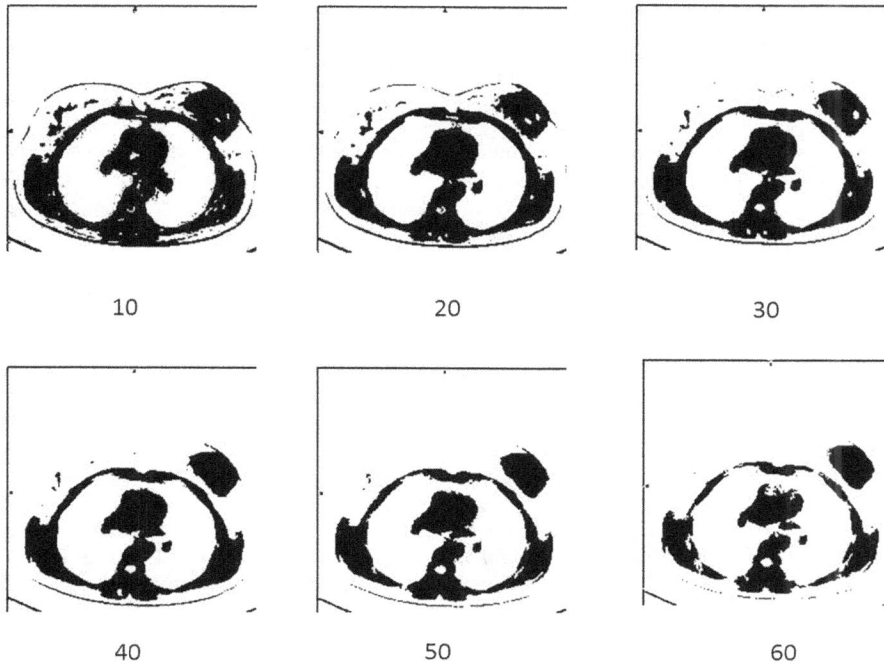

FIGURE 3.10 Shows internal markers images with various threshold values.

the image; the resultant image after the application of the edge detector is called the gradient image. In our study, we have used a Sobel edge detector to create a gradient image.

It is difficult to achieve a perfect segmentation using a single procedure, even under the most favourable conditions. Successful segmentation algorithms typically use a carefully constructed combination of procedures to achieve useful results. In our study, we tried to segment solid tumours in lymphoma, lung, breast, and liver malignancies from a single segmentation method using a watershed algorithm and achieved perfect segmentation in 85% of the representative images.

REFERENCES

[1] Ziessman H. A., O'Malley J. P., and Thrall J. H. *Nuclear Medicine The Requisites* (4th Edition) 2014, Elsevier Mosby, pages 227–264.

[2] Weber G. and Cantero A. Glucose-6-phosphatase activity in normal, precancerous, and neoplastic tissues. *Cancer Research* 1955; 15:105–108.

[3] Weber G. and Morris H. P. Comparative biochemistry of hepatomas. III. Carbohydrate enzymes in liver tumors of different growth rates. *Cancer Research* 1963; 23:987–994.

[4] Messa C., Choi Y., Hoh C. K., Jacobs E. L., Glaspy J. A., Rege S., et al. Quantification of glucose utilization in liver metastases: parametric imaging of FDG uptake with PET. *Journal of Computer Assisted Tomography* 1992; 16:684–689.

[5] Okazumi S., Isono K., Enomoto K., Kikuchi T., Ozaki M., Yamamoto H., et al. Evaluation of liver tumors using fluorine-18-fluorodeoxyglucose PET: characterization of tumor and assessment of effect of treatment. *The Journal of Nuclear Medicine* 1992; 33:333–339.

[6] Torizuka T., Tamaki N., Inokuma T., Magata Y., Sasayama S., Yonekura Y., et al. In vivo assessment of glucose metabolism in hepatocellular carcinoma with FDG-PET. *Journal of Nuclear Medicine* 1995; 36:1811–1817.

[7] Singh K. K. and Singh A. Study of Image Segmentation Algorithms for Different Types of Images. *International Journal of Computer Science Issues* 2010; 7(5).

[8] Dass R., Priyanka, and Devi S. Image Segmentation Techniques. *IJCT* 2012; 13(1):66–70.

[9] Acharjya P. P., Sinha A., Sarkar S., Dey S., and Ghosh S. A new approach of watershed algorithm using distance transform applied to image segmentation. *International Journal of Innovative Research in Computer and Communication Engineering* April 2013; 1(2).

[10] Stanislav L. Stoev RaFSi – A Fast Watershed Algorithm Based on Rain falling Simulation Computer Science Department

[11] John M. Gauch Image Segmentation and Analysis via Multiscale Gradient Watershed Hierarchies. *IEEE Transactions on Image Processing* January 1999; 8(1):69.

[12] Seal A. et al. Watershed: An Image Segmentation Approach. *(IJCSIT) International Journal of Computer Science and Information Technologies* 2015; 6(3): 2295–2297.

[13] Drever L. A., Roa W., McEwan A., and Robinson D. Comparison of three image segmentation techniques for target volume delineation in positron emission tomography. *Journal of Applied Clinical Medical Physics* 2007 Mar 9; 8(2):93–109.

[14] Geets et al A new gradient-based method and hierarchical cluster analysis for segmenting FDG-PET image. *European Journal of Nuclear Medicine and Molecular Imaging* 2007; 34:1427–1438.

[15] Ray S. et al. Comparison of two –dimensional and three-dimensional iterative watershed segmentation methods in hepatic tumor volumetrics. *Medical Physics* 2008 Dec; 35(12):5869–5881.

[16] Wang X., Li C., Eberl S., Fulham M. et al. Automated liver segmentation for whole-body low-contrast CT images from PET-CT scanners. *IEEE Engineering in Medicine and Biology Society* 2009; 2009:3565–3568.

[17] Campadelli P., Casiraghi E., and Esposito A. Liver segmentation from computed tomography scans a survey and a new algorithm. *Artificial Intelligence in Medicine* 2009; 45(2–3):185–196.

[18] Ballangan C., Chan C., Wang X., and Feng D. D. The impact of reconstruction algorithms on semi-automatic small lesion segmentation for PET: A phantom study. *Conference of the IEEE Engineering in Medicine and Biology Society* 2011; 2011:8483–3610. 1109/IEMBS.2011.6092093

[19] Zhang X., Tian J., Xiang D., Li X., and Deng K. Interactive liver tumor segmentation from ct scans using support vector classification with watershed. *Conference of the IEEE Engineering in Medicine and Biology Society* 2011; 10.1109/IEMBS.2011.6091484

[20] Jobin Christ M. C. and Parvathi R. M. S. Segmentation of Medical Image using Clustering and Watershed Algorithms American. *Journal of Applied Sciences* 2011; 8(12):1349–1352. ISSN 1546-9239

[21] Ballangan C., Wang X., Fulham M., Eberl S., and Feng D. D. Lung tumor segmentation in PET images using graph cuts. *Computer Methods and Programs in Biomedicine* 2013 March; 109(3):260–268.

[22] Bangara N. and Deepa A. Tumor Detection by Color Segmentation of PET/CT Liver Images. *JETWI* 2014; 6(1):148–156.

[23] Altunbas C., Howells C., and Proper M. Evaluation of threshold and gradient based (18)F-fluoro-deoxy-2-glucose hybrid positron emission tomographic image segmentation methods for liver tumor delineation. *Practical Radiation Oncology* 2014 Jul-Aug; 4(4):217–225.

[24] Arens A. I. J., Troost E. G. C., Hoeben B. A. W., Grootjans W., and Lee J. A. et al. Semiautomatic methods for segmentation of the proliferative tumor volume on sequential FLT PET/CT images in head and neck carcinomas and their relation to clinical outcome. *European Journal of Nuclear Medicine and Molecular Imaging* 2014 May; 41(5):915–924. doi: 10.1007/s00259-013-2651-0. Epub 2013 Dec.

[25] Zhao J., Ji G., Qiang Y., Han X. et al. A new method of Detecting Pulmonary Nodules with Improved Watershed Algorithm. *PLOS one* 2015 Apr 8; 10(4):e0123694.

[26] Meyer, F. Topographic distance and watershed lines. *Signal Processing* July 1994; 38:113–125.

[27] Grau V., Mewes A. U. J., Alcaniz M., Kikinis R., and Warfield S. K. Improved watershed transform for medical image segmentation using prior information. *IEEE Transactions on Medical Imaging* 2004; 23(4):447–458.

4 Medical Image Fusion

Transforms Techniques-Based Comparative Analysis for Brain Disease

B. Rajalingam and R. Santhoshkumar
Department of Computer Science and Engineering, St. Martin's
Engineering College, Secunderabad, Telangana, India

P. Deepan
Department of Computer Science and Engineering, St. Peter's
Engineering College, Hyderabad, Telangana, India

P. Santosh Kumar Patra
Department of Computer Science and Engineering, St. Martin's
Engineering College, Secunderabad, Telangana, India

CONTENTS

4.1 INTRODUCTION

The ever-increasing sophistication of medical imaging and information-processing technology has led to the creation of a wide variety of medical images that can be used in clinical diagnosis [1]. Applications for the images include disease diagnosis, surgery, and radiation therapy. Although each modality of medical imaging provides unique information about the human body, including its organs and cells, each modality has a specific set of applications [2,3]. Therefore, in many real-world clinical scenarios, a single sensor image is unable to offer sufficient information to the treating physicians [4,5]. When trying to gain more thorough information about diseased tissue or organs, it is typically necessary to merge the medical images obtained from various diagnostic modalities [6,7]. The difference between anatomical and functional images is shown in Table 4.1.

These results demonstrate how no single imaging modality can reliably and quickly detect or localise a cancerous lesion in its entirety. Image-fusion technologies are technologies that can

DOI: 10.1201/9781003333081-4

TABLE 4.1

Anatomical and Functional Images Differences

Anatomical Imaging (CT, MRI)	Functional Imaging (PET, SPECT)
Physical structure of the body	Activity of the body
Detects the changes in the body structure and confirms the presence of a mass	Shows the extent of the disease
Cannot diagnosis the disease earlier	Reveals the disease earlier
Cannot detect whether the mass is benign or malignant	Can detect whether a mass is benign or malignant
Difficult to detect abnormalities	Comparatively easy to detect abnormalities

instantly integrate multiple types of medical images [8,9]. These technologies can be used to combine data sets efficiently [10]. Not only does the fused image provide a more accurate and exhaustive characterization of a destination, but it also reduces the uncertainty and duplication in the image caused by the sensor [11,12]. In image-guided diagnosis and medical condition evaluation, the use of image fusion improves accuracy. Due to their downsampling, these transformations are not shift-invariant, which indicates that the fusion is susceptible to registration issues. This result is because downsampled data has shift invariance [13,14]. Over-complete wavelet transforms, such as the DTCWT, have been proposed to address the DWT's shift invariance and directionality limitations [15]. On the other hand, a 2-D wavelet-based DTCWT cannot accurately depict abrupt transitions like line and curve singularities because it is isotropic. There are only three directions in which the wavelet can record data simultaneously [16].

4.1.1 Non-Subsampled Shearlet Transform (NSST)

Shearlet transform: Case in point: It has a rapid decline in the spatial domain and is confined very precisely. Shearlets are sufficient to fulfill the requirements of the parabolic scaling law. This transform is sensitive to shifts in the direction that it is going. The number of directions has a factor of two increase for each progressively lower scale, making the total number of directions 48. However, it does not possess the property of being shift invariant, which is the origin of the pseudo Gibbs phenomena, as well as other inefficiencies in the fusion results. Other inefficiencies can be attributed to the fact that it is not fusion invariant, to avoid the problems discussed earlier. The NSST method generates the most accurate and efficient sparse approximations of visual input that are feasible. It is based on an affine structure that uses composite dilations as its primary building block. When functioning in a two-dimensional space (n = 2), the composite dilation-based affine system for a continuous wavelet L2 (R2) may be described as follows: the defined as,

$$\{\Psi_{ast}(x) = |\det M_{asl}|^{1/2} \ \Psi(M_{as}^{-1} \ x - t): t \in \mathrm{R}^2\} \tag{4.1}$$

here,

$$A_a = \begin{pmatrix} a & \sqrt{as} \\ 0 & \sqrt{a} \end{pmatrix} for \ a > 0, \quad s \in R, t \in R^2 \tag{4.2}$$

The analyzing elements are called shearlets. Here, a is scaling parameter, s is shear parameter, and t is translation parameter. The matrix M_{as} can be written as

$$M_{as} = B_s A_a \tag{4.3}$$

Where, B_s is the shear matrix, A_a is the parabolic scaling matrix.

$$A_a = \begin{pmatrix} a & 0 \\ 0 & \sqrt{a} \end{pmatrix}, \quad B_s = \begin{pmatrix} 1 & s \\ 0 & 1 \end{pmatrix} \tag{4.4}$$

Then shearlet transform of a function f is defined as

$$STf(a, s, t) = \langle f, \Psi_{ast} \rangle \tag{4.5}$$

The discrete version of shearlet transform $\hat{\Psi}_{jlk}$ ($j \geq 0$, $-2^j \leq 1 \leq 2^j - 1$, $k \in Z^2$) is obtained from sampling of continuous shearlet transform (a,s,t).

Discrete shearlet transform decomposition thus allows for multiscale subdivision and directional localization to be studied separately. A non-subsampled pyramid transform is used to achieve multiscale subdivision of the shearlet transform. As a result, the smoothness that surrounds singularities is no longer caused by the pseudo Gibbs phenomenon. Shift-invariant shearing filters are used for directional localisation in the second step. For low-frequency subbands, it divides the frequency plane into many trapezoidal high-frequency bands. To further break down the low frequency subband, a pyramid transform is used. Once the necessary level of breakdown is reached, this cycle is continued until it has been successfully completed.

NSST has the potential to be more effective than fundamental transformations, as previously stated (e.g. wavelet, contourlet). Wavelet and contourlet transforms suffer from restricted directionality and high computing complexity, while NSCT can address the fundamental deficiency of the earlier ones (such as shift variance).

NSST can better manage small changes in different directions (within an image) thanks to the use of NSLP and several shearing filters, which use the non-subsampled laplacian pyramid (NSLP). Before using direction filtering to obtain different subbands in various directions, NSLP, which has the virtue of being able to scale in many directions and multiple scales at once, must be used to deconstruct a picture into low- and high-frequency components. This sort of transformation is unusual in that it employs the shear matrix, also known as the ShF, for direction filtering. When the decomposition level is set to m = 3, an image is partitioned into m + 1 subbands, for a total of 4 subbands (one large fishing spoon and three half-fishes). The size of each subband is identical to what it was in the original picture (thus ensuring shift-invariance). The NSST makes use of a three-level decomposition mechanism, which is depicted in Figure 4.1.

This is how shearlet transform differs from the other MGA tools in terms of its distinguishing characteristics:

- It generates a condensed waveform that is well localised on various scales and orientations. The mathematical structure of shearlets is complex. A benefit of having it in the picture is that its representation is ideal when populated for images that include edges. It does not impose any restrictions on the number of directions and does not place any constraints on the size of the support for shearing. It offers a sincere segmentation method of edges in the two-dimensional space.
- Unlike curvelets, shearlets are linked to an interpretation structure that does not undergo any changes. When compared to the other MGA tools, the arithmetic of the inverse transform requires nothing more than the characterizations of shearing filters. In this procedure, composite inversion is not required at any point.

4.1.2 DESCRIPTION OF NSCT

The idea behind the contourlet is to use square-shaped brush strokes and a large number of small "dots" to create a super sparse expansion for very smooth contours, overcoming the limitation of the

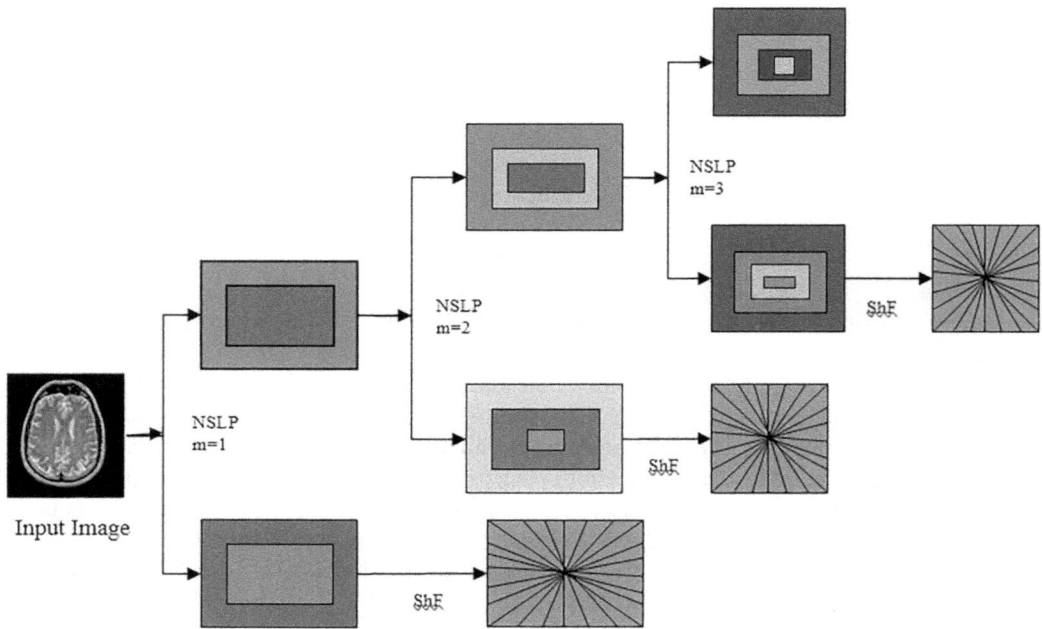

FIGURE 4.1 Image decomposition framework of shearlet transforms.

wavelet in this regard. For multi-scale decomposition, contourlet uses the Laplacian pyramid (LP), and for directional decomposition, it uses the directional filter bank (DFB). Each level of decomposition can have a different number of directions, which is much more flexible than wavelet's three. Unfortunately, downsamplers and upsamplers are included in both LP and DFB versions of the original contourlet [17]. During image decomposition and reconstruction, NSCT does away with downsamplers and upsamplers. A breakdown of the NSCT decomposition framework can be seen in Figure 4.2. NSDFB and NSPFB are non-subsampled pyramid filter banks used in NSCT. Two-channel non-subsampled 2-D filter banks are used to create the NSPFB [18]. In a DFB tree structure, each two-channel filter bank has downsamplers and upsamplers that can be turned off and upsamplers that can be turned on. The NSCT has both contourlet and shift-invariance properties in addition to its own. Image fusion makes it simple to find relationships between subbands because the sizes of the different subbands are identical when it is introduced. Designing fusion rules can benefit from this feature [19,20].

4.2 PROPOSED HYBRID ALGORITHM (NSCT-NSST)

Many hybrid image-fusion strategies are proposed in this paper to overcome the limitations of conventional picture-fusion systems [21]. The first approach offered combines the DTCWT with the non-subsampled shearlet transform (NSST). One of the proposed methods (DTCWT-NSST) −1 is seen in Figure 4.3.

4.2.1 An Overview of Proposed (NSCT-NSST) Algorithm

Method 1 uses DTCWT and NSST techniques on multimodal medical images as inputs. Steps below describe the procedure:-

Step 1. The two images provided as input should be analysed.
Step 2. A 256 × 256 resizing of the images is performed on the inputs.

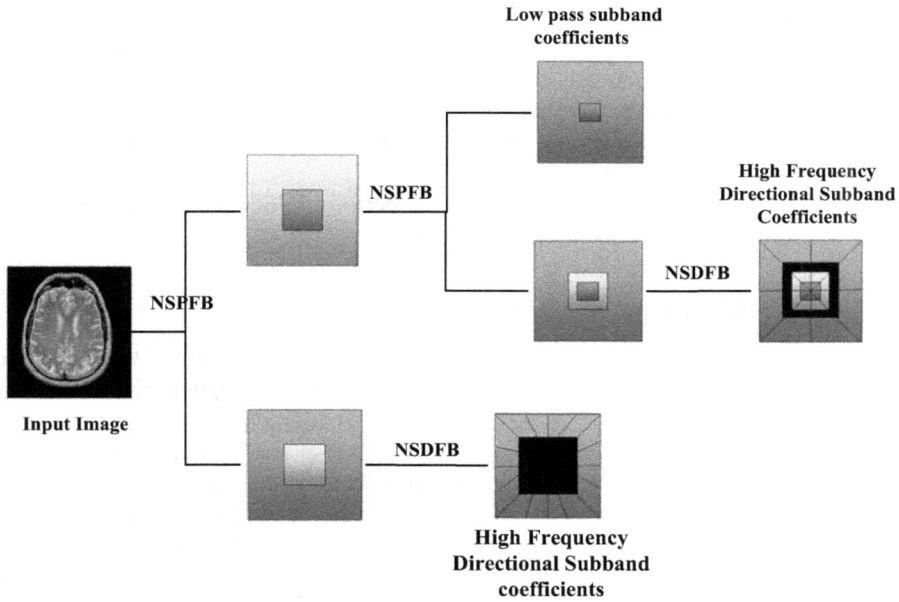

FIGURE 4.2 Decomposition framework of the NSCT.

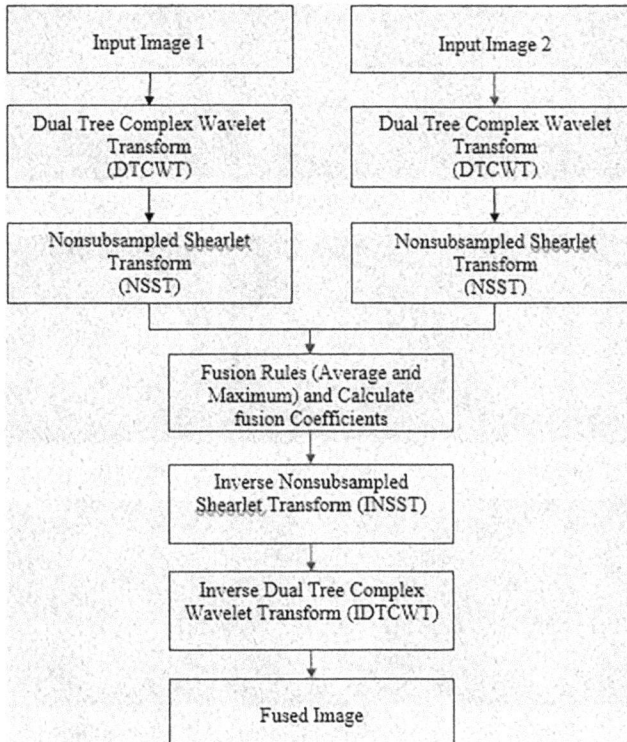

FIGURE 4.3 Block diagram of the proposed hybrid-fusion algorithm (DTCWT NSST)-1.

Step 3. The input photos are broken down into sets of complex coefficients using the dual-tree complex wavelet transform. For both coefficient sets, thresholds are generated independently for each decomposition level and for each source picture.

Step 4. Each of the deconstructed photos should have an NSST.

Step 5. In case of low frequency coefficients, use the very average fusion rule, and for high frequencies, the maximum fusion rule.

Step 6. To obtain the final proposed fused image, perform INSST followed by IDTCWTon the inverse transform of the fused image.

4.2.2 APPLYING NSST TO THE NSCT DECOMPOSED IMAGE

Using fusing rules based on the regional energies can satisfy the vision system well since the visual cortex is not attentive to a single pixel but is attentive to the edge, orientation, and surface texture of the image. High sub-band fusion rules, on the other hand, are extremely complex, and this complexity affects computation speed [22]. To achieve a satisfactory level of fusion effect and calculation speed, the NSST-DTCWT has more low frequency sub-band coefficients, which can easily grab image structure, which makes it simple to use the fusion rules in low and high frequency sub-band coefficients [23]. Various medical images can be combined to create a fused image if the two images are of different types. An initial NSST-DTCWT decomposition of image X/Y into decomposition coefficients is performed. Fusion images are constructed using the absolute value of the coefficients. Equations (3.7) and (3.8) explain the maximum and average fusion rules:

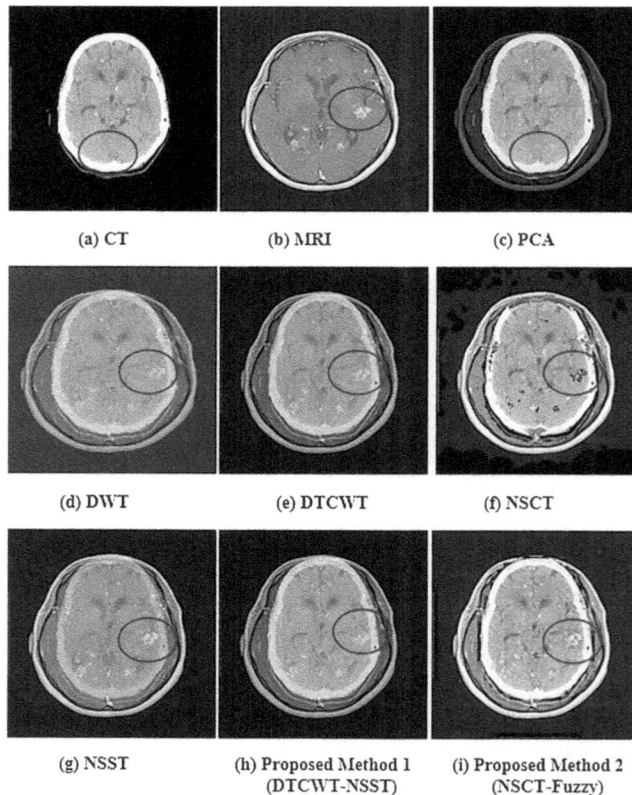

(a) CT   (b) MRI   (c) PCA

(d) DWT   (e) DTCWT   (f) NSCT

(g) NSST   (h) Proposed Method 1   (i) Proposed Method 2
                      (DTCWT-NSST)   (NSCT-Fuzzy)

FIGURE 4.4 Experimental results for neurocysticercosis disease affected images (Set 1).

$$C_F = \begin{cases} C_i^1, & if \quad C_i^1 > C_i^2 \\ C_i^2, & if \quad C_i^1 < C_i^2 \end{cases} \qquad (4.6)$$

$$C_F = \frac{1}{2}(C_i^1 + C_i^2) \qquad (4.7)$$

when X,Y are input images, CF is the combined coefficient, and finally, inverse NSST and inverse DTCWT are used to reconstruct the fused image using the merged coefficients.

4.3 RESULTS AND DISCUSSION

Patients infected with neurocysticercosis or other degenerative or neoplastic diseases are tested for the proposed HMMIF technique using a cross mixing of MRI, PET, CT and SPECT of the brain. These images are collected from the single patient because of their anatomical or functional similarities to one another, as well as the fact that they were taken at the same time [24,25]. There are several existing techniques, and the proposed hybrid image-fusion techniques have produced promising results, which can be seen in Figures 4.4–4.7. MRI/PET and SPECT images are combined from six separate sets of computed tomography (CT) and magnetic resonance imaging (MRI). A set of patient medical imaging data from a CT or MRI scanner is used as the first set of

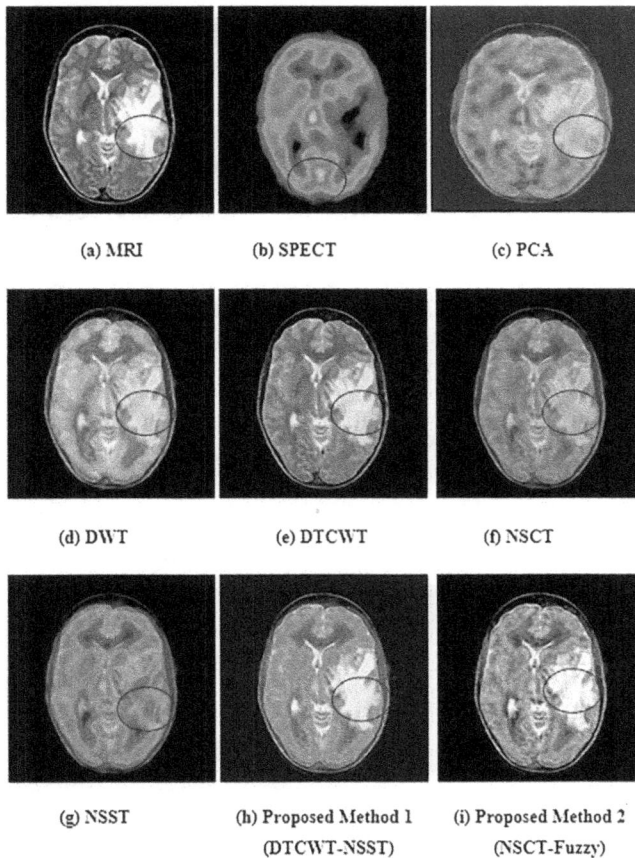

(a) MRI (b) SPECT (c) PCA

(d) DWT (e) DTCWT (f) NSCT

(g) NSST (h) Proposed Method 1 (DTCWT-NSST) (i) Proposed Method 2 (NSCT-Fuzzy)

FIGURE 4.5 Experimental results for metastatic bronchogenic carcinoma disease affected images (Set 2).

input images. MRI/SPECT brain pictures impacted by metastatic bronchogenic carcinoma illness are included in the second batch of input images. The third and fourth sets of input images exhibit MRI/SPECT images of astrocytic and anaplastic tumours, respectively.

The fifth and sixth sets of input pictures exhibit brain imaging altered by Alzheimer's and moderate Alzheimer's disease, respectively, using MRI/SPECT and MRI/PET. For the identical input pictures, fusion results have been obtained using PCA, DTCWT, NSCT, NSST, and the suggested hybrid approach combining DTCWT-NSST and NSCT-type 2 fuzzy. Both quality and amount of analysis are superior to other classic fusion methods provided in this paper. Every one of the cross-entropy measures are compared to the conventional and recommended hybrid-fusion processes, as shown in Tables 4.2 and 4.3.

The IQI, mSSIM, and EQM should likewise have the highest possible value and be as near to "1" as possible. Finally, a lower cross entropy value denotes a higher-quality fused output image. For an image-fusion approach to work, all of these conditions must be satisfied. In addition to the new hybrid-fusion approach just mentioned, algorithms like PCA, DWT, DTCWT, NSCT, and NSST have also been put to the test. Using fusion criteria, techniques such as averaging low-pass subband coefficients and selecting the highest possible high-pass subband coefficient value can be put into practise. Qualitative and quantitative data are analysed in this evaluation of the proposed approach.

Figures 4.8 and 4.9 provide the fusion factor and IQI for six sets of fused image pairings, some of which include CT-MRI, MRI-SPECT, and PET-MRI, among others. These figures may be found at the bottom of this section. The results of the tests are analysed using principal component analysis,

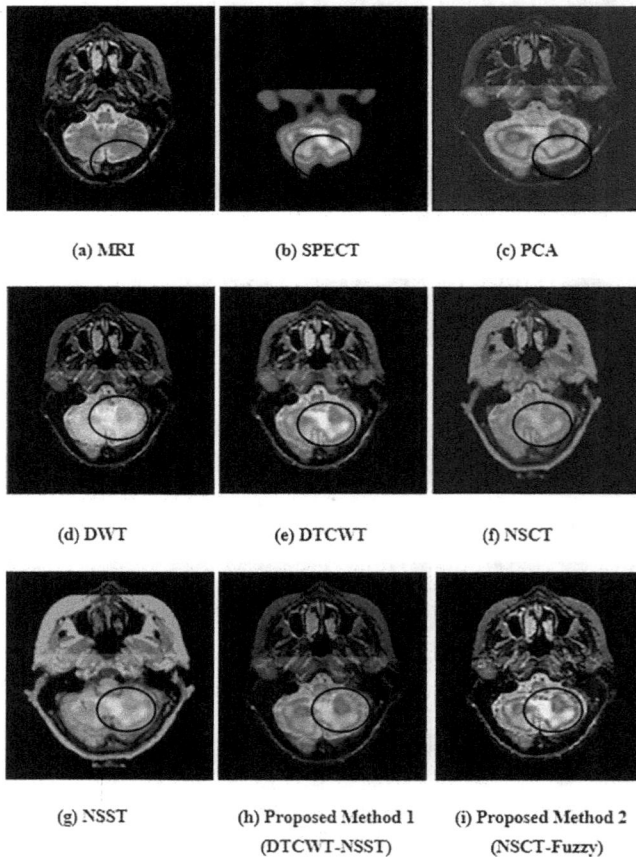

(a) MRI   (b) SPECT   (c) PCA

(d) DWT   (e) DTCWT   (f) NSCT

(g) NSST   (h) Proposed Method 1   (i) Proposed Method 2
                 (DTCWT-NSST)   (NSCT-Fuzzy)

FIGURE 4.6 Experimental results for Alzheimer's disease affected images (Set 5).

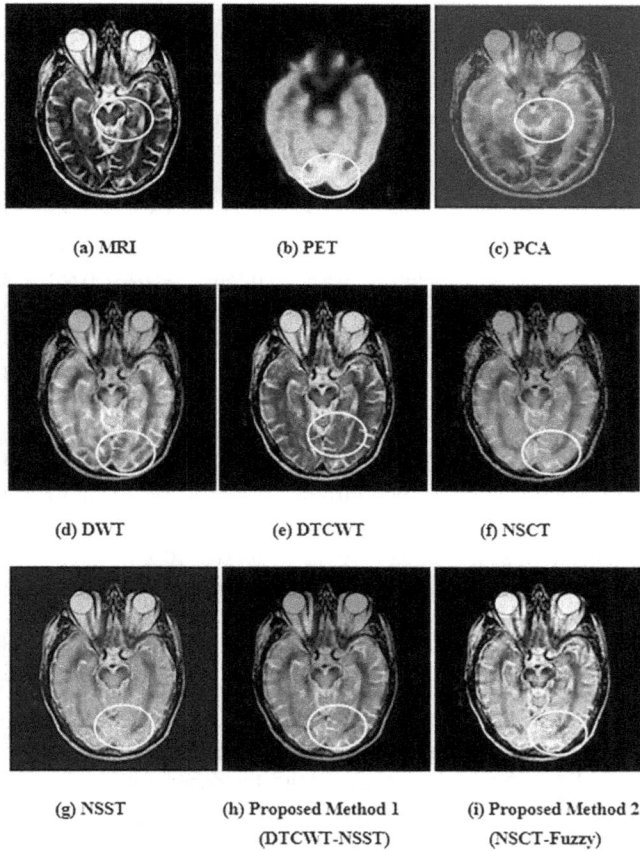

(a) MRI
(b) PET
(c) PCA

(d) DWT
(e) DTCWT
(f) NSCT

(g) NSST
(h) Proposed Method 1
(DTCWT-NSST)
(i) Proposed Method 2
(NSCT-Fuzzy)

FIGURE 4.7 Experimental results for Alzheimer's disease affected images (Set 6).

TABLE 4.2
Performance Metrics Comparative Analysis for Different Fusion Methods (Set 1, Set 2)

Study Set	Metrics Algorithm	FusFac	IQI	Mssim	CE_n	EQM	MI	PSNR	STD
Set 1	PCA	1.582	0.498	0.542	2.502	0.432	1.820	24.03	20.34
	DWT	1.716	0.508	0.572	2.072	0.499	1.899	25.90	22.23
	DTCWT	1.862	0.511	0.522	1.928	0.508	1.903	26.30	24.39
	NSCT	2.012	0.530	0.549	1.898	0.537	2.030	28.60	26.50
	NSST	2.161	0.552	0.575	1.807	0.571	2.230	29.88	28.34
	Proposed 1 (NSCT-NSST)	2.998	0.872	0.839	0.981	0.857	2.530	32.30	30.20
	Proposed 2 (NSCT-Fuzzy)	3.201	1.021	0.962	0.887	0.982	2.630	34.20	32.39
Set 2	PCA	2.062	0.451	0.418	2.051	0.510	2.230	19.02	24.54
	DWT	2.571	0.454	0.482	2.152	0.517	2.330	20.30	26.34
	DTCWT	2.671	0.518	0.489	2.098	0.529	2.494	23.67	27.45
	NSCT	2.712	0.534	0.505	2.189	0.564	5.594	25.30	34.45
	NSST	3.011	0.507	0.524	1.878	0.557	2.630	26.80	39.33
	Proposed 1 (NSCT-NSST)	4.851	0.712	0.792	0.953	0.878	3.230	34.09	57.45
	Proposed 2 (NSCT-Fuzzy)	5.012	0.837	0.871	0.865	0.941	3.420	35.07	58.99

TABLE 4.3

Performance Metrics Comparative Analysis for Different Fusion Methods (Set 3, Set 4)

Study Set	Metrics Algorithm	FusFac	IQI	Mssim	CE_n	EQM	MI	PSNR	STD
Set 3	PCA	1.520	0.506	0.439	2.710	0.452	2.203	24.30	20.30
	DWT	1.851	0.528	0.491	2.312	0.491	2.356	25.05	21.20
	DTCWT	1.902	0.551	0.521	2.251	0.517	2.367	27.70	24.30
	NSCT	1.997	0.599	0.556	2.004	0.551	2.554	29.20	25.40
	NSST	2.014	0.603	0.590	1.898	0.571	2.650	30.30	26.83
	Proposed 1 (DCWT-NSST)	3.828	0.871	0.819	0.961	0.871	3.120	36.30	30.40
	Proposed 2 (NSCT-NSST)	4.019	0.901	0.901	0.758	0.941	3.203	37.02	31.02
Set 4	PCA	1.582	0.501	0.409	2.691	0.421	2.030	19.09	22.32
	DWT	1.786	0.589	0.514	2.445	0.501	2.182	23.76	25.32
	DTCWT	1.790	0.601	0.536	2.271	0.56	2.473	27.80	28.40
	NSCT	1.858	0.688	0.498	2.025	0.591	2.783	29.40	30.23
	NSST	1.989	0.690	0.508	1.698	0.609	2.990	32.73	33.35
	Proposed 1 (DCWT-NSST)	2.833	0.881	0.781	0.931	0.881	3.690	40.45	39.40
	Proposed 2 (NSCT-NSST)	2.989	0.931	0.851	0.862	0.961	3.589	42.30	37.50

discrete-wavelet transform, discrete time continuous-wavelet transform, NSCT, and NSST techniques in that order. The fusion factor and IQI value of the DTCWT-NSST and NSCT-Type 2 fuzzy techniques that have been established are much higher than those of the other conventional ways currently in use. This is the case when contrasted with the other traditional methods.

The comparative examination of the mSSIM and cross entropy for six sets of image pairings, such as CT-MRI, MRI-SPECT, and MRI-PET, is depicted in Figures 4.10. The findings of the experiments are analysed using PCA, DWT, DTCWT, NSCT, and NSST methodologies respectively. In comparison to the other traditional methods that are currently in use, the values obtained by the suggested DTCWT-NSST and NSCT-Type 2 fuzzy methods for mSSIM are higher, but the values obtained for cross entropy are lower.

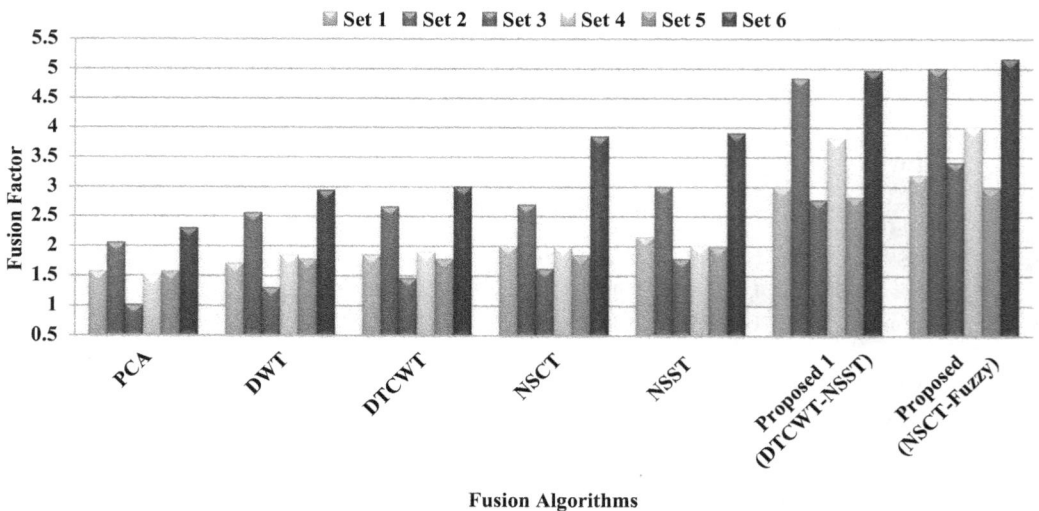

FIGURE 4.8 Comparative analysis for fusion factor.

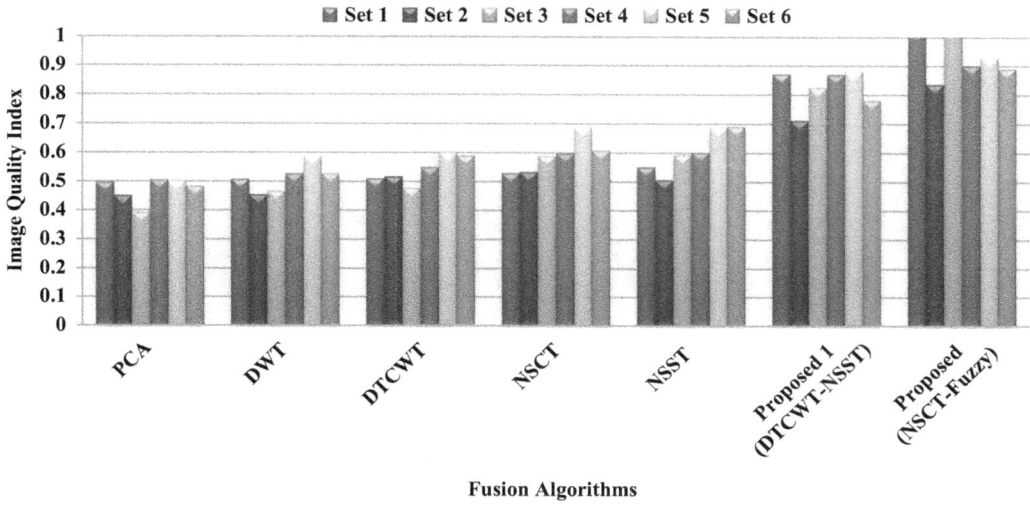

FIGURE 4.9 Comparative analysis for image quality index.

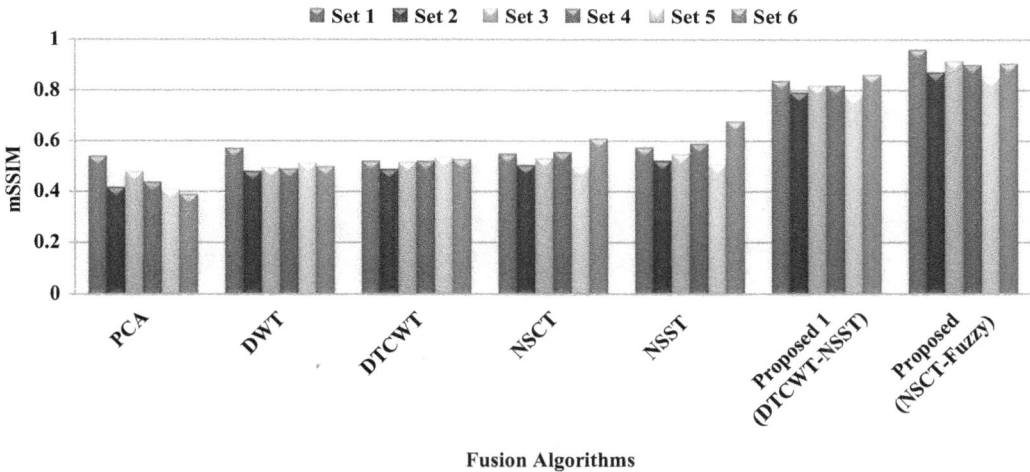

FIGURE 4.10 Comparative analysis for mean structural similarity index.

The comparative study of the EQM and MI for six sets of image pairings, such as CT-MRI, MRI-SPECT, and PET-MRI, is depicted in Figures 4.11 and 4.12. The findings of the experiments are analysed using PCA, DWT, DTCWT, NSCT, and NSST methodologies respectively. The DTCWT-NSST and the NSCT-Type 2 fuzzy that have been proposed both have a greater value for the EQM and the MI in comparison to the other standard techniques currently in use.

Figures 4.11 and 4.12 provide a comparison of the PSNR and standard deviation for six different image pairings, including CT-MRI, MRI-SPECT, and PET-MRI. PCA, DWT, DTCWT, NSCT, and NSST are used to analyse the results of the experiments. The PSNR and standard deviation of the newly created DTCWT-NSST and NSCT-Type 2 fuzzy techniques are higher than those of other existing classic methods. Table 4.4 shows the comparison of the suggested approaches to the existing methods.

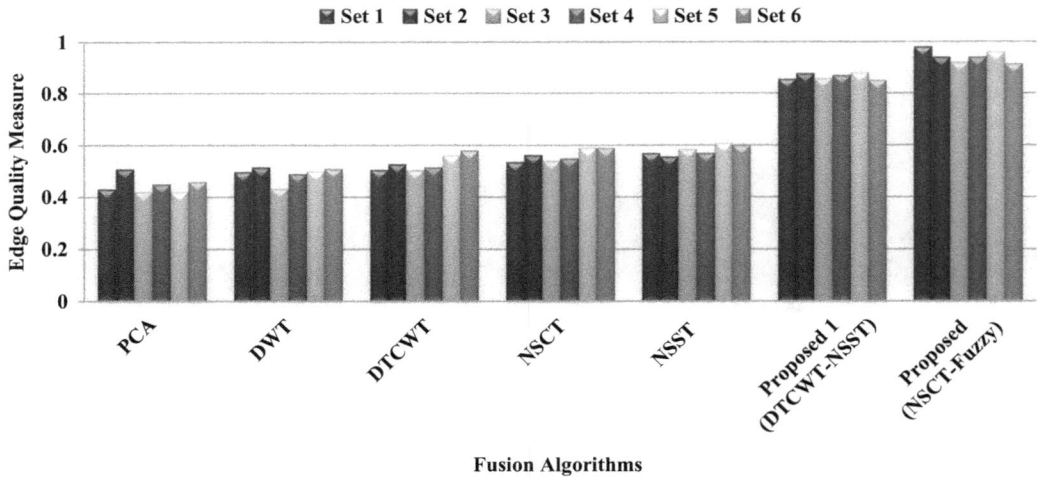

FIGURE 4.11   Comparative analysis of edge quality measure.

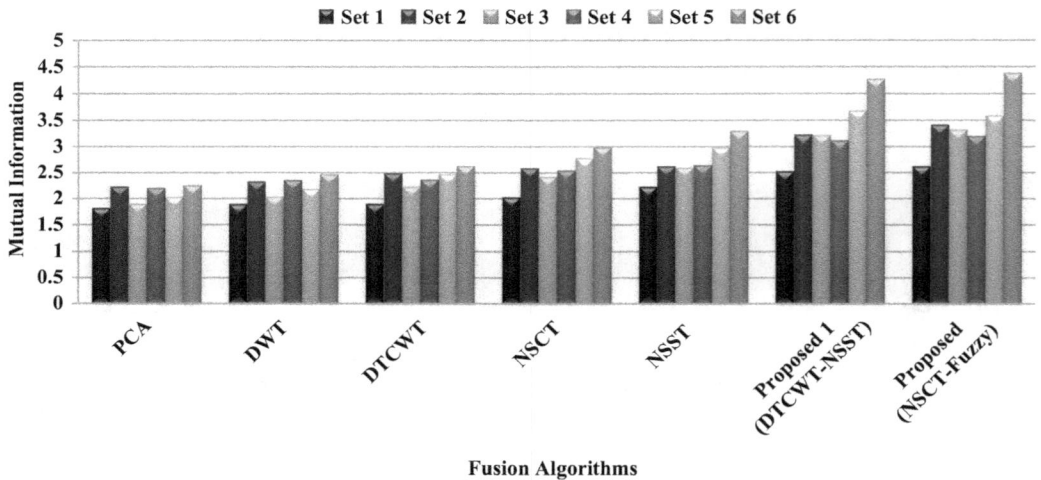

FIGURE 4.12   Comparative analysis for mutual information.

TABLE 4.4

Comparison of the Performance Metrics of the Proposed Methods with Existing Methods

Metrics Methods	Mutual Information	Standard Deviation	A
Jingming xia, et al. 2018	2.242	51.44	0.5887
Yong yang, et al. 2016	3.663	43.29	0.6197
Proposed Method 1 (DTCWT-NSST)	4.278	57.45	0.878
Proposed Method 2 (NSCT-Fuzzy)	4.389	58.99	0.941

4.4 CONCLUSION

The use of fusion criteria allows for the implementation of methods such as the averaging of the low-pass sub-band coefficients and the selection of the highest possible value for the high-pass subband coefficient. When fusing low-frequency coefficients, the maximum fusion rule is used, whereas fusing high-frequency coefficients calls for the average fusion rule to be used. The quality of the fusion has been evaluated using eight different performance parameters. According to the findings, the values of the proposed hybrid image fusion technique produce the highest possible values for four parameters. while the values for the proposed techniques produce the lowest possible values for cross entropy. According to their subjective assessment score (3.5 out of 4) for technique 1 (DTCWT-NSST) and method 2 (NSCT-Type 2 Fuzzy), respectively, the radiologist has analysed the fused output pictures and compared them to their input images.

REFERENCES

[1] A. Moin, V. Bhateja, and A. Srivastava. Weighted PCA Based Multimodal Medical Image Fusion in Contourlet Domain, 2016, Vol. 439, pp. 597–606.

[2] H. Li, X. He, D. Tao, Y. Tang, and R. Wang. Joint medical image fusion, denoising and enhancement via discriminative low-rank sparse dictionaries learning. *Pattern Recognition* Vol. 79, 2018, pp. 130–146.

[3] J.-J. Zonga, and T.-S. Qiu. Medical image fusion based on sparse representation of classified image patches. *Biomedical Signal Processing and Control, Elsevier*, Vol. 34, 2017, pp. 195–205.

[4] K. Wang. Rock Particle Image Fusion Based on Sparse Representation and Non-subsampled Contourlet Transform. *Optik, Elsevier*, Vol. 178, 2019, pp. 513–523.

[5] M. Manchanda, and R. Sharma. An improved multimodal medical image fusion algorithm based on fuzzy Transform. *Journal of Visual Communication and Image Representation*, Vol. 51, 2018, pp. 76–94.

[6] V. Bhateja, H. Patel, A. Krishn, A. Sahu, and A. Lay-Ekuakille. Multimodal Medical Image Sensor Fusion Framework Using Cascade of Wavelet and Contourlet Transform Domains. *IEEE Sensors Journal*, Vol. 15, 2015, No. 12, pp. 6783–6790.

[7] X. Liu, K. Chen, T. Wu, D. Weidman, F. Lure, and J. Li. Use of multi-modality imaging and artificial intelligence for diagnosis and prognosis of early stages of alzheimer's disease. *Translational Research, Elsevier*, Vol. 194, 2018, pp. 56–67.

[8] R. Santhoshkumar, M. KalaiselviGeetha, and J. Arunnehru. SVM-KNN based Emotion Recognition of Human in Video using HOG feature and KLT Tracking Algorithm. *International Journal of Pure and Applied Mathematics*, Vol. 117, No. 15, 2017, pp. 621–624, ISSN: 1314-3395.

[9] R. Santhoshkumar, and M. KalaiselviGeetha. Deep Learning Approach: Emotion Recognition from Human Body Movements. *Journal of Mechanics of Continua and Mathematical Sciences (JMCMS)*, Vol. 14, No. 3, June 2019, pp. 182–195, ISSN: 2454–7190.

[10] R. Santhoshkumar, and M. KalaiselviGeetha. Vision based Human Emotion Recognition using HOG-KLT feature. *Advances in Intelligent System and Computing, Lecture Notes in Networks and Systems*, Vol. 121, pp. 261–272, ISSN: 2194-5357, Springer 10.1007/978-981-15-3369-3_20

[11] R. Santhoshkumar, and M. KalaiselviGeetha. Human Emotion Prediction Using Body Expressive Feature, *Microservices in Big Data Analytics, IETE Springer Series*, ISSN 2524-5740, 2019, (Springer), 10.1007/978-981-15-0128-9_13

[12] R. Santhoshkumar, and M. KalaiselviGeetha. Emotion Recognition System for Autism Children Using Non-verbal Communication. *International Journal of Innovative Technology and Exploring Engineering (IJITEE)*, Vol. 8, No. 8, June 2019, pp. 159–165, ISSN: 2278-3075.

[13] P. Deepan, and L. R. Sudha. Remote Sensing Image Scene Classification using Dilated Convolutional Neural Networks. *International Journal of Emerging Trends in Engineering Research*, Vol. 8, 2020, No. 7, pp. 3622–3630. ISSN: 2347-3983, (Scopus Indexed).

[14] P. Deepan, and L. R. Sudha. Comparative Analysis of Remote Sensing Images using Various Convolutional Neural Network. *EAI End. Transaction on Cognitive Communications*, 2021. ISSN: 2313-4534, 10.4108/eai.11-2-2021.168714 (Other Journal).

[15] P. Deepan, and L. R. Sudha. Deep Learning and its Applications related to IoT and Computer Vision. *Artificial Intelligence and IoT: Smart Convergence for Eco-friendly Topography, Springer Nature*, 2021, pp. 223–244, (Springer Book Chapter) 10.1007/978-981-33-6400-4_11

[16] X.-Q. Luo, Z.-C. Zhang, B.-C. Zhang, and X.-J. Wu. Contextual Information Driven Multi-modal Medical Image Fusion. *IETE Technical Review, Taylor & Francis*, Vol. 34, 2016, No. 6, pp. 1–14.

[17] B. Rajalingam, R. Priya, and R. Bhavani. Hybrid Multimodal Medical Image Fusion Algorithms for Astrocytoma Disease Analysis. *Emerging Technologies in Computer Engineering: Microservices in Big Data Analytics, ICETCE 2019, CCIS, Springer*, Vol. 985, 2019, pp. 336–348

[18] B. Rajalingam, R. Priya, R. Bhavani. Hybrid Multimodal Medical Image Fusion Using Combination of Transform Techniques for Disease Analysis, *Procedia Computer Science*, Vol. 152, 2019, 150–157.

[19] G. Bhatnagar, Q. M. J. Wu, and Z. Liu. Human visual system inspired multi-modal medical image fusion framework. *Expert Systems with Applications, Elsevier*, Vol. 40, 2013a, No. 5, pp.1708–1720.

[20] G. Bhatnagar, Q. M. J. Wu, and Z. Liu. A new contrast based multimodal medical image fusion framework. *Neuro computing, Elsevier*, Vol. 157, 2015, No. 2015, pp. 143–152.

[21] B. Rajalingam, R. Priya, and R. Bhavani. Medical Image Fusion based on Hybrid Algorithms for Neurocysticercosis and Neoplastic Disease Analysis. *Journal of Mechanics of Continua and Mathematical Sciences*, Vol. 14, No. 4, 2019, pp. 171–187

[22] B. Rajalingam, R. Priya, and R. Bhavani. Multimodal Medical Image Fusion Using Hybrid Fusion Techniques for Neoplastic and Alzheimer's Disease Analysis. *Journal of Computational and Theoretical Nanoscience*, Vol. 16, 2019, pp. 1320–1331

[23] B. Rajalingam, R. Priya, and R. Bhavani. Hybrid Multimodality Medical Image Fusion Using Various Fusion Techniques with Quantitative and Qualitative Analysis. *Advanced Classification Techniques for Healthcare Analysis, IGI Global Publisher*, 2019, pp. 206–233.

[24] https://www.med.harvard.edu/aanlib (accessed 2017)

[25] https://radiopaedia.org/articles/neurocysticercosis (accessed 2017).

5 Artificial Intelligence and Medical Visualization

Nayankumar C. Ratnakar and Beenkumar R. Prajapati
L.M. College of Pharmacy, Gujarat University, Gujarat, India

Bhupendra G. Prajapati
Shree S.K. Patel College of Pharmaceutical Education & Research, Ganpat University, Gujarat, India

Jigna B. Prajapati
Acharya Motibhai Institute of Computer Application, Ganpat University, Gujarat, India

CONTENTS

5.1 INTRODUCTION

5.1.1 ARTIFICIAL INTELLIGENCE

Big data analytics and machine learning are having a deep influence on key aspects of current modern life, ranging from entertainment to healthcare. Netflix distinguishes which movies people prefer to watch, Amazon identifies which items most people like to buy from where, and Google tells which types of symptoms and situations the public is seeking. All this data pool can be used for very detailed particular profiling. These data are of great value for behavioral consideration and direction, and they have the potential for predicting healthcare data trends. There is great positivity that the use of different applications of AI can give substantial developments in all different areas

DOI: 10.1201/9781003333081-5

of healthcare, ranging from diagnostics to treatment. The AI algorithms are performing far better than humans in various jobs, like analyzing different medical images or correlating different symptoms and biomarkers from electronic records for the characterization and prediction of the disease (1). The term AI is used when a device does a thing the same as learning and problem-solving rational functions (2). AI is used in the computer science field, particularly for the formation of different systems execution tasks that required human behaviour intelligence using different methods (3).

In 1959, Arthur Samuel presented a term called machine learning (ML) to the computer field. ML is a subcategory of AI that uses different methods to allow the computer systems to study new data, short of being unambiguously programmed (4). Among the different techniques that come under ML, deep learning (DL) is one of the most gifted techniques in the broader AI domain represented in Figure 5.1.

DL is a representation-based learning method having numerous levels of representation. The main purpose of DL is to practice raw data to perform some sorting or recognition of tasks (5). To do so, machine learning is using different computational models and different algorithms. By using different algorithms, ML replicates the architecture of the biological neural networks in the brain; so, it's called artificial neural networks (ANNs) (6). Neural network architecture is designed in different layers composed of different interrelated nodes. Each node of the network completes a specific weighted sum or addition of the input data. Weights are dynamically optimized during the preliminary preparation phase. There are mainly three different kinds of layers: (1) the input layer, (2) output layer, (3) and hidden layer. The input layer generally receives input data. The output layer produces the data-processing results. The hidden layer generally extracts the different patterns followed within the data. There might be many hidden layers present according to the pattern of the algorithms. The performance of conventional artificial neuron networks is improved using the DL methods. Figure 5.2 describes classic ML and DL differences.

A deep artificial neuron network varies from the single or solo hidden layer by having a big number of hidden layers. This large number of hidden layers describes the specific depth of the neuron network (7). Convolutional neural networks have become very popular in computer-vision applications today among the different deep artificial neuron networks. In convolution neural network operations, the intensities of each pixel are calculated as the sum of each pixel of the original image by different convolution matrices. Different convolution matrices are also called kernels. For specific tasks, such as blurring, sharpening, or edge detection, different kernels are applied. Convolutional neural networks are like biologically derived networks behaving the same as the human brain cortex. The human brain cortex contains a complex structure of cells that are

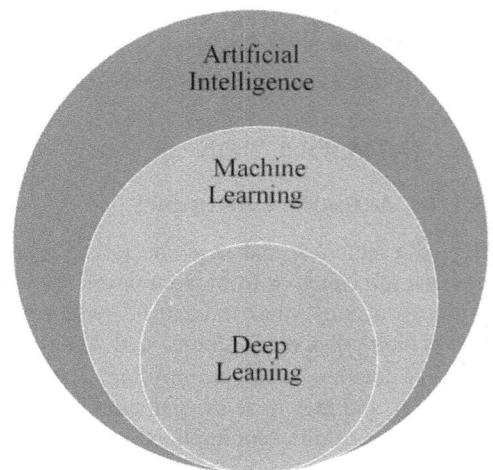

FIGURE 5.1   Artificial intelligence umbrella.

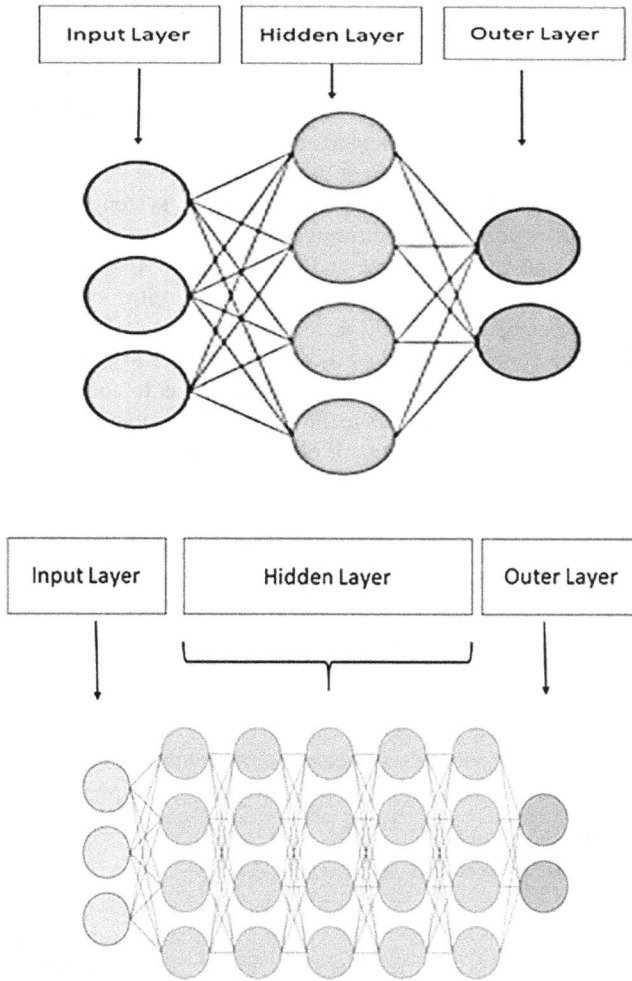

FIGURE 5.2   Classic machine-learning pattern and deep machine-learning pattern.

very sensitive to small regions of the visual field (8). The architecture of deep convolutional neural networks allows the composition of complex features from simpler features to interpret image raw data to detect specific features (8). Deep network architecture's complexity makes it demanding in relation to computational resources. With the development of the graphics processing unit, the application of the deep-learning application is possible. Perhaps there might be a high number of nodes required to detect complex relationships and patterns so that billions of parameters are optimized during the preliminary phase. Radiologists are already aware of computer-aided detection/diagnosis (CAD) systems, which were first introduced in chest x-ray and mammography applications in the 1960s (7). However, algorithms development advancements with easy access to different computational resources are allowing AI to be applied in radiological decision making at an advanced functional level (9).

5.1.2 Artificial Intelligence in Healthcare

Many countries have a shortage of experienced medical practitioners, even though demand for the healthcare services is increasing so fast. With a very high expectation of patients needing services, healthcare industries are also struggling to keep up with all advanced technological developments (10). Different healthcare services using health-tracking apps and web browsing are on demand due to the latest development in wireless technology and smart devices. So, it makes a new forms of healthcare delivery available from anywhere and anytime using remote interactions. It's a boon for underserved places that lack health specialists. It also helps to decrease costs and prevent unnecessary exposure to contagious illnesses at the hospitals. Tele-caller healthcare technology is also increasing in developing countries where the healthcare system is growing and healthcare infrastructure can be designed to meet the current needs (10).

One recent question is revolving worldwide and involves the active discussion about whether AI will replace the human healthcare practitioners in the future. But it is strongly believed that human healthcare physicians will not be replaced by different machines or software in the so-called predictable future, but they can certainly assist medical practitioners to make better clinical decisions and judgment in different areas of healthcare. Different methods to collect the different healthcare data and newer advancements in data analytics techniques have led to success in the application of AI in the healthcare industries. Different amounts of clinical questions and powerful data learning can solve clinically relevant information otherwise hidden in the massive amount of data that are critical in clinical decision making (11). Traditional healthcare ecology is understanding the importance of different AI-equipped data-mining tools in the next-generation healthcare technology. AI can make improvements to any different process within healthcare operation and delivery. An important driver for the implementation of AI applications in the healthcare system is its lower cost.

AI applications can cut annual US healthcare costs by USD 150 billion in 2026. A large part of these cost reductions from changing the healthcare model from a reactive to a proactive approach, particularly focusing on healthcare management rather than disease treatment. This approach will result in fewer hospitalizations, fewer doctor visits, and fewer treatments. AI-based technology will have an important role in helping people stay healthy with continuous monitoring that will give an earlier diagnosis, custom-made treatments, and more effective follow-ups (12).

5.2　FUNDAMENTS OF MEDICAL VISUALIZATION

5.2.1　Early Stage

Before AI systems, no trained data were available in the healthcare system. Data were collected from different clinical activities, such as screening, diagnosis, and treatment assignment. These clinically derived data are often available but have limitations including the demographic region, different medical records, different electronic recordings from specific medical devices, physical examinations notes, and clinical laboratory and images received (13).

In addition, physical examination notes and clinical laboratory results are the other two major data sources. We can differentiate them with a different image and genetic and electrophysiological data because these sources contain large portions of unstructured descriptive texts, e.g. clinical notes that are not directly analyzable. So, introducing artificial-intelligence-based technology mainly emphasizes translating the unstructured text to machine-recognizable electronic medical records. AI-based technologies are helping to extract different features from case reports to improve diagnosis accuracy (14).

5.2.2　Current Trends

One of the most capable areas of health innovation is the application of AI in medical imaging, including image processing and image interpretation (15). Indeed, AI may be useful for numerous applications starting from image procurement and processing to reporting, follow-up planning and checking, data storage, data mining, and many more. AI is projected to enormously impact radiologists' daily routines because of a wide range of these applications (16).

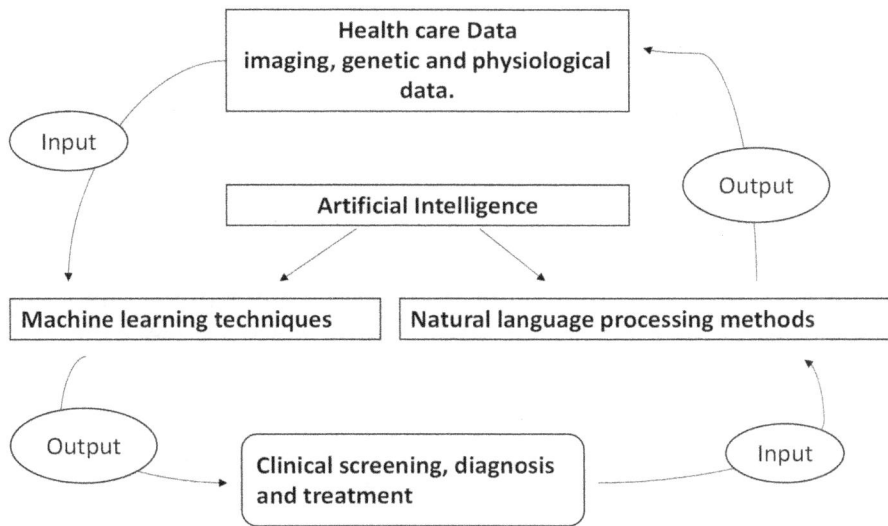

FIGURE 5.3 Artificial intelligence devices workflow.

AI models use sophisticated complex algorithms to learn from a larger number of healthcare data and then use the obtained results and insights to assist in clinical practice. It has learning and self-correcting abilities to improve its accuracy based on feedback through machine learning. An AI system can also provide up-to-date medical and clinical information from journals, textbooks, and clinical practices for proper patient care (17). The AI systems can help to reduce diagnostic and therapeutic errors that frequently occur in human clinical practice (18). The AI systems extract useful information from a large patient population to assist in making real-time inferences for health risk alerts and health outcome predictions (19).

Various AI devices are main categories into two major categories. The first category comprises ML techniques that investigate structured data such as imaging, genetic and physiological data. The ML procedures attempt to make a group of patients' behaviors and, from that, it decides the probability of the disease outcomes in the medical clinical applications (14). The second category includes the use of different natural language-processing methods that extract information from unstructured data, such as clinical notes or medical journals to enrich structured medical data. The natural language-processing procedures target turning texts into machine-readable structured data and then it can be analyzed by machine-learning techniques (20). For better presentation, the flow chart in Figure 5.3 describes the data generation through natural language-processing data enrichment and machine-learning data analysis to get a clinical decision (21).

5.3 AI TECHNIQUES IN MEDICAL VISUALIZATION

The human brain is created to discover and master things by itself, but a machine cannot do the same. In reality, the machine works precisely as it is delineated to perform. Machines take the input and produce output based on that input, and follow the instructions given, but a human brain could not think accordingly (22). The brain does not follow the extraneous instruction. It gets perception on its own, perceives many things via the nervous system, and makes its own decisions. For example, sensing the temperature of skin and odour, etc. (22).

The history of AI began with the gathering of scientists at Dartmouth College during the summer of 1956. Scientists discuss the possibility of creating an artificial brain. Alan Turing was a young British polymath who uncovered the mathematical possibility of AI. However, great challenges like the prerequisite of a computer that could store commands were not available at that time (23). An investment and interest in AI increased dramatically in the first two decades of the twenty-first century as machine learning was effectively used to solve myriad challenges in academia and industry (24).

AI in the future can perceive image acquisition and impulsive identification and investigate functions in the field of intelligent medical treatment. For example, an AI algorithm is used to detect skin cancer that can easily differentiate whether the skin mole is normal or melanoma. It can also apply to various eyeball images and can identify the sucrose cataract, normal cataract, or deepened myopia (25). AI is mushrooming exponentially over the last decade; high-pixel images are available with just a single click, from image acquisition to data reporting, investigation, data storage, data mining, and many others (8). Diagnostic medical imaging using AI is currently the subject of a thorough evaluation. The identification of imaging abnormalities using AI has demonstrated outstanding accuracy and sensitivity, and it holds out the prospect of improving tissue-based detection and characterization (26). The identification of minute changes with unknown significance, however, is a significant downside that arises with increased sensitivity (27).

According to a study on screening mammograms, artificial neural networks regularly exhibit higher sensitivity for aberrant results, especially for small lesions, even though they are not more accurate than doctors at detecting cancer (28). To ensure an efficient and secure integration into clinical practice at the outset of an AI-assisted diagnostic-imaging revolution, the medical community must foresee potential unknowns of this technology. Establishing AI's place in clinical medicine requires careful consideration of the risks it may present in light of its special capabilities. It won't be simple to distinguish between improved detection and overdiagnosis. To improve the quality and comparability of AI studies, a regular practice of external validation using non-sample data and well-specified cohorts is the fundamental of this assessment (29). Different medical-imaging modalities can be employed for a variety of clinical applications because of their distinctive qualities, varying responses to human body structure, and responses to organ tissue. Ultrasonic imaging, magnetic-resonance imaging (MRI), and computed tomography and projection imaging (such as x-ray imaging) is the most frequently employed image modalities for diagnostic analysis in clinics (MRI), as shown in Figure 5.4 (30).

5.3.1 ML in Medical Visualization

Machine learning in computer science and engineering is a fascinating field of research. It is regarded as a subset of AI since it makes it possible to conclude instances, a function of human intelligence. In

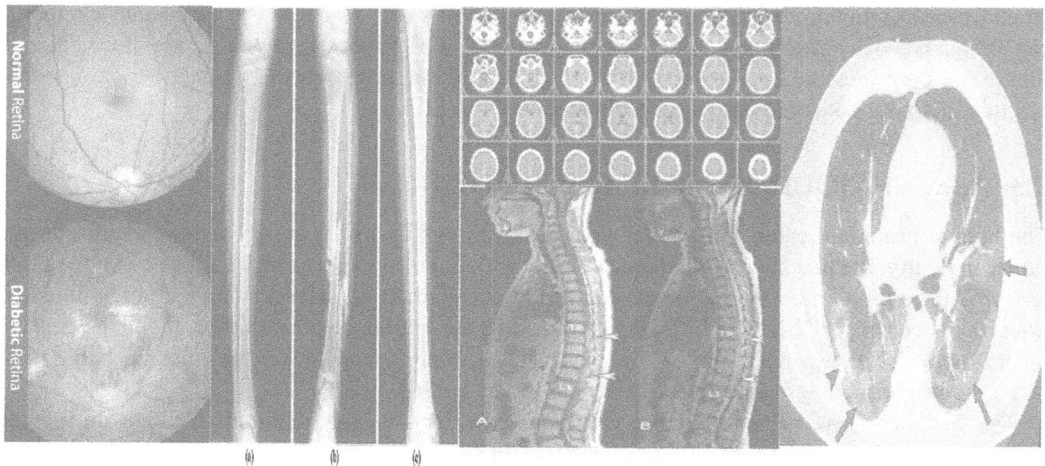

FIGURE 5.4   Image of fundus, x-ray, CT, MRI.

the realm of medical-imaging research, machine-learning techniques are frequently employed as efficient classifiers and grouping algorithms (31). It is obvious why having a machine conduct routine, well-defined work is appealing. Computers have a greater propensity for consistency and tenacity than humans do. Given recent research showing that computers are capable of learning and even mastering tasks that were once thought to be beyond their scope, machine-learning techniques may become useful in computer-aided diagnostic and decision-support systems. The finding that, periodically, machines may be capable of "understanding" patterns that are imperceptible to the human eye is even more remarkable. This discovery has dramatically and significantly increased curiosity in machine learning, especially in relation to how it may be applied to the analysis of medical images. For instance, it has been demonstrated that machine learning can diagnose numerous illnesses from medical photos as well as medical professionals (29).

5.3.1.1 What Is Machine Learning?

Whenever an ML algorithm is applied to a set of variables and some knowledge about those data, the system could learn from the training examples and use what it has learned to produce a forecast. If the algorithm system modifies its variable values to improve performance, i.e., more test cases are correctly detected, then it is considered to be performing that task (32). Unsupervised learning, reinforcement learning, and supervised learning are the three main categories of machine-learning techniques. Reinforcement learning (RL) is insufficient for medical applications since an RL system's choice will affect the patient's future health as well as their access to treatment choices. As a result, it is more difficult to predict long-term impacts (33).

If the training data set has labelled outputs that match the input data, that is the primary distinction between supervised and unsupervised learning. The difference between supervised and unsupervised learning is that the former infers a mathematical relationship between the inputs and the labelled outputs, while the latter infers a function that expresses hidden qualities found in the input data. Depending on the objective, the output data from supervised learning may have a categorical value or a numerical continuous value (34).

5.3.1.2 Algorithm of Machine Learning

The best feature weights can be determined using a variety of algorithms. These algorithms are based on various ways of modifying the feature weights and data presumptions. The following sections provide an overview of some of the most often used methods, including deep learning, decision trees, k-nearest neighbours, support-vector machines, and neural networks (35).

5.3.1.2.1 Neural Networks

Artificial neural networks (ANNs), also known as simulated neural networks, are the foundation of deep-learning algorithms (SNNs). By borrowing both their name and their physical makeup from the human brain, they mimic how organic neurons converse with one another. One or more hidden layers, an output layer, and a node layer are the components of an artificial neural network (ANN). The weight and threshold associated with each network, or artificial neuron, are connected to other nodes. A node is activated and starts sending data to the top layer of the network if its output rises beyond the specified threshold value. In any other case, no data is sent to the program's next layer. For neural networks to grow and improve their accuracy over time, training data is necessary. However, if they are calibrated for accuracy, these learning algorithms turn into helpful features in AI and computer science by allowing us all to rapidly categorize and cluster data. Tasks in voice recognition or picture identification can be done very quickly, rather than taking hours when human experts perform manual categorization. One of the most popular neural networks is used in Google's search algorithm (36).

5.3.1.2.2 K-nearest Neighbours

The k-nearest neighbours algorithm, often known as KNN or k-NN, is a supervised learning algorithm that makes predictions or classifications about the clustering of a single data point using proximity. It can be used to solve classification or regression problems, but because it is predicated on the discovery of similar points that are adjacent to one another, it is most usually used as a classification tool (37).

Classification issues are resolved by majority vote, which means that the term used most frequently to describe a given data piece is adopted. Although plural voting is the correct term, the descriptor "majority vote" is usually used in literature. The distinction between the two phrases arises from the fact that "majority voting" legally calls for a plurality of much more than 50%, which works best if there are only two options. If there are several classes, let's say four, you don't need 50% of the vote to decide which class wins; you might assign a class label with more than 25% of the vote (38).

5.3.1.2.3 Support-Vector Machines

The notion that the input data is converted to provide the biggest sector, or supporting vectors, between the two classes gives support vector machines their name. Support-vector machines allow for the free selection of the extent to which one desires a broad plane of separation versus the number of points that are wrong due to the wide plane (39).

These learning machines have been around for a while, but recently, they have gained more traction due to the addition of basic functions that can categorize cases that cannot be classified linearly by leveraging nonlinear relationships between points in different dimensions. This property distinguishes support vector-machine algorithms from many other machine-learning methods. An easy-to-understand example of the use of a nonlinear function is to convert data from an original space (the way the feature was collection and treatment instance, this same computed tomography attenuation) to a hyperdrive (the novel method the function is depicted example, the cosine of the CT absorption), where a hyperplane (a plane that appears to exist in that hyperdrive, with the concept of using the plane positioned to best detach the data points) (40).

5.3.1.2.4 Decision Tree

All of the machine-learning techniques that have been discussed so far have one significant drawback: it is typically impossible to extract the values used in the weights and activation functions to obtain information humans can understand. The important benefit of decision trees is that they provide rules that are understandable by humans for categorizing a particular case. The component of decision trees that relates to machine learning is the quick search for the various decision-point combinations that, when used, will produce the most accurate and simple tree. When the algorithm is run, one determines how critical it is to have accurate findings versus more choice points, as well as the maximal depth (i.e., the maximal number of decision points) and maximal breadth that is to be searched (41).

5.3.1.2.5 Naive Bayes Algorithm

Naive Bayes classifiers are a subset of classification algorithms based on the Bayes theorem. Instead of being a single algorithm, it is a collection of algorithms, and they are all predicated on the notion that just about every pairing of characteristics being classified is unrelated to every other pair (42).

5.3.1.3 Application of ML

5.3.1.3.1 ML in Skin Cancer Detection

AI integration in smartphone apps can instruct users on how to conduct skin examinations and relay the results to a doctor. Every kind of skin lesion is assigned a category, like "benign" and "malignant," either "naevi" or "melanoma," to construct a novel ML skin cancer algorithm (43). Deep-learning algorithms are instructed on an enormous number of photos from each class before being evaluated on a fresh image. Three basic steps make up the entire procedure. In stage 1, digitally enhanced macro or dermoscopic pictures tagged with the "ground truth" are the first images sent to the algorithm. In stage 2, convolutional layers divide the extracted features from the images. A

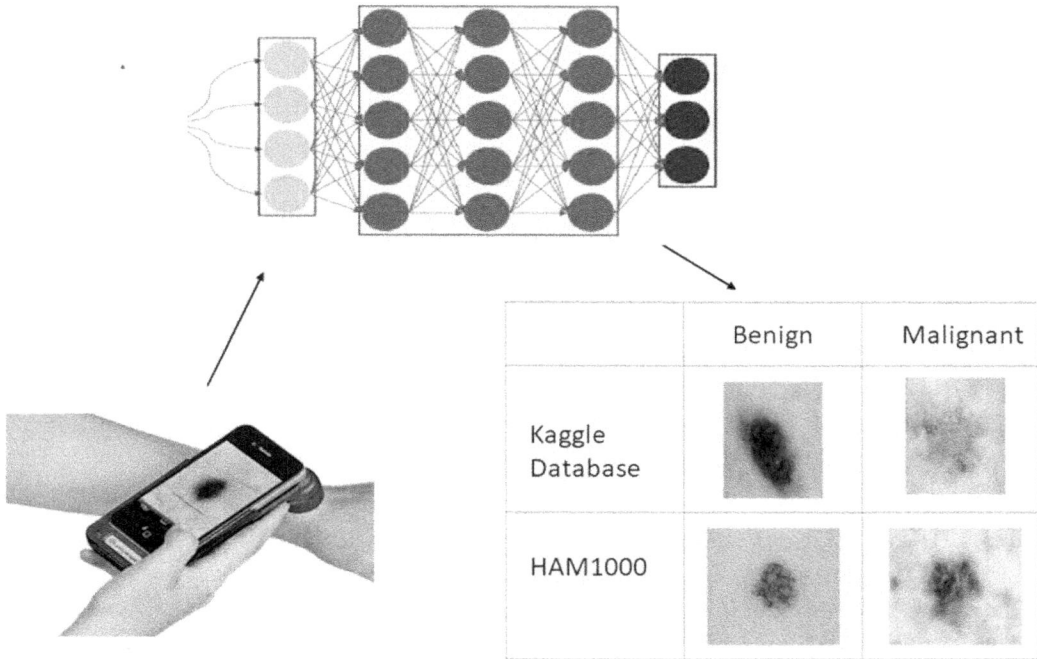

FIGURE 5.5 Detection of skin cancer using ML.

feature map is a levelled abstraction of the data's visual representation. Low-level properties like edges, corners, and forms are extracted in the first convolutional layer. Higher-level information is gathered by later convolutional layers to determine the kind of skin lesion. In stage 3, feature maps are used by the machine-learning algorithm to differentiate between different kinds of skin lesion patterns. An updated image can now be classified using deep learning (44). Detection of skin cancer using ML is shown in Figure 5.5.

5.3.1.3.2 *Machine Learning in COVID-19 Diagnosis*

Machine-learning and deep-learning algorithms have been proven to help analyze the enormous high-dimensional features of medical photos. Patients with COVID-19 exhibit CT or x-ray findings similar to other viruses and atypical pneumonia diseases. As a result, machine-learning and deep-learning techniques may make it simpler to automatically distinguish COVID-19 from those other pneumonia infections. Several methods, notably Ensemble, VGG-16, ResNet, InceptionNetV3, MobileNet v2, Xception, CNN, VGG16, Truncated Inception Net, and KNN, have been used to analyze chest images of COVID-19 patients. Notably, using these approaches to x-rays has resulted in positive results. This finding is especially important because x-rays are widely available and inexpensive. These methods can determine the degree of COVID-19 pneumonia, as well as the likelihood of short-term death, in addition to separating COVID-19 individuals from non-COVID pneumonia cases (45). The availability of publicly available libraries of CT and x-ray pictures of individuals with COVID-19 has made it simpler to deploy machine-learning algorithms to a huge number of clinical images and also to conduct all the training and validation processes (46).

More useful data for stratifying COVID-19 patients would come from an analysis of their clinical and demographic data, their relationship to aspects of CT and x-ray imaging, and the efficacy of machine-learning prediction approaches. Additionally, because deep-learning models are black boxes, one of their biggest problems in medical applications is the unpredictability of their results, which needs to be fixed (47).

5.3.1.3.3 Machine Learning in Diagnosing Breast Cancer

Machine learning can be used to aid with illness diagnosis in a healthcare context. It frequently uses ultrasound or x-ray pictures to aid in breast cancer screening. Methods using machine learning (ML) for identifying, evaluating, and categorizing breast cancer. Using machine learning, researchers were provided with a digital photo of fine-needle aspiration (FNA) of a breast tumor (ML) (48). A breast cancer diagnosis utilizing a combination of mammography and ML techniques has been made (49). Prostate cancer and breast cancer Gleason grades have been successfully determined by analyses employing histopathology images and automated grading systems (50,51). ML algorithms for automated breast cancer and prostate cancer diagnosis and classification on digital histopathology images has also been shown by several previously reported methods (52).

5.3.1.3.4 ML in Diagnosing Eye Diseases

Recently, there has been a noticeable rise in the use of AI methods for diagnostic imaging, from processing through interpretation. Recent articles on the use of AI in radiography, electro-encephalography, electrocardiogram (ECG), x-ray scanning, ultrasound imaging, and angiography employ MRI and CT more frequently than 50% of the time. Research efforts have focused on disorders with high prevalence, including cataracts, adult macular degeneration (AMD), glaucoma, as well as diabetic retinopathy (DR), among the uses of AI in ophthalmology. AI may be useful for decreasing clinical obligations as it allows doctors with less expertise to scan for diseases and identify them efficiently and fairly. AI has gained popularity in the field of ophthalmology since it may be used to uncover clinically meaningful features for diagnostic and predictive purposes. The efficiency of professionals and programs in diagnosing different eye-imaging modalities has been examined in several studies. Slit lamp images, optical coherence tomography (OCT), and fundus photography are a few of the AI methods utilized in ophthalmology (53).

5.3.1.3.4.1 Fundus photography
Normal FP typically involves the acquisition of pictures at one-field 45° to a posterior pole of a retina, and the complete retina can be observed at an angle of 230° (54). Wider spectrum FP detection is a recent discovery in the field of AI diagnostics, and its advancement calls for more complex algorithms (55). AI may be applied in medical contexts to analyze retinal images and diagnose illnesses. The Google Chips and Amazon DeepLens cameras allow the possibility to integrate cutting-edge algorithms within devices, which is a useful strategy in a range of medical fields (56). The first self-driving AI-based DR diagnostic system, IDx-DR, was approved by the United States Food and Drug Administration in 2018. Recent efforts have sought to automate pupillary tracking by integrating an actuator into the fundus camera. It has been shown that Google Brain can estimate participants' cardiovascular risk factors, like aging, systolic pressure, haemoglobin A1c, and sex, from a single fundus image, a feat that is unachievable for professional medical experts (57). More than 50,000 ocular pictures taken in a range of lighting conditions are available on Kaggle, one of the largest dataset model and data-processing competition websites in the world, with severity ratings ranging from 0 to 4. Additionally, EyePACS and MESSIDOR are the two most used photo datasets for DR classification (58). Figure 5.6 shows the application of DL algorithm for automatic detection of eye disorders.

5.3.1.3.4.2 Optical Coherence Tomography (OCT):
OCT is a non-invasive, non-contact optical image-based diagnostic method that aids in the diagnosis of several macular diseases and provides detailed data about retinal morphology (59). An ML technique was recommended to predict the need for anti-VEGF medicine based on OCT pictures obtained during the initial examination. AUCs of 0.77 and 0.07, respectively, were found for the groups having low and high treatment regimens (60).

Retinal OCT may provide insights for early detection of neurodegenerative inside the brain, including Alzheimer's disease, according to recent research that analyzed a unique mix of retinal OCT and MRI images (61).

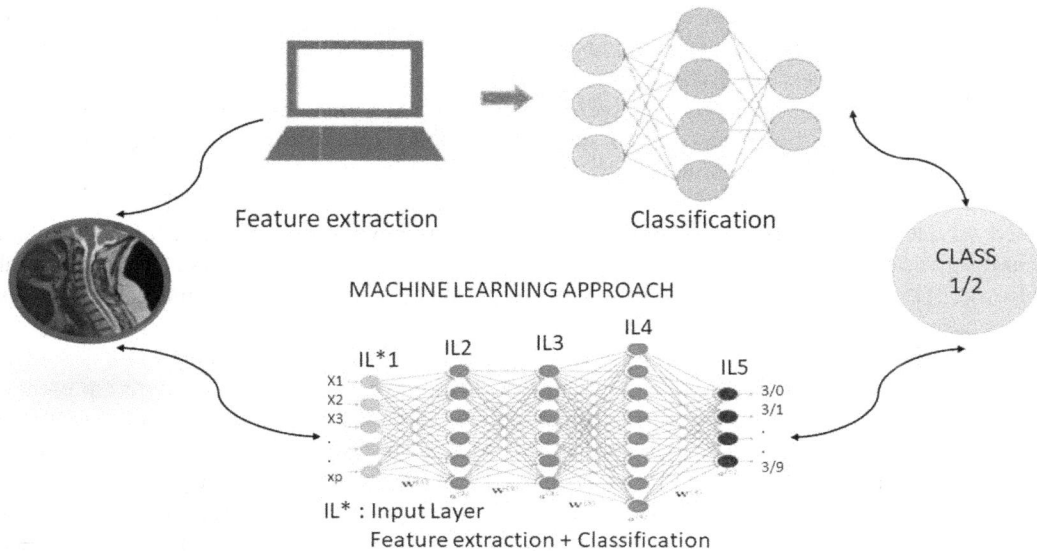

FIGURE 5.6 Application of DL algorithm for automatic detection of eye disorders.

5.3.1.3.4.3 Slit Lamp   Using just a slit lamp, an elevated light source, to project a narrow stream of light into the eye allows one to inspect the posterior and anterior segments of the eye. The bulk of the eye and its adnexa receive broad illumination as a means of facilitating general observation. Congenital cataracts are a significant contributor to childhood blindness, and their identification requires the use of slit-lamp images (62,63). The phenotypic of congenital cataracts are much more complex than senile cataracts. Both the variability of cataract patients and the complexity of their ocular pictures can be seen in slit-lamp images.

5.3.1.3.5   ML in Diagnosing Brain Disorder

AI models as an assisting tool for various frameworks of brain care, such as selecting candidates for surgical intervention, target description for the operative procedure, route description for corrective surgery, designing of tissue deformation for intra-operative support, and patient prognosis for postoperative assessment (64).

AI-enhanced brain care can help patients with a variety of neurological conditions, including epilepsy, brain tumours, lesions, Parkinson's disease, brain traumas, and cerebrovascular abnormalities. Techniques for natural language processing (NLP), including gradient boosting machine (GBM), sparse autoencoder (SAE), genetic algorithm (GA), ANN, SVM, fuzzy C-means, RF, and k-means, were all used. In addition, customized approaches and lesser ML algorithms were adopted. There were several utilizations of data types, such as magnetic resonance, computed tomography, IUS, DTI, HSI, EHR, MER, and functional near-infrared spectroscopy (fNIRS) (65).

5.3.2   Deep Learning in Medical Visualization

DL is an AI area that has expanded quickly in recent years. DL is essentially a subset of the larger family of machine learning that uses neural networks (similar to the neurons in our brains) to simulate behaviour resembling that of the human brain. To possibly find patterns and classify the information following those patterns, DL algorithms concentrate on mechanisms for information-processing patterns. DL uses larger data sets than ML does, and the prediction method is self-managed by the machines (66). Due to its many advantages, including its versatility, high performance, potent generalization capability, and wide range of applications, the science world has focused on DL. The development of increasingly powerful computers and the abundance of medical data have both greatly increased interest in this sector (67). The various invitations, challenges, conferences, or findings that are presented by research organizations worldwide demonstrate the interest in DL (68). As new developments are routinely produced, the numerous contributions increase the effectiveness of the current models (69). Additionally, the growth of DL has been aided in many scientific fields, including medicine, by the production of enormous amounts of digital data, robust computer facilities, graphics processing units (GPU), and cloud-based services. Deep learning can be thought of as an improvement over conventional artificial neural networks because it builds a network with multiple (more than two) layers (70). Deep neural networks (DNN) can find hierarchical feature representations in which the higher-level features can be inferred from the lower-level characteristics.

To determine the local anatomical properties, several medical image-processing techniques now in use rely on morphological feature representations. However, most of these feature representations were created manually, by specialists, and required a lot of time and work. Additionally, the properties of the designed images are frequently problem-specific and barely reusable, meaning they are not guaranteed to function for other image kinds. For instance, the imaging segmentation and registration methods created for T1-weighted 1.5-Tesla brain MR pictures do not apply to T1-weighted 7.0-Tesla images (71), let alone to images of other modalities or organs. The difference between ML and AI is shown in Figure 5.7.

Deep-learning-based AI has proven beneficial in several medical disciplines. It excels particularly in strictly delineated clinical tasks where the vast majority of the data necessary for the assignment is enclosed inside the data, depicted as a 1D signal (such as electrocardiography), 2D or 3D medical imaging (such as a fundus images picture or optical coherence tomography), or organized electronic medical record (72).

Because diagnoses in dermatology are primarily based on visual appearance, applications in this field are particularly well suited for AI. This idea was proven by a study in which the researchers trained a CNN to categorize lesions from images of skin illness (73). Malignant melanomas and carcinomas might be distinguished with an accuracy comparable to those of up to 21 board-certified dermatologists. In a second dermatology application, a CNN outperformed a panel of

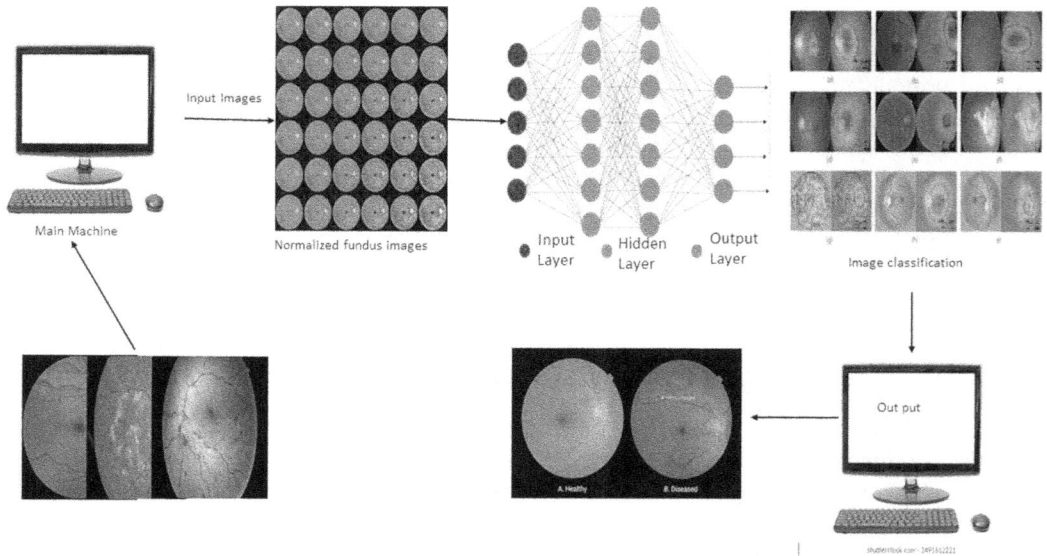

FIGURE 5.7   Classical difference between ML and AI.

doctors who conducted the same examination in a time-consuming manual approach or even outperformed them. This application concerned onychomycosis diagnosis (74).

5.4 AI SOFTWARE IN MEDICAL VISUALIZATION

As technology continues to revolutionize every aspect of healthcare, software utilizing AI, especially notably the component of AI referred to as ML, has emerged as an ever-significant part of a growing array of medical equipment. Medical devices having ML capability have drawn more attention in recent years. Over the past 10 years, the FDA has investigated and approved a rising number of devices that have been legally sold (via 510(k) clearance, granted De Novo request, or granted PMA) with ML, and it predicts that this trend will continue (75).

The best general-purpose AI imaging tools are Quibim, Enlitic, Butterfly Network, Lunit, ChironX, Aidoc, Contextflow, and 4Quant. Here is a list of some of the most recent AI/ML-based software that the USFDA has authorized is enlisted in, Table 5.1.

5.5 AI-BASED MEDICAL IMAGE SEGMENTATION FOR 3D PRINTING

A crucial part of many areas of medical research, instruction, and clinical practice is feature extraction for 3D printers and 3D visualization. Computerized quantifications and visualization techniques must be highly developed for medical picture segmentation. As AI technology has advanced, it is now possible to swiftly and correctly identify tumours or organs in medical imaging and automatically outline them (76). The process of extracting areas of interest (ROIs) using 3D image data, such as that from CT or MRI scans, is known as medical-image segmentation. The major objective of segregating this information is to locate the anatomical regions needed for a given study, such as simulating physical attributes or realistically putting implants with CAD designs inside of patients. Recent developments in AI-based software applications are making it simpler to execute common jobs like medical image segmentation, which is a time-consuming task (77).

From the segmented image medical experts can now design patient-specific medical gadgets to aid in surgery planning thanks to 3D printing (3DP). A variety of tools can be used to produce anatomical models from patient scans; however, research on the geometrical variance produced during the digital translation of images to models is few (78). Deep convolutional neural networks (DCNN) are used in AI-based segmentation in the AIMIS3D platform to automatically extract tumour and organ borders (79). Using DCNN, a new technique for computer-aided design (CAD) analysis, it is possible to automatically extract characteristics and monitor vast volumes of data to create quantitative choices (80). There is a growing belief that deep-learning research could be a viable replacement for manual, traditional approaches to image recognition and pattern classification issues.

5.5.1 SEGMENTATION TECHNIQUES

Automatic segmentation is typically offered by segmentation applications like Vital Images Advanced Visualization by Vitrea. To automatically or even partially automatically separate particular organs from surrounding tissues, it makes use of sophisticated algorithms. Auto-segmentation software uses a pre-set algorithm, which is based on the anatomical of interest to let the user choose which region to segment. The automatic and interactive segmentation technologies both contribute to the 3D models. From the models, many anatomical regions can be integrated. They are also generated like a STL file for further reworking and 3D printing. When geographic segmentation divides 3D objects, an arterial phase volume that displays the artery and a venous phase's volume that displays the veins are utilized (81).

TABLE 5.1

Most Recently USFDA Approved AI/ML-Based software

US FDA approval and 510(k) Clearance	AI Software	Inventors	Medical imaging category	Applications
06/17/2021, K203514	Precise Position	Philips Healthcare Co., Ltd.	CT Radiology	With the use of AI, Philips Precise Position helps swiftly and accurately situate patients for successful CT scans.
06/16/2021, K202718	Qmenta Care Platform Family	Mint Labs, Inc., D/B/A. QMENTA	Radiology	The imaging platform from QMENTA is an all-inclusive, fully integrated platform for end-to-end solutions. Every component necessary for an imaging study is included, including secure data gathering and storage, quantified image processing, centralized reviewing procedures, and study closeout.
06/10/2021, K203629	IDx-DR	Digital Diagnostics Inc.	Ophthalmic	An AI diagnostic tool called IDx-DR uses patient data to determine whether they have diabetic retinopathy on its own (including macular edema)
05/19/2021. K210237	CINA CHEST	Avicenna.AI	Radiology	CINA-PE and CINA-AD, including AI tools for detection and emergency triage of pulmonary embolism and aortic dissection
04/30/2021, K210001	HYPER AiR	Shanghai United Imaging Healthcare	Radiology	Fluorodeoxyglucose (FDG) PET scans' noise and contrast can be improved with the help of the image processing tool HYPER AiR, which is designed to be employed by radiologist and nuclear medicine specialists.
04/23/2021, K203502	MEDO-Thyroid	MEDO DX Pte. Ltd.	Radiology	Medo then analyses these to present the most relevant image of the lobes and nodules. Furthermore, it segments the lobes and the nodules and calculates the TI-RADS scoring.
04/23/2021, K203314	Cartesion Prime (PCD-1000A/3) V10.8	Canon Medical Systems Corporation	Radiology	AiCE-i for PET uses deep learning artificial neural network techniques that can analyse the statistical features of the signal and noise of PET data in order to enhance image quality and lower image noise for FDG whole body data. The AiCE algorithm can be used to denoise and enhance PET image quality.
04/20/2021, K203610	Automatic Anatomy Recognition	Quantitative Radiology Solutions, LLC	Radiology	Designed to work independently of a specific treatment planning system, AAR is deployed on a cloud-based platform.
04/19/2021, K203469	AI Segmentation	Varian Medical Systems	Radiology	AI segmentation is designed to produce fast, accurate and intelligent contouring to reproducibility of critical structure delineation. It reduces 80% contouring time than manual contouring
04/16/2021, K203517	Saige-Q	DeepHealth, Inc.	Radiology	The Saige-Q code represents the software's suspicion of any potential findings in mammography. Saige-Q additionally creates a preview image of the exam's most suspect image for tests that are flagged as suspicious. Radiologists can

Date, K-number	Product	Company	Specialty	Description
04/14/2021, K202992	BriefCase, RIB Fractures Triage (RibFx)	Aidoc Medical, Ltd.	Radiology	The rib fractures solution from Aidoc is a treatment and notification tool designed for use with CT image processing. It flags and notifies users of potential positive rib fracture findings.
04/02/2021, K202441	Eclipse II with Smart Noise Cancellation	Carestream Health, Inc.	Radiology	Cares Stream is Smart Noise Cancellation uses deep, convolutional neural network technology to give exceptional CNN-based noise reduction, improving image quality, preserving fine detail, improving contrast-to-noise ratio, and making radiographs simpler to read.
03/31/2021, K210071	SIS System (Version 5.1.0)	Surgical Information Sciences, Inc.	Radiology	SIS System is designed for viewing, presenting, and documenting medical imaging. It has a variety of features for image analysis, image compression, and intraoperative functional planning. The 3D outputs can be used with orthogonal image guided surgery or other devices for further processing and visualization.
03/31/2021K203443,	MAGNETOM Vida, MAGNETOM Sola, MAGNETOM Lumina, MAGNETOM Altea with syngo MR XA31A	Siemens Medical Solutions USA, Inc.	Radiology	With the 1.5T Open Bore MAGNETOM Altea system, you can perform MRI services with complete assurance in terms of output, reproducibility, and patient happiness.
03/31/2021, K203258	Syngo. CT Lung CAD VD20	Siemens Healthcare GmbH	Radiology	In order to help radiologists, identify solid pulmonary nodules while reviewing chest CT scans, Syngo CT Lung CAD was created.
03/24/2021, K203225	Aquilion ONE (TSX-306A/3) VI0.4	Canon Medical Systems Corporation	Radiology	Utilize the strength of one-beat cardiac and AI increased image sharpness in combination with PIQE to overcome the difficulties of coronary artery visualization in stents and badly calcified vessels.
03/23/2021, K210209	Viz ICH	Viz.Ai, Inc.	Cardiology	Automated Detection and Triage of Suspected ICH
03/19/2021, K203235	VBrain	Vysioneer Inc.	Radiology Brain	Vbrain is the first AI device to receive FDA clearance for tumor auto contouring in radiation therapy.
03/09/2021, K203256	Imbio RV/LV Software	Imbio, LLC	Cardiology	Imbio RV/LV Analysis helps physicians quickly assess potential ventricular dilation by automatically processing CTPA scans to measure the maximal diameters of the right and left ventricles of the heart, and reporting the resulting RV/LV ratio.
03/05/2021, K202300	Optellum Virtual Nodule Clinic, Optellum Software, Optellum Platform	Optellum Ltd	Radiology Pulmonary	The world's first AI-based early lung cancer decision support software.

(Continued)

TABLE 5.1 (Continued)
Most Recently USFDA Approved AI/ML-Based software

US FDA approval and 510(k) Clearance	AI Software	Inventors	Medical imaging category	Applications
02/25/2021, K202990	NinesMeasure	Nines, Inc.	Radiology Pulmonary	The novel lung nodule assessment tool Nines Measure, created with AI, can hasten the diagnosis of several respiratory illnesses.
01/07/2021, K202414	BrainInsight	Hyperfine Research, Inc.	Radiology Brain	Hyperfine BrainInsight offers automated AI tools for brain imaging that give clinicians useful quantitative biomarker information. These tools may help to improve patient care and lessen the workload of neuroradiological specialists by eliminating the need for manual measurements.
12/07/2020, K201039	HepaFat-AI	Resonance Health Analysis Services Pty Ltd.	Radiology Hepatic	HepaFat-AI analyses MRI datasets automatically to determine the amount of liver fat in patients, giving medical professionals a comprehensive, multi-metric solution to utilize in the evaluation of patients with confirmed or suspected fatty liver disease. Doctors get access to several variables about a patient's liver function via a single short, non-invasive MRI scan.
12/04/2020, K202487	HealthJOINT	Zebra Medical Vision Ltd.	Radiology Joints	The Zebra Health Joint is intended to assist clinicians in the preoperative planning of the surgical procedure
11/20/2020, K200873	HALO	NICo-Lab B.V.	Radiology Neurology	HALO is to process and analyze contrast-enhanced CT angiograms of the brain obtained in an acute situation to make it easier for patients suspected of having a stroke to have their brain vasculature evaluated
10/11/2020, K202501	Quantib Prostate	Quantib BV	Radiology Prostate	The MRI prostate reporting procedure is improved by Quantib Prostate, which is readily accessible from the radiologist's reading station and makes use of deep learning algorithms.
09/16/2020, K201369	AVA (Augmented Vascular Analysis)	See-Mode Technologies Pte. Ltd.	Vascular	AVA analyses each image in a vascular ultrasound scan using deep learning with a single click, delivering highly accurate vascular reports in under a minute. No need for hand drawings.
07/30/2020, K193283	AI-Rad Companion Prostate MR	Siemens Medical Solutions USA Inc	Biopsy Prostate	MRI scans of the prostate are automatically segmented using the AI-Rad Companion Prostate MR for Biopsy Support, which also allows radiologists to mark any areas they believe to be suspicious.

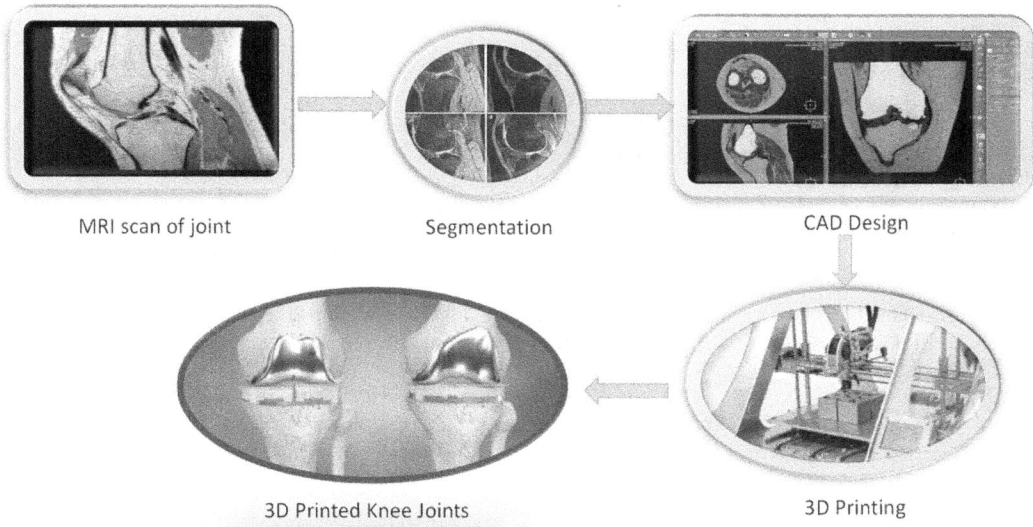

MRI scan of joint   Segmentation   CAD Design

3D Printed Knee Joints   3D Printing

FIGURE 5.8 AI-based segmentation approaching in 3D printed Knee Joints.

5.5.2 APPLICATION OF AI-BASED SEGMENTATION FOR 3D PRINTING

A platform-independent, extensible, 3-dimensional, automated-segmentation image-processing application has made significant progress. The lumbar spine, cancer, arteries, and nearby nerves were divided and visualized as 3D objects using CT images of the osteosarcoma. The lumbar spine might be printed in 3D to demonstrate how tumour tissue has infiltrated and destroyed the bone cortex. In breast cancer, the tumour target position must be precisely irradiated during radiation therapy. Nevertheless, with each treatment, the patient's position could alter and the breast could move to other locations. A plastic breast bra that was 3D printed was utilized to limit breast mobility and reduce breast position shift, which was quantitatively assessed on CT images. The 3D conversion was done using CT breast cancer patient images (82). The segmentation pattern of joint bone is shown for 3D printing in Figure 5.8.

5.6 CONCLUSION

The AI-enabled medical visualization can lead to more accurate & speedy outcomes. The image processing in medical visualization can make better image structuring & advance image data interpreting. AI subset as machine learning & deep learning can provide better more relevant image data analysis for diagnosis or treatment as discussed for skin cancer detection, COVID-19 diagnosis, diagnosing breast cancer, eye diseases, diagnosing brain disorder. The image-data recording becomes more sophisticated using AI. The dataset is a key important factor for any AI-enabled system. AI-based medical image segmentation for 3D printing is a major advancement in medical image visualization for better medical-oriented services. The various application of AI-based segmentation for 3-D printing assist in better outcomes.

REFERENCES

[1] Miller DD, Brown EW Artificial Intelligence in Medical Practice: The Question to the Answer? *The American Journal of Medicine*. 2018;131(2):129–133.

[2] Kirch DG, Petelle K Addressing the Physician Shortage: The Peril of Ignoring Demography. *JAMA.* 2017;317(19):1947–1948.

[3] Chartrand G, Cheng PM, Vorontsov E, Drozdzal M, Turcotte S, Pal CJ, et al. *Deep Learning: A Primer for Radiologists.* 2017;37(7):2113–2131.

[4] Lee JG, Jun S, Cho YW, Lee H, Kim GB, Seo JB, et al. Deep Learning in Medical Imaging: General Overview. *Korean Journal of Radiology.* 2017;18(4):570–584.

[5] LeCun Y, Bengio Y, Hinton G Deep learning. *Nature.* 2015;521(7553):436–444.

[6] King BF, Jr. Guest Editorial: Discovery and Artificial Intelligence. *AJR American Journal of Roentgenology.* 2017;209(6):1189–1190.

[7] Erickson BJ, Korfiatis P, Akkus Z, Kline TL *Machine Learning for Medical Imaging.* 2017;37(2): 505–515.

[8] Pesapane F, Codari M, Sardanelli F Artificial intelligence in medical imaging: threat or opportunity? Radiologists again at the forefront of innovation in medicine. *European Radiology Experimental.* 2018;2(1):35.

[9] Reuter-Oppermann M, Kühl N Artificial Intelligence for Healthcare Logistics: An Overview and Research Agenda. In: Masmoudi M, Jarboui B, Siarry P, editors. *Artificial Intelligence and Data Mining in Healthcare.* Cham: Springer International Publishing; 2021, p. 1–22.

[10] Bohr A, Memarzadeh K The rise of artificial intelligence in healthcare applications. *Artificial Intelligence in Healthcare.* 2020:25–60. doi: 10.1016/B978-0-12-818438-7.00002-2. Epub 2020 Jun 26.

[11] Kolker E, Özdemir V, Kolker E How Healthcare Can Refocus on Its Super-Customers (Patients, n =1) and Customers (Doctors and Nurses) by Leveraging Lessons from Amazon, Uber, and Watson. *OMICS: A Journal of Integrative Biology.* 2016;20(6):329–333.

[12] Jiang F, Jiang Y, Zhi H, Dong Y, Li H, Ma S, et al. Artificial intelligence in healthcare: past, present and future. *Stroke and Vascular Neurology.* 2017;2(4):230.

[13] Gillies RJ, Kinahan PE, Hricak H Radiomics: Images Are More than Pictures, They Are Data. *Radiology.* 2015;278(2):563–577.

[14] Darcy AM, Louie AK, Roberts LW Machine Learning and the Profession of Medicine. *JAMA.* 2016;315(6):551–552.

[15] Lakhani P, Prater AB, Hutson RK, Andriole KP, Dreyer KJ, Morey J, et al. Machine Learning in Radiology: Applications Beyond Image Interpretation. *Journal of the American College of Radiology: JACR.* 2018;15(2):350–359.

[16] Kushniruk A, Borycki E The Human Factors of AI in Healthcare: Recurrent Issues, Future Challenges and Ways Forward. In: Househ M, Borycki E, Kushniruk A, editors. *Multiple Perspectives on Artificial Intelligence in Healthcare: Opportunities and Challenges.* Cham: Springer International Publishing; 2021, p. 3–12.

[17] Lee CS, Nagy PG, Weaver SJ, Newman-Toker DE Cognitive and system factors contributing to diagnostic errors in radiology. *AJR American Journal of Roentgenology.* 2013;201(3):611–617.

[18] Castro VM, Dligach D, Finan S, Yu S, Can A, Abd-El-Barr M, et al. Large-scale identification of patients with cerebral aneurysms using natural language processing. *Neurology.* 2017;88(2):164.

[19] Neill DB Using Artificial Intelligence to Improve Hospital Inpatient Care. *IEEE Intelligent Systems.* 2013;28(2):92–95.

[20] Murff HJ, FitzHenry F, Matheny ME, Gentry N, Kotter KL, Crimin K, et al. Automated identification of postoperative complications within an electronic medical record using natural language processing. *JAMA.* 2011;306(8):848–855.

[21] Shanu N, Ganesh RS Use of Deep Learning in Biomedical Imaging. In: Parah SA, Rashid M, Varadarajan V, editors. *Artificial Intelligence for Innovative Healthcare Informatics.* Cham: Springer International Publishing; 2022, p. 3–33.

[22] Signorelli CM Can Computers Become Conscious and Overcome Humans? 2018;5.

[23] Kaplan A, Haenlein M Siri, Siri, in my hand: Who's the fairest in the land? On the interpretations, illustrations, and implications of artificial intelligence. *Business Horizons.* 2019;62(1):15–25.

[24] Popenici SAD, Kerr S Exploring the impact of artificial intelligence on teaching and learning in higher education. *Research and Practice in Technology Enhanced Learning.* 2017;12(1):22.

[25] Xu M, Jia C Application of Artificial Intelligence Technology in Medical Imaging. *Journal of Physics: Conference Series.* 2021;2037(1):012090.

[26] Kim H-E, Kim HH, Han B-K, Kim KH, Han K, Nam H, et al. Changes in cancer detection and false-positive recall in mammography using artificial intelligence: a retrospective, multireader study. *The Lancet Digital Health.* 2020;2(3):e138–e148.

[27] van den Heuvel TLA, van der Eerden AW, Manniesing R, Ghafoorian M, Tan T, Andriessen TMJC, et al. Automated detection of cerebral microbleeds in patients with traumatic brain injury. *NeuroImage: Clinical*. 2016;12:241–251.

[28] Becker AS, Marcon M, Ghafoor S, Wurnig MC, Frauenfelder T, Boss A Deep Learning in Mammography: Diagnostic Accuracy of a Multipurpose Image Analysis Software in the Detection of Breast Cancer. *Investigative Radiology*. 2017;52(7).

[29] Liu X, Faes L, Kale AU, Wagner SK, Fu DJ, Bruynseels A, et al. A comparison of deep learning performance against health-care professionals in detecting diseases from medical imaging: a systematic review and meta-analysis. *The Lancet Digital Health*. 2019;1(6):e271–e297.

[30] Liu X, Gao K, Liu B, Pan C, Liang K, Yan L, et al. Advances in Deep Learning-Based Medical Image Analysis. *Health Data Science*. 2021;2021:8786793.

[31] Wang S, Summers RM Machine learning and radiology. *Medical Image Analysis*. 2012;16(5):933–951.

[32] Suzuki K Pixel-Based Machine Learning in Medical Imaging. *International Journal of Biomedical Imaging*. 2012;2012:792079.

[33] Gottesman O, Johansson F, Komorowski M, Faisal A, Sontag D, Doshi-Velez F, et al. Guidelines for reinforcement learning in healthcare. *Nature Medicine*. 2019;25(1):16–18.

[34] Alloghani M, Al-Jumeily D, Mustafina J, Hussain A, Aljaaf AJ A Systematic Review on Supervised and Unsupervised Machine Learning Algorithms for Data Science. In: Berry MW, Mohamed A, Yap BW, editors. *Supervised and Unsupervised Learning for Data Science*. Cham: Springer International Publishing; 2020. p. 3–21.

[35] Sarker IH Machine Learning: Algorithms, Real-World Applications and Research Directions. *SN Computer Science*. 2021;2(3):160.

[36] Jung S-K, Kim T-W New approach for the diagnosis of extractions with neural network machine learning. *American Journal of Orthodontics and Dentofacial Orthopedics*. 2016;149(1):127–133.

[37] Laaksonen J, Oja E, editors. Classification with learning k-nearest neighbors. Proceedings of International Conference on Neural Networks (ICNN'96); 1996. 3-6 June 1996.

[38] Uddin S, Haque I, Lu H, Moni MA, Gide E Comparative performance analysis of K-nearest neighbour (KNN) algorithm and its different variants for disease prediction. *Scientific Reports*. 2022;12(1):6256.

[39] Pisner DA, Schnyer DM Chapter 6 - Support vector machine. In: Mechelli A, Vieira S, editors. *Machine Learning*. Academic Press; 2020. p. 101–121.

[40] Kurilová V, Goga J, Oravec M, Pavlovičová J, Kajan S Support vector machine and deep-learning object detection for localisation of hard exudates. *Scientific Reports*. 2021;11(1):16045.

[41] Goswami S, Pramanick R, Patra A, Rath SP, Foltin M, Ariando A, et al. Decision trees within a molecular memristor. *Nature*. 2021;597(7874):51–56.

[42] Chen H, Hu S, Hua R, Zhao X Improved naive Bayes classification algorithm for traffic risk management. *EURASIP Journal on Advances in Signal Processing*. 2021;2021(1):30.

[43] Das K, Cockerell CJ, Patil A, Pietkiewicz P, Giulini M, Grabbe S, et al. Machine Learning and Its Application in Skin Cancer. *International Journal of Environmental Research and Public Health*. 2021;18(24).

[44] Das K, Cockerell CJ, Patil A, Pietkiewicz P, Giulini M, Grabbe S, et al. Machine Learning and Its Application in Skin Cancer. 2021;18(24):13409.

[45] Mohammad-Rahimi H, Nadimi M, Ghalyanchi-Langeroudi A, Taheri M, Ghafouri-Fard S Application of Machine Learning in Diagnosis of COVID-19 Through X-Ray and CT Images: A Scoping Review. 2021;8.

[46] Ozsahin I, Sekeroglu B, Musa MS, Mustapha MT, Uzun Ozsahin D Review on Diagnosis of COVID-19 from Chest CT Images Using Artificial Intelligence. *Computational and Mathematical Methods in Medicine*. 2020;2020:9756518.

[47] Singh A, Sengupta S, Lakshminarayanan V Explainable Deep Learning Models in Medical Image Analysis. 2020;6(6):52.

[48] Wolberg WH, Street WN, Mangasarian OL Machine learning techniques to diagnose breast cancer from image-processed nuclear features of fine needle aspirates. *Cancer Letters*. 1994;77(2):163–171.

[49] Akselrod-Ballin A, Chorev M, Shoshan Y, Spiro A, Hazan A, Melamed R, et al. Predicting Breast Cancer by Applying Deep Learning to Linked Health Records and Mammograms. *Radiology*. 2019;292(2):331–342.

[50] Petrolis R, Ramonaitė R, Jančiauskas D, Kupčinskas J, Pečiulis R, Kupčinskas L, et al. Digital imaging of colon tissue: method for evaluation of inflammation severity by spatial frequency features of the histological images. *Diagnostic Pathology*. 2015;10(1):159.

[51] Nir G, Karimi D, Goldenberg SL, Fazli L, Skinnider BF, Tavassoli P, et al. Comparison of Artificial Intelligence Techniques to Evaluate Performance of a Classifier for Automatic Grading of Prostate Cancer From Digitized Histopathologic Images. *JAMA Network Open*. 2019;2(3): e190442-e.

[52] Mosquera-Lopez C, Agaian S, Velez-Hoyos A, Thompson I Computer-Aided Prostate Cancer Diagnosis From Digitized Histopathology: A Review on Texture-Based Systems. *IEEE Reviews in Biomedical Engineering*. 2015;8:98–113.

[53] Tong Y, Lu W, Yu Y, Shen Y Application of machine learning in ophthalmic imaging modalities. *Eye and Vision*. 2020;7(1):22.

[54] Vujosevic S, Benetti E, Massignan F, Pilotto E, Varano M, Cavarzeran F, et al. Screening for Diabetic Retinopathy: 1 and 3 Nonmydriatic 45-degree Digital Fundus Photographs vs 7 Standard Early Treatment Diabetic Retinopathy Study Fields. *American Journal of Ophthalmology*. 2009;148(1): 111–118.

[55] Kaines A, Oliver S, Reddy S, Schwartz SD Ultrawide Angle Angiography for the Detection and Management of Diabetic Retinopathy. *International Ophthalmology Clinics*. 2009;49(2).

[56] Göbl R, Navab N, Hennersperger C SUPRA: open-source software-defined ultrasound processing for real-time applications. *International Journal of Computer Assisted Radiology and Surgery*. 2018;13(6):759–767.

[57] Poplin R, Varadarajan AV, Blumer K, Liu Y, McConnell MV, Corrado GS, et al. Prediction of cardiovascular risk factors from retinal fundus photographs via deep learning. *Nature Biomedical Engineering*. 2018;2(3):158–164.

[58] Al Turk L, Wang S, Krause P, Wawrzynski J, Saleh GM, Alsawadi H, et al. Evidence Based Prediction and Progression Monitoring on Retinal Images from Three Nations. *Translational Vision Science & Technology*. 2020;9(2):44-.

[59] Huang D, Swanson EA, Lin CP, Schuman JS, Stinson WG, Chang W, et al. Optical Coherence Tomography. *Science*. 1991;254(5035):1178–1181.

[60] Bogunović H, Waldstein SM, Schlegl T, Langs G, Sadeghipour A, Liu X, et al. Prediction of Anti-VEGF Treatment Requirements in Neovascular AMD Using a Machine Learning Approach. *Investigative Ophthalmology & Visual Science*. 2017;58(7):3240–3248.

[61] Ong Y-T, Hilal S, Cheung CY, Venketasubramanian N, Niessen WJ, Vrooman H, et al. Retinal neurodegeneration on optical coherence tomography and cerebral atrophy. *Neuroscience Letters*. 2015;584:12–16.

[62] Lin D, Chen J, Lin Z, Li X, Wu X, Long E, et al. 10-Year Overview of the Hospital-Based Prevalence and Treatment of Congenital Cataracts: The CCPMOH Experience. *PloS one*. 2015; 10(11):e0142298.

[63] Wu X, Long E, Lin H, Liu Y Prevalence and epidemiological characteristics of congenital cataract: a systematic review and meta-analysis. *Scientific Reports*. 2016;6(1):28564.

[64] Burgos N, Colliot O Machine learning for classification and prediction of brain diseases: recent advances and upcoming challenges. *Current Opinion in Neurology*. 2020;33(4).

[65] Segato A, Marzullo A, Calimeri F, De Momi E Artificial intelligence for brain diseases: A systematic review. *APL Bioengineering*. 2020;4(4):041503.

[66] Janiesch C, Zschech P, Heinrich K Machine learning and deep learning. *Electronic Markets*. 2021;31(3):685–695.

[67] Anaya-Isaza A, Mera-Jiménez L, Zequera-Diaz M An overview of deep learning in medical imaging. *Informatics in Medicine Unlocked*. 2021;26:100723.

[68] Dong S, Wang P, Abbas K A survey on deep learning and its applications. *Computer Science Review*. 2021;40:100379.

[69] Wason R Deep learning: Evolution and expansion. *Cognitive Systems Research*. 2018;52:701–708.

[70] Shen D, Wu G, Suk H-I Deep Learning in Medical Image Analysis. *Annual Review of Biomedical Engineering*. 2017;19(1):221–248.

[71] Wu G, Kim M, Wang Q, Gao Y, Liao S, Shen D, editors. Unsupervised Deep Feature Learning for Deformable Registration of MR Brain Images. *Medical Image Computing and Computer-Assisted Intervention – MICCAI* 2013;2013 2013//; Berlin, Heidelberg: Springer Berlin Heidelberg.

[72] Litjens G, Kooi T, Bejnordi BE, Setio AAA, Ciompi F, Ghafoorian M, et al. A survey on deep learning in medical image analysis. *Medical Image Analysis*. 2017;42:60–88.

[73] Esteva A, Kuprel B, Novoa RA, Ko J, Swetter SM, Blau HM, et al. Dermatologist-level classification of skin cancer with deep neural networks. *Nature*. 2017;542(7639):115–118.

[74] Han SS, Park GH, Lim W, Kim MS, Na JI, Park I, et al. Deep neural networks show an equivalent and often superior performance to dermatologists in onychomycosis diagnosis: Automatic construction of onychomycosis datasets by region-based convolutional deep neural network. *PloS one.* 2018;13(1):e0191493.

[75] Health, C for D. and R. What are examples of software as a medical device? *FDA.* 2020. https://www.fda.gov/medical-devices/software-medical-device-samd/what-are-examples-software-medical-device

[76] Jia G, Huang X, Tao S, Zhang X, Zhao Y, Wang H, et al. Artificial intelligence-based medical image segmentation for 3D printing and naked eye 3D visualization. *Intelligent Medicine.* 2022;2(1):48–53.

[77] What is medical image segmentation and how does it work? | synopsys. (n.d.). Retrieved August 21, 2022, from https://www.synopsys.com/glossary/what-is-medical-image-segmentation.html

[78] Fogarasi M, Coburn JC, Ripley B Algorithms used in medical image segmentation for 3D printing and how to understand and quantify their performance. *3D Printing in Medicine.* 2022;8(1):18.

[79] Hu P, Wu F, Peng J, Bao Y, Chen F, Kong D Automatic abdominal multi-organ segmentation using deep convolutional neural network and time-implicit level sets. *International Journal of Computer Assisted Radiology and Surgery.* 2017;12(3):399–411.

[80] Sun L, Wang J, Hu Z, Xu Y, Cui Z Multi-View Convolutional Neural Networks for Mammographic Image Classification. *IEEE Access.* 2019;7:126273–126282.

[81] Geiger, S (n.d.). Medical 3d printing application guide | data segmentation for medical imaging. *Proto3000.* Retrieved August 21, 2022, from https://proto3000.com/applications/application-guide-data-segmentation-for-medical-3d-printing/

[82] Yu HJ, Chen J-H, Mehta RS, Nalcioglu O, Su M-Y MRI measurements of tumor size and pharmacokinetic parameters as early predictors of response in breast cancer patients undergoing neoadjuvant anthracycline chemotherapy. *Journal of Magnetic Resonance Imaging.* 2007;26(3):615–623.

6 Machine-Learning Models for Early Diagnosis of Depressive Mental Affliction

Chandra Mani Sharma
CRDT, IIT Delhi, New Delhi, India

Rahul Ramanathan Krishnamoorthy
University of Illinois, Urbana Champaign, USA

Vijayaraghavan M. Chariar
CRDT, IIT Delhi, New Delhi, India

CONTENTS

DOI: 10.1201/9781003333081-6

6.1 INTRODUCTION

Depression is a common mental health disorder that causes people to feel sad for long periods and lose interest in things they used to enjoy or find rewarding. It is a disease that can disrupt one's productivity in daily activities, sleep, and appetite. Globally, mental disorders represent the greatest burden of noncommunicable diseases. They are accountable for a significant number of disability-adjusted life years (DALYs) lost by populations. Depression is one of the most prevalent mental disorders. Early detection of depression can enhance the efficacy of treatment. This study aims to use machine learning to identify early signs of depression by analyzing people's daily activities. Multiple machine-learning models were trained on a dataset containing both real and synthetic samples. The process of data collection has two components. The first section consisted of a questionnaire based on the Hamilton Depression Rating Scale (HDRS). The other section consisted of 18 questions regarding daily activities and behavior. To eliminate inconsistencies, the raw dataset was sanitized, normalized, and preprocessed. The dataset was then used to train classification models using a variety of machine-learning algorithms, including K-Nearest Neighbors (KNN), support-vector machines (SVM), decision trees (DT), linear discriminant analysis (LDA), and Gaussian Naive Bayes. We examined the efficacy of the synthetic minority oversampling technique (SMOTE) and random undersampling in preventing overfitting, which could occur if the dataset was unbalanced. Various performance metrics, including precision, specificity, sensitivity, AUC-ROC score, f-score, etc., were used to evaluate the techniques. Combining a decision tree classifier with SMOTE produced the best results. The accuracy score was increased to 84.7 percent using hyperparameter optimization and grid search, and the AUC-ROC was raised to 0.934.

Depression impairs cognitive and social functioning, leading to decreased performance in the workplace and elsewhere [1]. It even affects the quality of interpersonal relationships, especially with family [2,3]. Hence, early identification and treatment of depression can help improve one's life. Early detection and appropriate treatment of the disease can promote remission, prevent relapse, and reduce the burden of the symptoms on the individual.

The majority of mental health disorders are diagnosed by expert clinicians, although there are self-reporting or assessment tools for certain diseases (such as depression and anxiety disorders). The specialists utilize a variety of rating scales based on disease diagnostic manuals such as DSM-V, ICD-10 Ch. 5, etc. With an acute shortage of mental health professionals and an ever-increasing prevalence of mental disorders, there is an urgent need to automate the task of diagnosing mental disease so that healthcare providers can screen large numbers of individuals in less time. Artificial intelligence and machine learning may help accomplish this goal. In addition to clinician-administered tests, there are self-reporting instruments for some mental health disorders, such as depression disorders. The available screening tools focus solely on how a person feels, without examining other behavioral characteristics. However, behavioral assessment may provide useful hints for exploring in greater depth why a person feels a certain way and what types of daily challenges are being faced. It can aid in both disease diagnosis and the prescription of an effective treatment.

The purpose of this study was to use machine-learning techniques to infer the onset of depression based on certain behavioral cues from a person's daily activities. For this purpose, a dataset capturing 18 critical activity parameters of an individual, along with HDRS scales, was used. The dataset was cleaned and standardized so that more accurate predictions could be made. Several machine-learning models were trained on this dataset using a variety of algorithms, and their performance was compared. The best-performing algorithm was used as a model for a system with a graphical user interface that was built with Python's KivyMD package. A person can put in their values for the 18 traits, and if depression is found, they will be notified so they can get help from a trained professional.

6.2 LITERATURE REVIEW

As a result of technological advancements, artificial intelligence is permeating the mental health and well-being space. This area of study has increasingly become the focus of a variety of disciplines. To get an idea of the increasing interest in the area, we analyzed several research publications in the Google Scholar database. Advanced search options were used to retrieve the results for each of the years starting in 2011 and ending in 2021. The search string was "depression detection using machine learning." Furthermore, under advanced options, some extra key words were supplied, including deep learning, depression, SVM, KNN, classification, ANN, major depressive disorder, etc. Figure 6.1 shows an increasing trend in the number of research publications during recent years.

There is an ongoing effort to use machine learning to make early depression diagnoses using a variety of data. These studies have varying characteristics which they use to identify people with depression, like audio files [4], surveys [5,6], MRI scans [7,8] and even comments on social media sites [9,10]. Artificial neural networks (ANN), support-vector machines (SVM), k-nearest neighbors (KNN), decision trees, and random forests are among the most frequently employed machine-learning algorithms for this purpose. Some studies, like that by Nemesure et al. [11], even used a combination of algorithms whose output was used as an input in a higher-level classifier. There are a few limitations to the datasets used by the studies conducted in this field. Rubin-Falcone et al. [7] used MRI scans, which can be expensive and hence would not be an ideal method to identify depression at an early stage in a way that is accessible to most people. Islam et al. [9] used some advanced software like NCapture and LIWC, which has the same problem of accessibility as Rubin-Falcone et al.'s MRI scans. Furthermore, several studies used datasets of a small group of participants or even a small number of characteristics to compare. Even those by Nemesure et al. [11] and

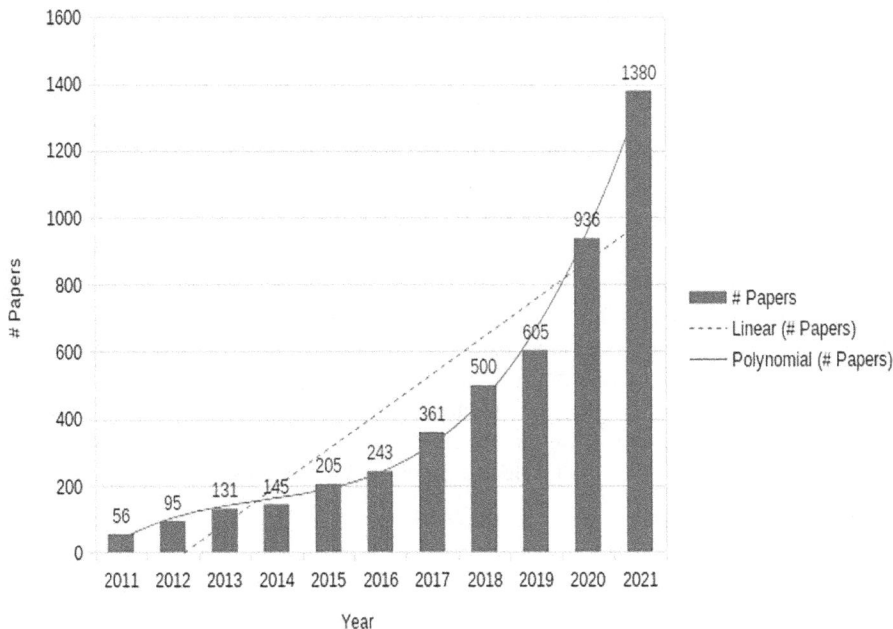

FIGURE 6.1 Number of research papers on depression detection using ML in Google Scholar.

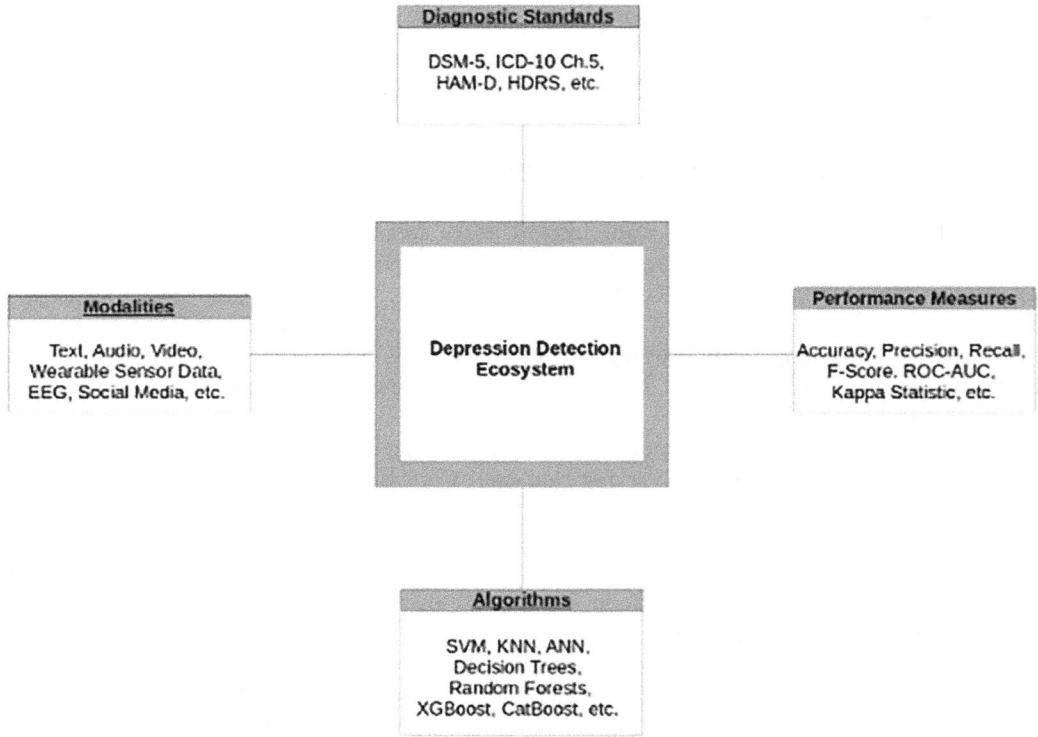

FIGURE 6.2   Essential components of a typical depression detection ecosystem.

Kasthurirathne et al. [12], which use very large datasets, collect data from hospitals and universities, may be unable to capture a variety of instances in the population. This inability limits the generalizability of the results. Additionally, the datasets tend to be heavily imbalanced since the population of those depressed is much lower than the healthy population. Na et al. [13] tried to address this issue by using the Synthetic Minority Oversampling Technique (SMOTE). However, the several synthetic samples created could pose a problem when created without considering the majority class, which can lead to the creation of ambiguous examples. Apart from accuracy, various metrics are used to measure the efficacy of the machine-learning algorithm. Most studies use the area under the receiver-operating characteristic curve (AUC-ROC), which is one of the most widely used evaluation metrics for such classification models. Precision, sensitivity, and specificity are other parameters related to the AUC-ROC, which are frequently mentioned. Some studies even highlight the use of a confusion matrix to obtain false positive and false negative statistics. Other metrics include the F1 score [9,14], the Brier score [15], and the mean kappa index [8]. However, given that the AUC-ROC is one of the most reliable performance-measuring metrics, this study will use it to measure the machine-learning model's efficacy. Furthermore, the precision, recall, and F1 score will also be used. Figure 6.2 shows the essential components of a depression-detection system.

Several studies have been conducted to identify people with depression using machine learning, as shown in Table 6.1 below.

6.2.1   DIAGNOSTIC TOOLS AND SCALES FOR DEPRESSION

A number of scales and tools are used for depression screening. Some of them are used by a qualified practitioner, while others can be used as a self-assessment tool.

TABLE 6.1

Comprehensive Comparison of Existing Literature According to Type of Mental Health Disorder, Dataset Used, Machine-Learning Algorithm and Performance Metrics

Reference	Type of Mental Health Disorder	Dataset	Best Reported Algorithm	Performance Evaluation Metrics
Rubin-Falcone et al. (2017) [7]	Major Depressive Disorder (MDD) and Bipolar	They conducted their own patient survey and used sMRI brain images.	Support Vector Machine, 75%	Area Under Curve, Confusion Matrix
Islam et al. (2018) [9]	Depression	Collected data from Facebook comments using NCapture and analyzed them using LIWC software.	Decision Tree	Precision, Recall and F-measure
Haque et al. (2021) [5]	Child Depression	Young Minds Matter survey, Australia.	Random Forest, 95%	Precision, Area Under Curve
Cacheda et al. (2019) [10]	Depression	Data collected by eRisk 2017 of social media platform reddit	Random Forest	Early Risk Detection Error
Priya et al. (2020) [14]	Depression	Self-collected data based on the questionnaire	Random Forest	F1 Score
Jiménez-Serrano et al. (2015) [6]	Postpartum Depression	Data from seven Spanish hospitals on postpartum women's depression	Naïve Bayes	F-Score, Specificity, Sensitivity, Area Under Curve
Nemesure et al. (2021) [11]	Generalized Anxiety Disorder and Major Depressive Disorder	Data of 4184 students from the University of Nice Sophia-Antipolis	XGBoost was used as a higher-level classifier, with Random Forest, SVM, KNN, and a Neural Network as inputs.	Area Under Curve
Espinola et al. (2021) [8]	Major Depressive Disorder	Data from Thirty-three individuals (11 males) over the age of 18; 22 with a history of MDD and 11 without.	Random Forest model with 100 trees, 87.5%	Mean Kappa Index, Sensitivity and Specificity
Bhakta et al. (2016) [16]	Depression in Senior Citizens	—	Bayesian Classifier and Decision Tree, 95%	Area Under Curve, Precision
Tasnim et al. (2019) [4]	Depression	Audio collections AVEC 2013 and AVEC 2017 Audio/Visual Emotion Challenge	Deep Neural Network	Precision, Recall, Mean Absolute Error, Root Mean Squared Error
Yan et al. (2020) [17]	Major Depressive Disorder	Patients from Xijing hospital	Support Vector Machine, 95%	Area Under Curve
Kasthurirathne et al. (2019) [12]	Depression	Data of 84,317 adult patients, collected at Eskenazi Health, Indianapolis, Indiana	Random Forest	Sensitivity, Area Under Curve, and Specificity
Zhang et al. (2021) [15]	Postpartum Depression	Two EHR datasets containing data on 15,197 women and 53,972 women from single-site and multiple sites, respectively.	A range of ML algorithms, including XGBoost, random forest, multilayer Perceptron, etc.	Area Under Curve, Sensitivity, Specificity, Brier Score
Na et al. (2020) [13]	Depression	Used data from the Korea Welfare Panel Study (KoWePS)17	Random Forest	Area Under Curve, Confusion Matrix

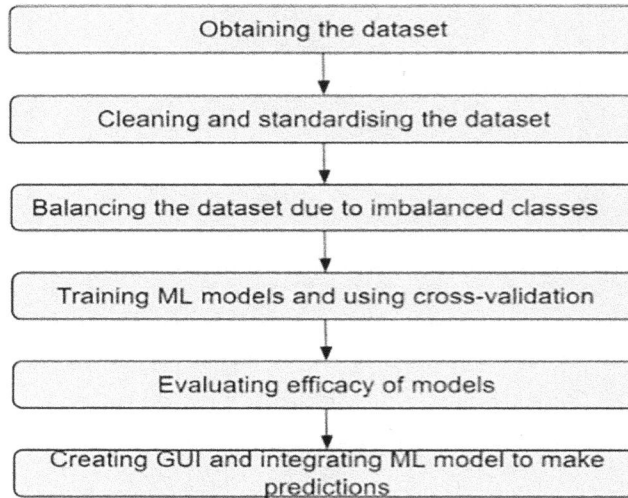

FIGURE 6.3   Outlining the process of the methodology used in the research.

6.3 MATERIALS AND METHODS

The steps taken to achieve the final result of an application that can identify people with depression are outlined in Figure 6.3.

6.3.1 DATASET

The process of data collection has two components. The first section consisted of a questionnaire based on the Hamilton Depression Rating Scale (HDRS). The other section consisted of 18 questions regarding daily activities and behavior. About 2000 of these entries were found through surveys, and the other 3000 were synthesized. The dataset contains two parts: one part with 18 general traits and attributes of people who consented to the study, and the other part is the class of depressed or healthy individuals identified using the Hamilton Depression Rating Scale (HDRS).

6.3.2 CLEANING AND STANDARDIZING THE DATASET

Given that the dataset was obtained via survey, a few missing values had to be filled. For characteristics that could have decimal values, the mean was used to fill the blank spaces. For characteristics with integer values, the mode was used to fill blank spaces. Inputs of characteristics, which are words, were arbitrarily assigned consecutive integer values. The scaler function in the Scikitlearn Python library was used to standardize the dataset.

6.3.3 BALANCING THE DATASET

The dataset contains 3885 entries for individuals classified as healthy and 1225 entries for individuals classified as depressed, as illustrated in Figure 6.4. The ratio of depressed to healthy entries is 35:111, indicating that the dataset is clearly imbalanced. This imbalance may result in a more inaccurate machine-learning model. As a result, the SMOTE function [18] from the imblearn Python library was used to balance the data. Additionally, a combination of SMOTE and random undersampling was used to balance the dataset, taking the majority class into account. When these two functions were pipelined together, the RandomUnderSampler function in imblearn was used with a sampling strategy of 0.5 and SMOTE with a sampling strategy of 0.4.

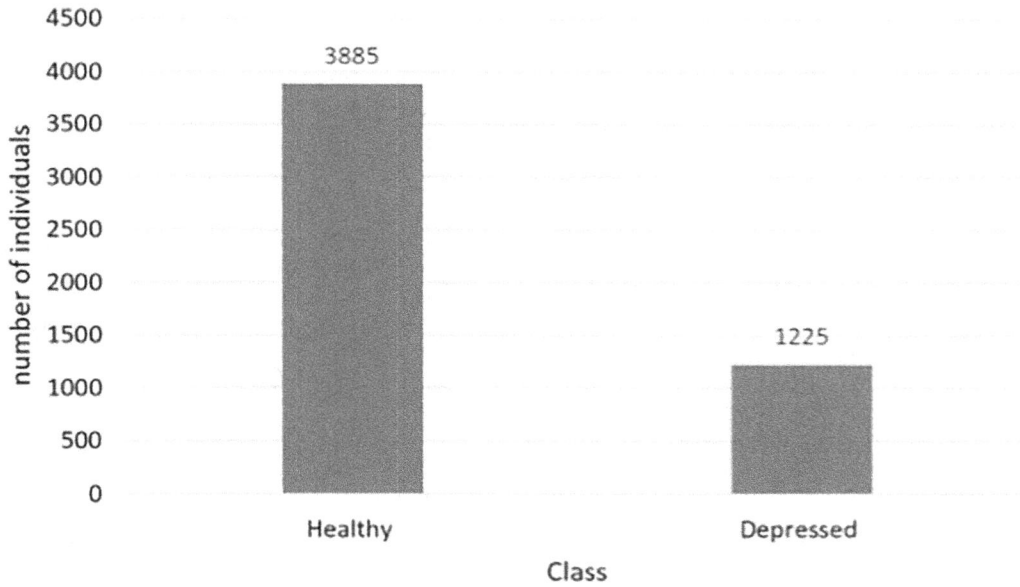

FIGURE 6.4 Distribution of data by class.

6.3.4 TRAINING AND CROSS-VALIDATION

Linear discriminant analysis, K-neighbors classifier, decision tree classifier, Gaussian NB, and SVM were the five machine-learning algorithms that were trained and compared.

6.3.4.1 K-Nearest Neighbors Classifier

K nearest neighbors is a simple but critical machine-learning algorithm. It is the most frequently used algorithm for classification and pattern-recognition tasks, which makes it an excellent candidate for this research. This algorithm first determines the number of neighbors (K) and then computes the euclidean distance between data points to determine the K nearest neighbors. The model operates by assigning a new data point to the category with the greatest number of neighbors [19]. This algorithm is straightforward to implement and performs better when dealing with large datasets. However, the computational cost associated with determining the value of K and calculating the euclidean distance between data points is considerable. Finally, because KNN may fail to perform well when there are too many features, dimensionality reduction techniques such as feature selection can be used.

6.3.4.2 Decision Tree

The name implies the use of a tree-like flowchart to generate predictions via various feature-based splits. This classification technique divides a population into branch-like segments that form an inverted tree with a root node, internal nodes, and leaf nodes. The algorithm is non-parametric, which enables it to efficiently handle large, complex datasets without imposing a complex parametric structure [20]. They are capable of handling both continuous and categorical variables, which are both present in the dataset used in this study.

6.3.4.3 Linear Discriminant Analysis

Linear discriminant analysis is extremely efficient at solving multiple classification problems with well-separated classes. The method's intuition is to find a subspace with a lower dimension than the original data sample dimension, in which the original problem's data points are "separable" [21]. LDA's fundamental concept is to project data points onto a line to maximize scatter between classes and minimize scatter within each class, resulting in easily distinguishable classes. It is a linear projection computation. LDA assumes that the data points have a Gaussian distribution and that, when plotted, they form a bell-shaped curve.

6.3.4.4 Gaussian Naive Bayes

Gaussian Naive Bayes is a classification technique founded on Bayes' theorem, which presupposes predictor independence. It takes each data point and assigns it to the class to which it is most similar. Rather than calculating that proximity using the euclidean distance from the class means, the GNB considers not only the distance from the mean but also its relationship to the class variance [22]. When this assumption of independence held true, this model outperformed others and required less data to train. However, in practice, it is nearly impossible for all of a dataset's features to be completely independent of one another.

6.3.4.5 Support-Vector Machine

The support-vector machine (SVM) is a supervised machine-learning algorithm that is typically used to solve classification problems. Each data point is plotted in an n-dimensional space using this algorithm, where n is the number of features in a given dataset. The machine is based on separating hyperplanes defined by data classes [23]. This algorithm performs well with multidimensional data and is particularly effective at obtaining a distinct margin of separation. However, when dealing with large datasets, the required training time increases, increasing the model's computational cost. Additionally, it does not work well with datasets that contain a high level of noise and have a high degree of overlap between the target classes. With a test size of 30% and an arbitrary random state of 6, the train-test-split function from the Scikit Learn library was used. Finally, a 10-fold cross validation was used to determine the algorithms' performance on the dataset.

6.4 EXPERIMENTAL RESULTS

6.4.1 TOOLS AND SET-UP

The following is a list of Python libraries used to create the machine-learning algorithm along with the application:

6.4.1.1 Scikit Learn

Scikit Learn is a large Python library that enables the easy implementation of a wide variety of machine-learning algorithms. It includes packages for several commonly used machine-learning algorithms, including DT, KNN, LDA, GNB, and SVC. Additionally, this module was used to improve the consistency of the dataset by importing the standard scaler function.

6.4.1.2 Imblearn

Imbalanced-learn is a Python module that helps balance significantly skewed datasets due to distinct majority and minority classes. This library contains the random undersampler and the synthetic minority oversampling technique (SMOTE), which were used to balance the dataset due to the clear majority of healthy individuals.

6.4.1.3 Numpy

Numpy provides a number of techniques for processing data from large multi-dimensional arrays and includes a number of mathematical functions. It was primarily used in this project to calculate the mean of the area under the curve to evaluate the machine-learning models' efficacy.

6.4.1.4 Pandas

Pandas is a widely used library for data analysis. It was primarily used to clean the data in this project so that it could be easily standardized and trained using the Scikit learn package.

6.4.1.5 Joblib

Joblib is a Python library that simplifies the process of saving and loading data-related Python objects. It was used in this project to store the final machine-learning model that was used in the application, preventing it from having to be trained each time. This aided in time savings but was computationally inefficient.

6.4.1.6 Kivy

Kivy is a simple Python library that enables the development of cross-platform applications for Windows, macOS, Android, iOS, and Linux. It was used to create a user interface through which a user could input data to be cross-referenced by the machine-learning algorithm, which would then provide an output. Kivy has its own syntax and is easily integrated into Python.

The computer system used in the experiment had an Intel i5 processor, 8 GB of RAM, and the Windows 10 Pro operating system.

6.4.2 EVALUATING THE EFFICACY OF MODELS

The following five metrics were used to evaluate and select the most suitable model to use in the application:

6.4.2.1 Accuracy

It is the percentage of classifications the model correctly predicts. It is obtained after testing and a 10-fold cross-validation.

6.4.2.2 AUC-ROC

The receiver operating characteristics curve is a probability curve, and the area under the curve is a measure of how well the model can distinguish between classes. The higher the AUC, the better the model is at distinguishing classes. This value was obtained after undergoing a 10-fold cross validation.

6.4.2.3 Precision

It is the ratio of the true positives to the sum of the true and false positives.

6.4.2.4 Recall

It is the ratio of true positives to the sum of true positives and false negatives.

6.4.2.5 F1 score

It is the weighted harmonic mean of precision and recall. A better model will have an F1 score closer to 1.

Table 6.2 displays the results obtained from the original dataset without SMOTE class balancing. As the majority of samples belong to class 0, all models become skewed toward this class (class 0). The GNB classifier has the highest accuracy (76.40%) in this instance. It also results in the highest AUC-ROC score (0.757). Regarding class 0 and class 1 precision, DT and GNB are the best performers for their respective classes. Nevertheless, it is evident from the recall metric that all classifiers perform poorly in terms of depression detection due to class 1's low recall value. The DT classifier exhibits the highest recall value in this instance.

To mitigate the impact of class imbalance on poor class 1 recall, we employ the SMOTE technique for class balancing. The performance of classifiers after application of SMOTE is depicted in Table 6.3. It results in an improvement in overall performance, particularly the precision and recall values for depression class (class 1). The DT classifier achieves the best accuracy, AUC score, class 1 precision, and F1-score values in this instance. The GNB classifier achieves the highest class 1 recall rate.

TABLE 6.2

Performance Metrics of Models Trained on Imbalanced Dataset Without Using SMOTE or Random Undersampling

ML Model	Accuracy	AUC-ROC	Precision		Recall		F1-Score	
			0	1	0	1	0	1
GNB	76.4%	0.757	0.77	**0.51**	0.98	0.08	0.86	0.13
SVC	76.0%	0.520	0.76	0.00	**1.00**	0.00	**0.87**	0.00
LDA	75.9%	0.748	0.79	0.52	0.94	0.21	0.86	0.30
DT	75.3%	0.665	**0.83**	0.48	0.84	**0.46**	0.84	**0.47**
KNN	71.5%	0.512	0.76	0.24	0.92	0.08	0.83	0.12

TABLE 6.3

Performance Metrics of Models Trained Using Only SMOTE

ML Model	Accuracy	AUC-ROC	Precision		Recall		F1-Score	
			0	1	0	1	0	1
DT	83.5%	0.839	0.82	**0.83**	**0.83**	0.82	**0.82**	**0.83**
GNB	74.2%	0.831	**0.85**	0.68	0.57	**0.90**	0.68	0.78
LDA	70.4%	0.768	0.72	0.69	0.65	0.75	0.69	0.72
KNN	66.4%	0.729	0.69	0.65	0.60	0.73	0.64	0.69
SVC	51.6%	0.523	0.51	0.53	0.61	0.43	0.55	0.48

In the literature, random undersampling for the majority class has been used extensively as an adjunct to SMOTE. The random undersampling and SMOTE combination was evaluated. The results are displayed in Table 6.4. However, random undersampling does not improve the performance of the ML algorithms tested; rather, it degrades it. The accuracy of DT classifiers decreases from 83.50% to 75.50%.

The joblib library was used to create a.sav file with the machine learning model. Using the Kivy library, a GUI was created with prompts so that a user could input their values for the 18 characteristics. These values were compared and evaluated by the model, which produced an output that was reflected on the user interface and indicated whether they were depressed or healthy.

TABLE 6.4

Performance Metrics of Models Trained Using SMOTE and Random Undersampling

ML Model	Accuracy	AUC-ROC	Precision		Recall		F1-Score	
			0	1	0	1	0	1
DT	75.5%	0.733	**0.80**	0.63	0.83	**0.59**	0.81	**0.61**
GNB	71.8%	**0.773**	0.76	**0.65**	0.88	0.44	**0.82**	0.53
LDA	69.9%	0.752	0.74	0.61	0.88	0.36	0.80	0.45
SVC	66.7%	0.541	0.67	0.00	**1.00**	0.00	0.80	0.00
KNN	62.9%	0.581	0.70	0.43	0.79	0.32	0.74	0.37

6.5 DISCUSSION

Tables 6.2, 6.3, and 6.4 above show the results obtained before and after balancing the dataset using SMOTE and random undersampling. Overall, the decision tree algorithm with SMOTE had the best efficacy. It had the highest accuracy of 83.5% and an AUC-ROC of 0.839. Furthermore, the precision, recall, and F1 score were consistently high, around 0.82 or 0.83. This result shows that the model can, a lot of the time, figure out who is depressed and healthy. The decision tree algorithm can be further optimized using the GridSearchCV function found in the Scikit Learn library. It is a function that is fit with different hyperparameters for the decision tree to find the optimal combination. The criterion parameter had two options: gini and entropy. Max depth was arbitrarily assigned a range of 1–15, min samples per leaf 1–10, and min samples per split 1–15. After a few attempts, the combination that yielded the highest accuracy had criterion as entropy, max depth as 14, min samples leaf as 2, and min samples split as 14. The accuracy of this algorithm was 84.7%, and the AUC-ROC was 0.934.

This model was imported using the joblib library, and a GUI was created using the kivy library. Shown below is a picture of the user interface in which a user would input their values for the 18 characteristics. After clicking the submit button, the values would be cross-referenced with the model, and one of the two following outputs would be displayed.

6.6 LIMITATIONS

Although the machine-learning model works with relatively high accuracy and AUC-ROC, there are a few limitations to this project. First, the dataset can be improved on by adding more characteristics so that a correlation between them, and depression can be identified for more accurate identification. Furthermore, a larger dataset using surveys from people all around the world can be used to improve the applicability of the project. This, however, will necessitate a significant number of resources, which may not be readily available.

Second, other machine-learning algorithms can be explored, too. This research only considered popular algorithms and left out others like random forest and deep neural networks, which may yield more accurate results. Furthermore, other forms of cross validation like K-fold cross validation or LOOCV should be considered too to find the optimal method.

6.7 CONCLUSION

This paper has demonstrated that machine learning can be used to identify people with depression with an accuracy of 84.7%. Using a large dataset of over 5000 entries, training a decision tree algorithm has proven effective in detecting depression in a way that is easily accessible by people via a smartphone or a laptop. Depression is a disease for which appropriate treatment after early detection can help reduce the effect of symptoms and even encourage remission. However, it must be acknowledged that this form of detection is not perfect and can be improved. Future work could include using multiple algorithms whose output could be used as an input for a higher-level algorithm. Also, more characteristics could be found so that the machine-learning algorithm can be trained more accurately.

REFERENCES

[1] Lépine, J. P., & Briley, M. (2011). The increasing burden of depression. *Neuropsychiatric Disease and Treatment*, 7(Suppl 1), 3.
[2] Gotlib, I. H., & Hammen, C. L. (Eds.). (2008). *Handbook of Depression*. Guilford Press.
[3] Gao, S., Calhoun, V. D., & Sui, J. (2018). Machine learning in major depression: From classification to treatment outcome prediction. *CNS Neuroscience & Therapeutics*, 24(11), 1037–1052.

[4] Tasnim, M., & Stroulia, E. (2019, May). Detecting depression from voice. In *Canadian Conference on Artificial Intelligence* (pp. 472–478). Cham: Springer.

[5] Haque, U. M., Kabir, E., & Khanam, R. (2021). Detection of child depression using machine learning methods. *PLoS One*, *16*(12), e0261131.

[6] Jiménez-Serrano, S., Tortajada, S., & García-Gómez, J. M. (2015). A mobile health application to predict postpartum depression based on machine learning. *Telemedicine and e-Health*, *21*(7), 567–574.

[7] Rubin-Falcone, H., Zanderigo, F., Thapa-Chhetry, B., Lan, M., Miller, J. M., Sublette, M. E., … & Mann, J. J. (2018). Pattern recognition of magnetic resonance imaging-based gray matter volume measurements classifies bipolar disorder and major depressive disorder. *Journal of Affective Disorders*, *227*, 498–505.

[8] Espinola, C. W., Gomes, J. C., Pereira, J. M. S., & dos Santos, W. P. (2021). Detection of major depressive disorder using vocal acoustic analysis and machine learning—an exploratory study. *Research on Biomedical Engineering*, *37*(1), 53–64.

[9] Islam, M., Kabir, M. A., Ahmed, A., Kamal, A. R. M., Wang, H., & Ulhaq, A. (2018). Depression detection from social network data using machine learning techniques. *Health Information Science and Systems*, *6*(1), 1–12.

[10] Cacheda, F., Fernandez, D., Novoa, F. J., & Carneiro, V. (2019). Early detection of depression: social network analysis and random forest techniques. *Journal of Medical Internet Research*, *21*(6), e12554.

[11] Nemesure, M. D., Heinz, M. V., Huang, R. *et al.* (2021). Predictive modeling of depression and anxiety using electronic health records and a novel machine learning approach with artificial intelligence. *Scientific Reports*, *11*, 1980. 10.1038/s41598-021-81368-4

[12] Kasthurirathne, S. N., Biondich, P. G., Grannis, S. J., Purkayastha, S., Vest, J. R., & Jones, J. F. (2019). Identification of patients in need of advanced care for depression using data extracted from a statewide health information exchange: A machine learning approach. *Journal of Medical Internet Research*, *21*(7), e13809.

[13] Na, K. S., Cho, S. E., Geem, Z. W., & Kim, Y. K. (2020). Predicting future onset of depression among community dwelling adults in the Republic of Korea using a machine learning algorithm. *Neuroscience Letters*, *721*, 134804.

[14] Priya, A., Garg, S., & Tigga, N. P. (2020). Predicting anxiety, depression and stress in modern life using machine learning algorithms. *Procedia Computer Science*, *167*, 1258–1267.

[15] Zhang, Y., Wang, S., Hermann, A., Joly, R., & Pathak, J. (2021). Development and validation of a machine learning algorithm for predicting the risk of postpartum depression among pregnant women. *Journal of Affective Disorders*, *279*, 1–8.

[16] Bhakta, I., & Sau, A. (2016). Prediction of depression among senior citizens using machine learning classifiers. *International Journal of Computer Applications*, *144*(7), 11–16.

[17] Yan, B., Xu, X., Liu, M., Zheng, K., Liu, J., Li, J., … & Li, B. (2020). Quantitative identification of major depression based on resting-state dynamic functional connectivity: a machine learning approach. *Frontiers in Neuroscience*, *14*, 191.

[18] Chawla, N. V., Bowyer, K. W., Hall, L. O., & Kegelmeyer, W. P. (2002). SMOTE: synthetic minority over-sampling technique. *Journal of Artificial Intelligence Research*, *16*, 321–357.

[19] Triguero, I., Maillo, J., Luengo, J., García, S., & Herrera, F. (2016, December). From big data to smart data with the k-nearest neighbours algorithm. In *2016 IEEE International Conference on Internet of Things (iThings) and IEEE Green Computing and Communications (GreenCom) and IEEE Cyber, Physical and Social Computing (CPSCom) and IEEE Smart Data (SmartData)* (pp. 859–864). IEEE.

[20] Song, Y. Y., & Ying, L. U. (2015). Decision tree methods: applications for classification and prediction. *Shanghai Archives of Psychiatry*, *27*(2), 130.

[21] Xanthopoulos, P., Pardalos, P. M., & Trafalis, T. B. (2013). Linear discriminant analysis. In *Robust Data Mining* (pp. 27–33). New York, NY: Springer.

[22] Raizada, R. D., & Lee, Y. S. (2013). Smoothness without smoothing: why Gaussian naive Bayes is not naive for multi-subject searchlight studies. *PLoS One*, *8*(7), e69566.

[23] Basu, A., Walters, C., & Shepherd, M. (2003, January). Support vector machines for text categorization. In *The 36th Annual Hawaii International Conference on System Sciences, 2003. Proceedings of the* (pp. 7-pp). IEEE.

7 Non-Invasive Technique of Breast Cancer Diagnosis Using Interpretation of Fractal Dimension of Cells Nuclei in Buccal Epithelium

D. Klyushin, O. Kravets, and K. Golubeva
Taras Shevchenko National University of Kyiv, Ukraine

N. Boroday
Institute for Problems of Cryobiology and Cryomedicine of the National Academy of Sciences of Ukraine

CONTENTS

7.1 INTRODUCTION

According to the World Cancer Research Fund International, breast cancer is the most common cancer among women and the most common cancer overall. Therefore, an important question arises of creating a method for the early diagnosis of breast cancer. Such a method should be simple, cheap, accurate, and non-traumatic. Currently, common diagnostic methods, such as clinical review, mammography, and aspiration biopsy, do not always show high accuracy and can be traumatic.

DOI: 10.1201/9781003333081-7

Our work is focused on considering the machine-learning methods for diagnosing breast cancer obtaining features using fractal analysis of the distribution of chromatin in Feulgen-stained images of buccal epithelial nuclei (Andreichuk et al. 2021; Klyushin et al. 2021).

7.2 MALIGNANT-ASSOCIATED CHANGES IN BUCCAL EPITHELIUM

Malignant-associated changes in cells distant from a tumor were discovered by H. Nieburg (Nieburgs, Herman, and Reisman 1962, Nieburgs 1968). He discovered the lability of X-chromatin in somatic cells depending on functional changes in the body and the general somatic environment. If there was a malignant tumor in an organism, changes in the content of X-chromatin in the buccal epithelium and peripheral blood neutrophils were observed. Oncologists have found that the number of cells with X-chromatin correlates with impaired functionality of the heterocyclic X chromosome.

Tumor-associated changes were manifested as increases in nuclei of epitheliocytes and the size of zones of limited chromatin with light halo. Similar phenomena were found in the nuclei of cells of other organs. Obrapalska et al. (1973) reported that tumor-associated changes in the buccal epithelium were observed in more than 70% of cancer patients. Increasing of DNA content in the nuclei of epitheliocytes in patients with melanoma was found in comparison with the control group of practically healthy people. In addition, in patients with melanoma, a decreasing amount of X-chromatin was found compared with patients who had benign tumors or healthy people. In women with breast cancer, increasing of DNA content and the size of the interphase nuclei of the buccal epithelium was recorded. At the same time, it was reported in (Ogden, Cowpe, and Green 1990) that in men with bronchial epithelioma and healthy men, the difference between the amount of DNA in buccal epithelial epithelial cells was not insignificant.

The buccal epithelium is a popular target for early disease detection (Rathbone, Drummond, and Tucker 1994; Rosin 1992; Prasad, Mukundan, and Krishnaswamy 1995). It is a fairly accurate reflects health of a person. For example, by the proportion of nuclei with negative electrical charge of the buccal epithelium and the speed of nuclei movement during microelectrophoresis, one can determine the a person's biological age and other indicators. Using the buccal epithelium, the genetic effects caused by a toxic environment can be assessed. For example, under the influence of genotoxic carcinogens (in particular, tobacco), the number of micronuclei in exfoliative cells can increase 10 times compared to the control (Nair et al. 1991; Tolbert, Shy, and Allen 1992). Therefore, a change in the number of micronuclei can be considered a marker of various pathologies. For example, after chemotherapy or radiation therapy, the number of micronuclei in the oral cavity of cancer patients increases. The same phenomenon has been observed in people chewing carcinogenic gums (Adhraryn, Dave, and Trivedi 1991) or exposed to mutagenic influences (Sarto et al. 1990).

Chromatin makes it possible to assess the level of buccal epithelium differentiation in patients with gastric or duodenal ulcers. This assessment uses indicators such as the index of maturation, differentiation, and the karyopyknotic index. Changes of the normal differentiation of the buccal epithelium are a sign of some disorders. Cellular atypia of the buccal epithelium strongly correlates with precancerous and neoplastic changes and makes it possible to almost accurate diagnose these diseases. Also, changes of the buccal epithelium differentiation can occur due to metabolic and hormonal disturbances, as well as mechanical influences and chemical reactions (Schonwetter, Stolzenberg, and Zasloff 1995).

Palcic et al. (1994) found that changes in DNA content and chromatin texture in the nucleus are associated with the appearance of malignant neoplasms. These changes were found in normal cells outside the tumor. Presumably, this is how normal cells react to malignant changes in organs (in particular, in the mammary gland). This finding allowed the authors to suggest that tumor-associated changes are strongly pronounced near the tumor and fade or disappear as they move away from it, or after it disappears due to a surgical operation. On this basis, the authors proposed the use of quantitative cytospectrophotometry for the diagnosis of early forms of cancer and its prognosis.

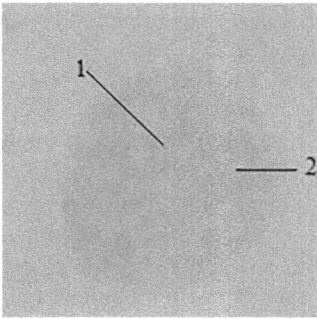

FIGURE 7.1 Condensed and decondenced hromatine in a nucleus of buccal epithelium (1—heterochromatin, 2—euchromatin).

Ogden et al. (1990) attempted to evaluate the effect of a tumor on the buccal epithelium to characterize processes in organs distant from the tumor. Changes in the size of nuclei and nuclear membranes, as well as chromatin heterogeneity, were found in almost 80% of patients with various tumors. However, the researchers were unable to identify clear patterns, with the exception of an increase in the nuclei of buccal epithelium cells and a change in the nuclear-cytoplasmic ratio. Nevertheless, they confirmed the effect of tumors on the condition of the buccal epithelium.

The traditional object of study of genomic DNA has been blood, but recently, researchers have increasingly focused their attention on the DNA of buccal epithelial cells. An analysis of the literature demonstrates that a malignant tumor has a hidden effect on many body systems, causing a corresponding reaction, in particular, in the buccal epithelium.

As well-known the nucleus chromatin is classified as condensed or decondensed. The level of chromosome decondensation can vary. Complete decondensed chromatine is called euchromatin, and completely condensed chromatin is called heterochromatin. Heterochromatin may be intensely stained with Feulgen stain and may be definitely registered using a light microscope (Figure 7.1).

Lieberman-Aiden et al. (2009) found that DNA in the cell nucleus is packed into a globule that looks like a folded three-dimensional Peano curve. This finding led to intensive research into the fractal properties of cells. Currently, the fractal dimension of cells is used to assess their heterogeneity in endometrial hyperplasia and highly differentiated endometrioid carcinoma (Bikou et al. 2016) to assess survival in melanoma (Bedin et al. 2010), leukemia (Adam 2006) and other diseases (Losa 2012; Metze 2010, 2013). Note that the fractal properties of cells have previously aroused the interest of many researchers (Einstein et al. 1998; Ohri, Dey, and Nijhawan 2004; Losa and Castelli 2005), but in these studies, tumor cells, and not buccal epithelium, were studied. Researchers observed that increasing of the average DNA content in the nucleus is a marker of malignant tumor (Boroday et al. 2016; Klyushin et al. 2021). Therefore, given the presence of tumor-associated changes in the buccal epithelium, it can be assumed that these changes, among other things, can affect the fractal dimension of cell nuclei in cancer patients. We prove this hypothesis in this work.

7.3 BREAST CANCER DIAGNOSIS USING MACHINE LEARNING

There are many modern approaches to the problem of diagnosing breast cancer. For example, works (Yan et al. 2018; Yang et al. 2019; Patil et al. 2019) focus on the use of convolutional neural networks (CNN) and recurrent neural networks (RNN) for diagnosing breast cancer based on histopathological images collected by biopsy. Moreover, in the works (Yang et al. 2019; Patil et al. 2019), the methods are given, which can be interpreted and important for medical diagnosis. Another example can be the work (Punitha, Al-Turjman, and Thompson 2021), which uses an artificial neural network connected to a bee algorithm for cancer diagnosis to select the best features and parameters, as well as a dataset with images that were obtained by fine-needle biopsy. The work (Yifan, Jialin and Boxi 2021) uses the same data as (Punitha, Al-Turjman, and Thompson 2021), but uses the Adaboost and Random

Forest methods for diagnostics. Another work (Hu, Whitney, and Giger 2020) is also an example of breast cancer diagnostics based on multiparametric magnetic resonance imaging. Features are extracted from images using a convolutional neural network, and then classification is carried out using the support-vector machine.

The work (Khamparia 2021) is focused on the consideration of artificial neural networks that will be further trained on mammography images. Another example is the work (Kavitha 2022), in which neural networks and deep-learning methods are used to diagnose breast cancer using mammography images. All the works cited as examples show high accuracy. But these works are based on data collected by dangerous and expensive diagnostic methods. So biopsy and high-definition mammography can be traumatic or harmful to health due to radiation exposure. Therefore, the question arises of finding a safer and cheaper method for the early diagnosis of breast cancer.

7.4 MATERIALS AND METHODS

We investigated the control group (29 woman), patients with breast cancer at the second stage (68 woman), and the patients with fibroadenomatosis (33 woman). Diagnoses were confirmed histologically. The dataset consists of 20256 photos of interphase nuclei of buccal epithelium (6752 nuclei photographed without filter, through a yellow filter and through a violet filter).

Smears of oral mucosa cells were taken from the spinous layer and dried at temperature $21–22C°$, fixated in the Nikiforov mixture and Feulgen-stained with cold hydrolysis in 5 n HCl for 15 min. After dissolving content of a cell excepting DNA, Feulgen-stained chromatin was photographed by an Olympus analyzer, consisting of an Olympus BX microscope, a Camedia C-5050 digital zoom camera and a computer. As a rule, every smears consisted of 52 nuclei. The content of DNA-fuchsine in the nuclei was computed as a product of the optical density by area. For every nuclei, we obtained a photo 128×128 pixels.

To perform the binarization, we used the 3-sigma rule. The algorithm assumes that the pixels are divided on two classes (foreground and background). The foreground (image of a nucleus) is a set of pixels whose brightness differs from the average brightness less than by three values of standard deviation. Other pixels are considered as a background.

Next, comparing the values of brightness of each pixel using the 3-sigma rule, we classified points to the corresponding class. All pixel of the background considered to be black (Figure 7.2).

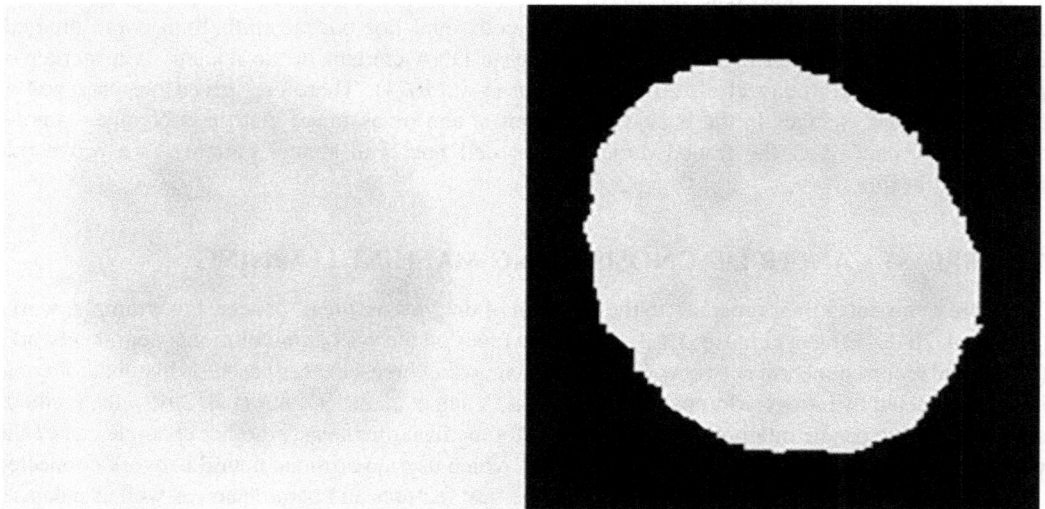

FIGURE 7.2 Nuclei after adaptive threshold pre-processing.

The background of the photos often contains artifacts (noise, spots, or other defects). The color brightness of such pixels is close to the brightness of the foreground, i.e., it is a mistake. Meantime, it is necessary to grant that the distribution of chromatin in the nucleus is heterogeneous. As a result, a nucleus looks like a pink foggy spot, consisting of dark regions (heterochromatin) and light regions (euchromatin).

Therefore, after selecting, a background on a binary image, we must restore the original color, but only for a foreground. For this purpose, we used the smoothing image. For removing artifacts, we compared the brightness of their pixels with surrounding pixels. If they were pixels of a background of an image, we paint the suspicious pixel by black color. Spots on a foreground were eliminated in a similar way, but in this case, we used not a small threshold, but a confidence interval constructed using the e-sigma rule. We compared the brightness of their pixels with surrounding pixels, also. If the brightness of suspicious pixels fell out of a confidence interval for the surrounding pixels, we assigned to the suspicious pixels the average brightness of surrounding pixels. Then, we computed the fractal dimension of an image.

7.5 FRACTAL ANALYSIS OF CHROMATIN

To determine the fractal dimension of an image, we used the Hurst exponent, connected with the fractal dimension D by the formula $H = 2 - D$ (Butakov and Grakovskiy 2005). For the Hurst exponent computed for a data sequence, at first, we mapped an image into a sequence of brightness of pixels using a space-filling Hilbert curve (Sagan 1994) passing though every pixel of an image and sequentially read the values of the color brightness of the pixels. Thus, we obtained three vectors of color brightness corresponding to three colors channel of the RGB color model.

1. Compute the standard deviation of values in current segment of a data sequence:

$$\delta_{m,N} = \sum_{i=1}^{m} (x_i - \bar{x}_N), \tag{7.1}$$

where N is the size of the segment (varying from 2 to the end the sequence), m is the upper limit of summing (from 1 to $N-1$), x_i is a brightness of a pixel, $\bar{x}_N$ is the mean brightness of the segment. Therefore, we compute $N-1$ values $\delta_{2,N}, \dots, \delta_{N-1,N}$.

2. Compute the range of standard deviations (7.1):

$$R = \max_{m=2,\dots,N} \delta_{m,N} - \min_{m=2,\dots,N} \delta_{m,N} \tag{7.2}$$

3. Normalize the range of deviation (7.2):

$$Q = \frac{R}{s}, \tag{7.3}$$

where s is the standard deviation of the whole data sequence.

4. Compute $\lg Q$ and $\lg N$ using (7.3) and the line dependence of $\lg Q$ on $\lg N$.
5. Compute the Hurst exponent as the tangent of the slope angle of the line dependence of $\lg Q$ on $\lg N$.

Thus, the dataset with the features used in the work contains the data on 97 patients (68 patients with breast cancer, 29 people from the control group). A patient is represented by three samples (for each of the RGB channels) of fractal dimensions for each image of the interphase nuclei of the patient's buccal epithelium.

To use the usual methods of machine learning, we add a few more features. This is necessary because each patient is represented only by a sample of fractal dimensions, which complicates the classification process. The main idea of expanding the number of features is to add different means and statistical values to the data, which are calculated for each sample. Therefore, for each sample of each patient, we calculate the following values.

- Arithmetic mean
- Geometrical mean
- Harmonic mean
- Median
- Standard deviation

Analyzing the graphs represented in Figures 7.3–7.5, it is possible to put forward the theory that the signs obtained from the blue channel are the most informative.

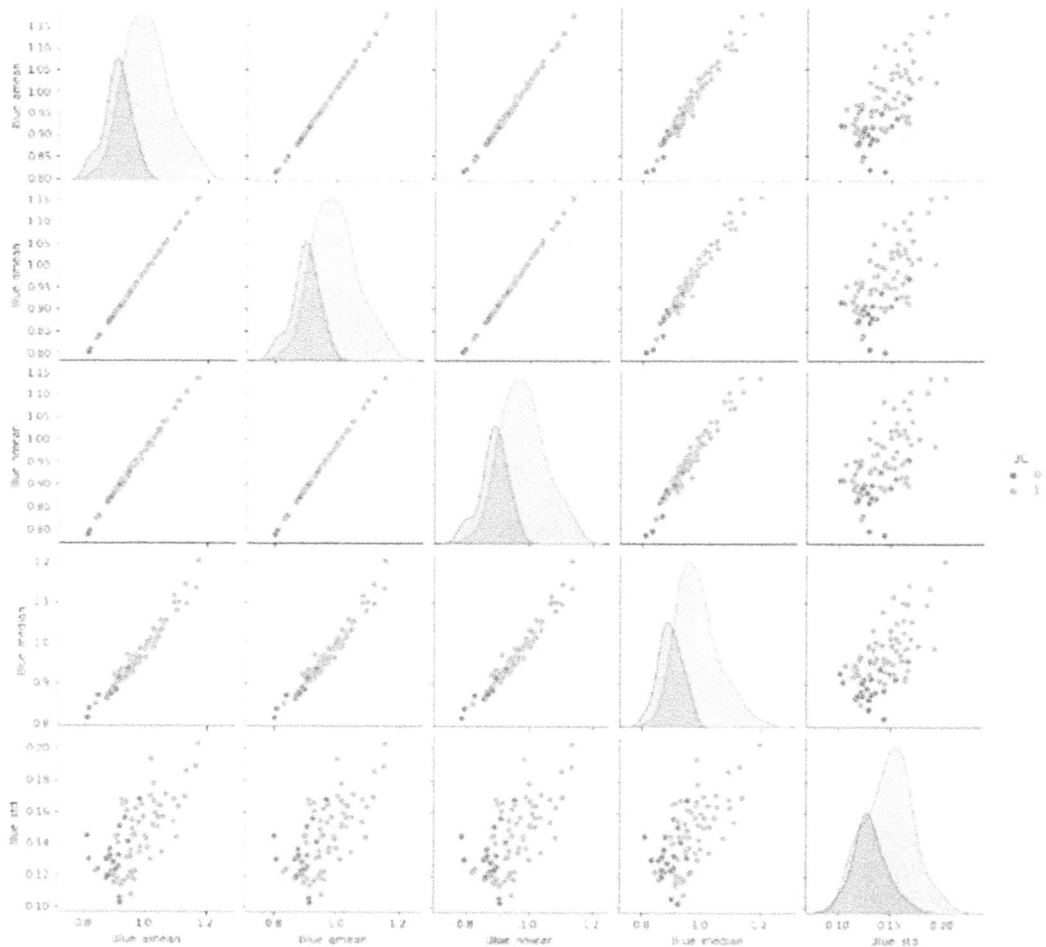

FIGURE 7.3 Comparative graphs for signs created by sampling the blue channel. The graph shows the distribution of the data, where the ordinate and abscissa axes have the corresponding signs. Diagonal contains graphs of the distribution of data by the corresponding feature. The parameter BC equal to 0 is the control group. BC equal to 1 is the group of patients with breast cancer.

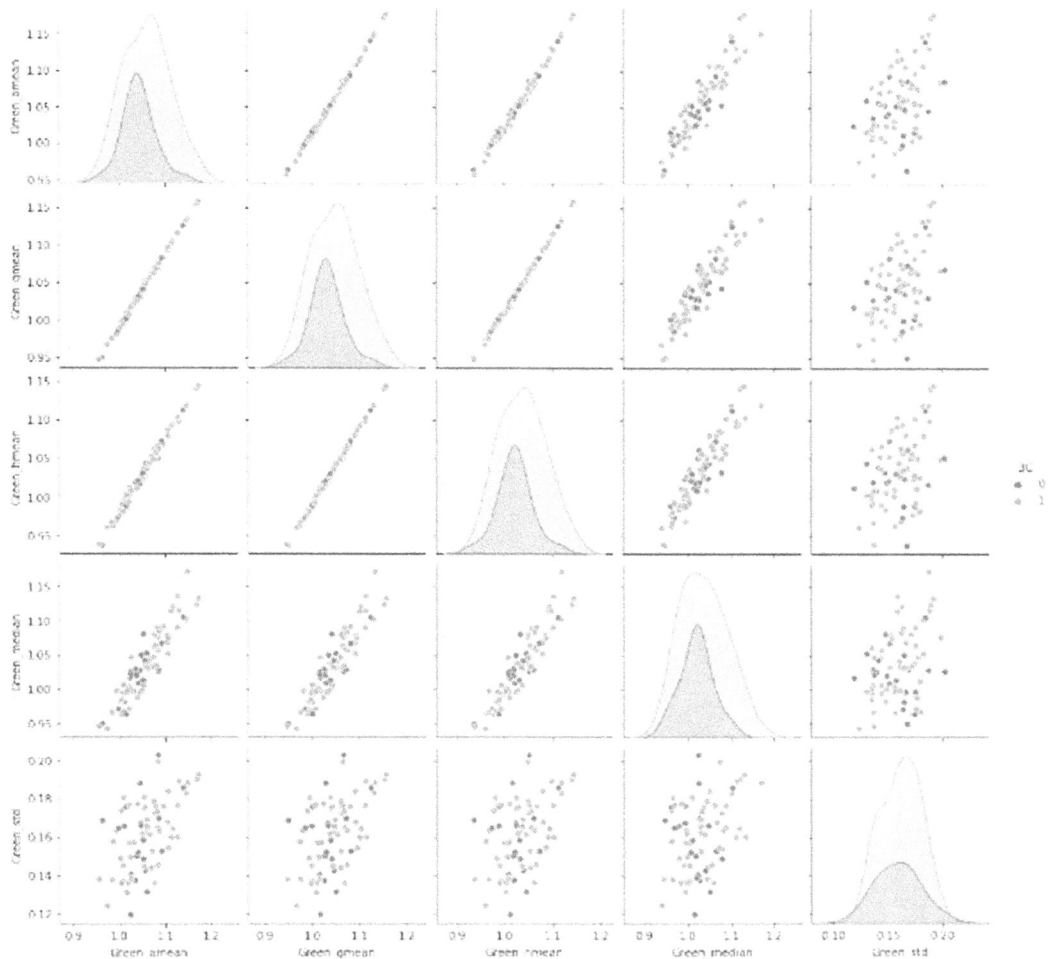

FIGURE 7.4 Comparative graphs for signs created by sampling the green channel. The graph shows the distribution of the data, where the ordinate and abscissa axes have the corresponding signs. Diagonal contains graphs of the distribution of data by the corresponding feature. The parameter BC equal to 0 is the control group, BC equal to 1 is the group of patients with breast cancer.

7.6   ALGORITHM ADABOOST

Consider the Adaboost algorithm (Zhu et al. 2009) for classifying patients with breast cancer. This powerful machine-learning algorithm is based on the sequential combination of simple classification algorithms in which each next one will correct the error of the previous ones. We have the following data for learning the algorithm: $(x_1, y_1), (x_2, y_2), \ldots, (x_n, y_n)$, where $x_i \in R^p$ is an input of the model, $\{1, 2, \ldots, K\}$ is an output of the model, and K is the number of classes. The purpose of the algorithm is to find a classification rule $C(x)$ using training data. For new x the rule $C(x)$ returns a label of class from the set $\{1, 2 \ldots, K\}$.

7.6.1   ALGORITHM ADABOOST-SAMME

1. Initialize weights of observations $w_i = \frac{1}{n}$, $i = 1, 2, \ldots, n$.

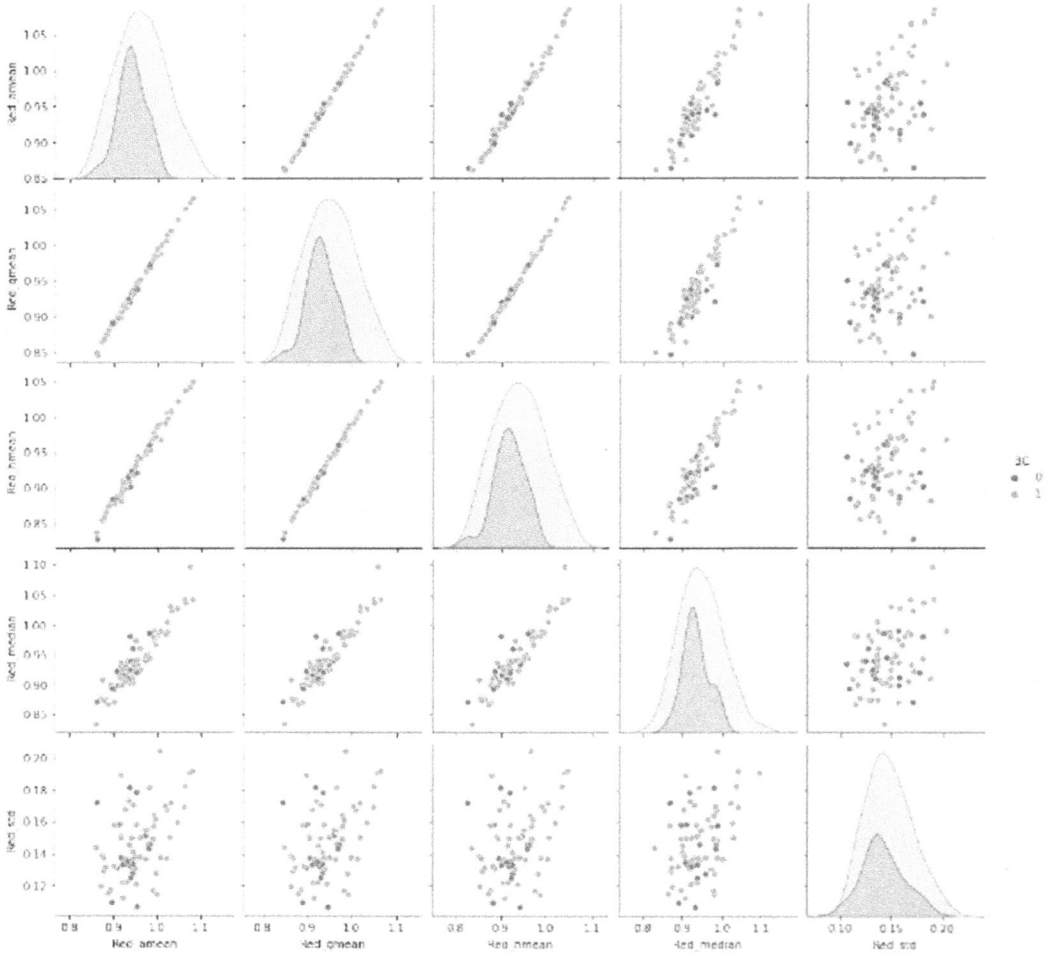

FIGURE 7.5 Comparative graphs for signs created by sampling the red channel. The graph shows the distribution of the data, where the ordinate and abscissa axes have the corresponding signs. Diagonal contains graphs of the distribution of data by the corresponding feature. The parameter BC equal to 0 is the control group. BC equal to 1 is the group of patients with breast cancer.

2. From $m = 1$ to M:

    2.1 Learn a simple classifier on training data using the weights w_i.

    2.2 Compute an error of the obtained classifier

$$err^{(m)} = lr \sum_{i=1}^{n} w_i I\,(y_i \neq T^{(m)}\,(x_i)) \Bigg/ \sum_{i=1}^{n} nw_i,$$

    where lr is a learning rate and I is an indicator function.

    2.3 Compute

$$\alpha^{(m)} = \log \frac{1 - err^{(m)}}{err^{(m)}} + \log(K - 1).$$

2.4 Update the weights of observations
For $i = 1, 2 \ldots ., n$.

$$w_i \leftarrow w_i \exp(\alpha^{(m)} I\,(y_i \neq T^{(m)}\,(x_i)))$$

2.5 Normalize new weights w_i.

As a result, we obtain the following classification function:

$$C\,(x) = \arg \max_k \sum_{m=1}^{M} \alpha^{(m)} I\,(T^{(m)}\,(x) = k).$$

7.6.2 DECISION TREE

The Decision Tree algorithm is usually used as a simple classifier in the Adaboost algorithm (Hastie, Tibshirani, and Friedman 2009). This machine-learning algorithm is known for being easy to interpret. The algorithm builds a tree at each node of which the data is split, according to the variable chosen by the algorithm. Each leaf of the tree belongs to one of the classes, according to which the classification is carried out.

Let our training data contain N observations: i.e. (x_1, y_1), (x_2, y_2), ..., (x_N, y_N), where $x_i = (x_{i1}, x_{i2}, \ldots, x_{ip})$. Class labels are $y_i \in \{1, 2, \ldots, K\}$, where K is the number of classes. Let we have a dividing on M regions $R_1, R_2, \ldots, R_M$ then at the node m, which represents the region R_m containing N_m training samples, we denote by

$$\hat{p}_{mk} = \frac{1}{N_m} \sum_{x_i \in R_m} I\,(y_k = k)$$

the proportion of class k at node m. We classify the observation at node m into the class $k\,(m) = \arg \max_k \hat{p}_{mk}$. It should be noted that when using observation weights, it is the proportions of classes in the nodes that will change.

In experiments with the Adaboost algorithm, the Gini index is used to select the optimal variable for splitting.

$$Q_m\,(T) = \sum_{k \neq k'} \hat{p}_{mk} \hat{p}_{mk'} = \sum_{k=1}^{K} \hat{p}_{mk}\,(1 - \hat{p}_{mk}),$$

where T is the constructed tree. For splitting, a variable is also chosen that minimizes the Gini index.

Another splitting criterion is the cross entropy K

$$Q_m\,(T) = - \sum_{k=1}^{K} \hat{p}_{mk} \log \hat{p}_{mk}.$$

A decision tree has many split-stopping criteria, but the Adaboost algorithm usually uses trees of depth 1 or trees of maximum depth 2.

7.6.3 TESTING ADABOOST

To conduct testing, we divided the dataset into two parts: a training sample (80%) and a test sample (20%) on which the resulting model will be evaluated. For the Adaboost algorithm, we tested with different sets of paired parameters, namely the number of classifiers and the learning rate. Note that the learning rate parameter lr is the weight that is applied to each classifier on every boosting iteration. Thus, when the learning rate is greater than one, the contribution of the generated classifiers to the final result increases, and when the learning rate is less than one, on the contrary, it decreases. With this approach, you need to maintain a trade-off between the speed of learning and the number of classifiers (Figures 7.6–7.8).

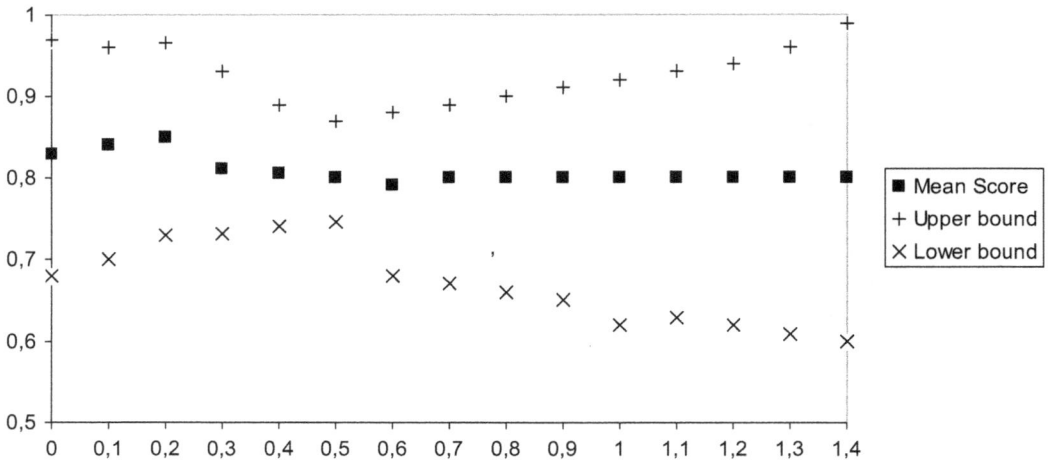

FIGURE 7.6 Graphs for selecting the optimal learning rate for the Adaboost algorithm based on Decision Tree with depth 1 with 150 classifiers. The abscissa shows the values of the learning rate parameter, and the ordinate shows the accuracy and its bounds.

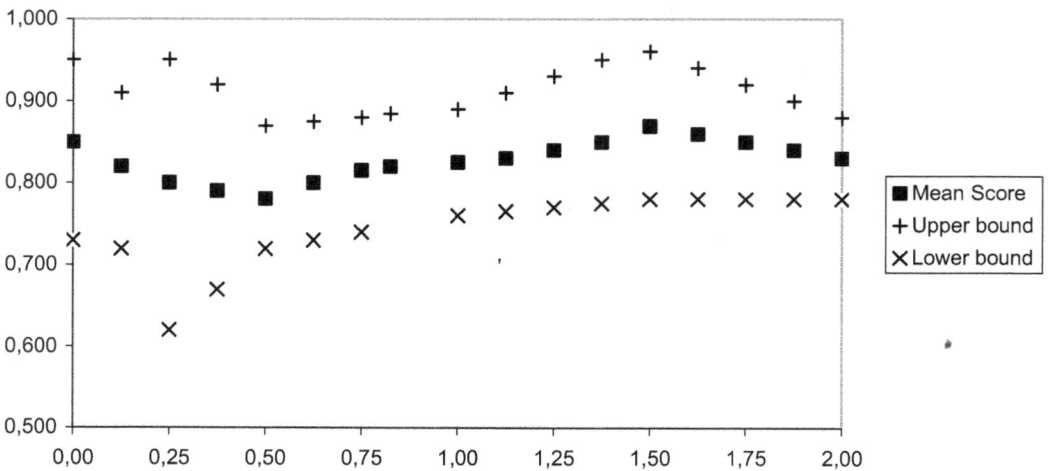

FIGURE 7.7 Graph for selecting the optimal learning rate for the Adaboost algorithm based on Decision Tree with depth 2 with 150 classifiers. The abscissa shows the values of the learning rate parameter, and the ordinate shows the accuracy and its bounds.

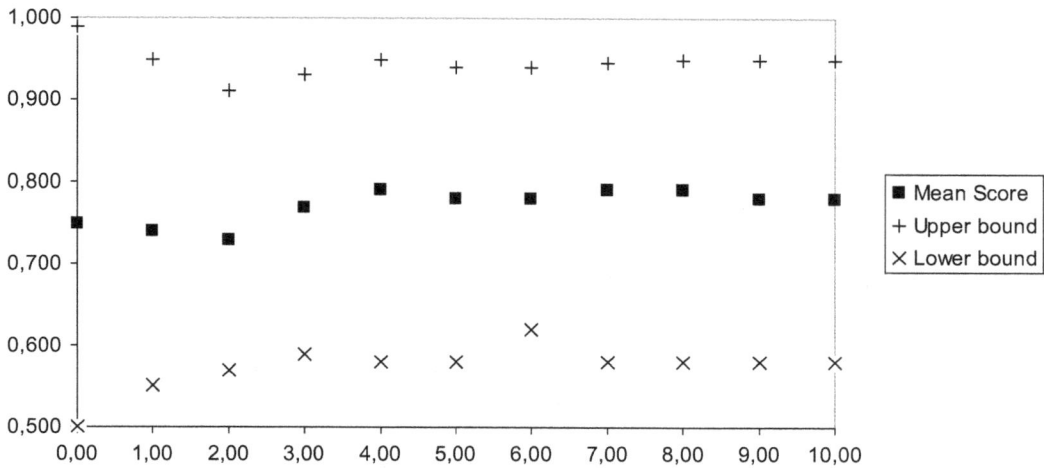

FIGURE 7.8 Depth fitting plot for the Decision Tree algorithm with the Gini splitting criterion, which is trained on the blue channel data. The abscissa shows the values of the max depth parameter, and the ordinate shows the accuracy.

We also performed cross-validation for each set of parameters with splitting the training data into five parts. The choice of the optimal set of parameters was carried out using the accuracy metric averaged over cross-validation.

After choosing the optimal parameters of the model, it is trained on the entire training sample. The final evaluation of the model is carried out on a test sample according to the metrics.

- $Accuracy = \dfrac{True\ Positive + True\ Negative}{True\ Positive + True\ Negative + False\ Positive + False\ Negative}$
- $Sensitivity = \dfrac{True\ Positive}{True\ Positive + False\ Negative}.$
- $Specificity = \dfrac{True\ Negative}{True\ Negative + False\ Positive}.$

For the Adaboost algorithm with the Decision Tree classifier with a maximum depth of 1, the following parameters turned out to be the best: the learning rate is 0.2, the number of classifiers is 150. The resulting model gives the following metric values on the test sample.

- Accuracy = 0.95
- Sensitivity = 0.92
- Specificity = 1.0

For the Adaboost algorithm with a Decision Tree classifier with a maximum depth of 2, the best learning speed is 1.5 and the number of classifiers is 150.

The resulting model gives the following metric values on the test sample.

- Accuracy = 0.85
- Sensitivity = 0.92
- Specificity = 0.71

7.6.4 CONCLUSIONS ON ADABOOST

The Adaboost algorithm with 150 decision trees with a depth of 1 and a learning rate of 0.2 showed the best results. Testing shows that the Adaboost algorithm works beautifully on the task at hand. Accuracy (95%), sensitivity (92%) and specificity (100%) obtained are superior to the results of some other diagnostic methods. For example, the sensitivity of mammography is approximately 87% (D'Orsi and Sickles 2017), while the specificity ranges between 93% and 88% (Nelson et al. 2016).

However, the Adaboost algorithm does not have a clear and transparent interpretation, which is important in the tasks of diagnosing diseases.

7.7 ALGORITHM RANDOM FOREST

Consider the Random Forest algorithm (Breiman 2021) for the problem of diagnosing breast cancer. The theory put forward earlier about the greater information content of the blue data channel will also be tested. The idea of the Random Forest algorithm is to build an ensemble of decision trees that are trained on different subsamples of the training data. The end result of the classification is the averaging of all the results of the constructed decision trees.

7.7.1 RANDOM FOREST

Training the Random Forest algorithm consists in applying the bootstrap aggregation (bagging) technique to Decision Tree algorithms. Assume that we have training data $X = (x_1, x_2, ..., x_n)$ with class labels $Y = (y_1, y_2, ..., y_n)$. Bootstrap aggregation B times selects a random subsample from the training sample and trains the Decision Tree algorithm on the newly received sample.

For $b = 1, ... , B$:

1. Create a subsample X_b, Y_b from the training sample X, Y.
2. Train Decision Tree f_b on the sample X_b, Y_b.

After training all Decision Tree algorithms for new data x, the results of all Decision Tree classifiers are averaged. That is, the class that has chosen the largest number of Decision Trees will be selected. This method is also called the simple voting method.

To test the hypothesis about the greater informativeness of the data obtained from the blue channel, the Random subspace method (Ho 1998) was used to select a subsample for training Decision Tree algorithms. The idea of the method is to project the training sample into subspaces (training sample space). Thus, subsamples with a smaller dimension are obtained, on which classifiers learn. For our task, we will divide the feature spaces into three subspaces for each of the channels (blue, green, red).

Also, in addition to the simple voting method, logistic regression was used for the Random Forest algorithm with the Random subspace method. Thus, logistic regression learned from the results of the three decision trees that were learned from each of the data channels. This makes it possible to find the most informative data channel by checking weights of logistic regression.

7.7.2 LOGISTIC REGRESSION

Logistic regression (Yang 2019) is a statistical classification algorithm that checks whether the input data belongs to one class or another.

Let we have a binary classification (then class 0 is a control group, and class 1 is a group of patients with breast cancer), and input data x. Then, the probability that x will belong to second class (class 1) is

$$P(G = 1 | X = x) = \sigma(\beta_0 + \beta_1^T x),$$

where G is a corresponding class and a sigmoid function has the form

$$\sigma(x) = \frac{1}{1 + e^{-x}}.$$

The learning of logistic regression is performed using minimization of a cost function $L(\beta)$ by gradient methods

$$L(\beta) = \sum_{i=1}^{N} \{y_i \log p(x_i; \beta) + (1 - y_i)p(x_i; \beta)\},$$

where N is the number of training samples, x is an input sample, y is a sample of class labels, $p(x_i; \beta) = P(G = 1|X = x_i; \beta)$.

7.7.3 TESTING RANDOM FOREST

For testing, we divided the dataset into two parts: a training sample (80%) and a test sample (20%) on which the resulting model will be evaluated. Let us consider several approaches with the Random Forest algorithm.

First, the Random subspace method was used to create three subspaces of training data for each of the channels. After that, the Decision Tree algorithm was trained on the data of each of the data channels. For each of the three trees, we carried out cross-validation by splitting the training data into five parts and selecting the parameters for the maximum depth of the tree and the algorithm splitting criterion (the Decision Tree parameters were chosen after the accuracy metric). As a result, the following results were obtained for each of the data channels (Figures 7.8–7.10).

Decision Tree trained on data from the blue channel.
Depth = 3.
Splitting criteria = Gini index.
Accuracy = 0.75

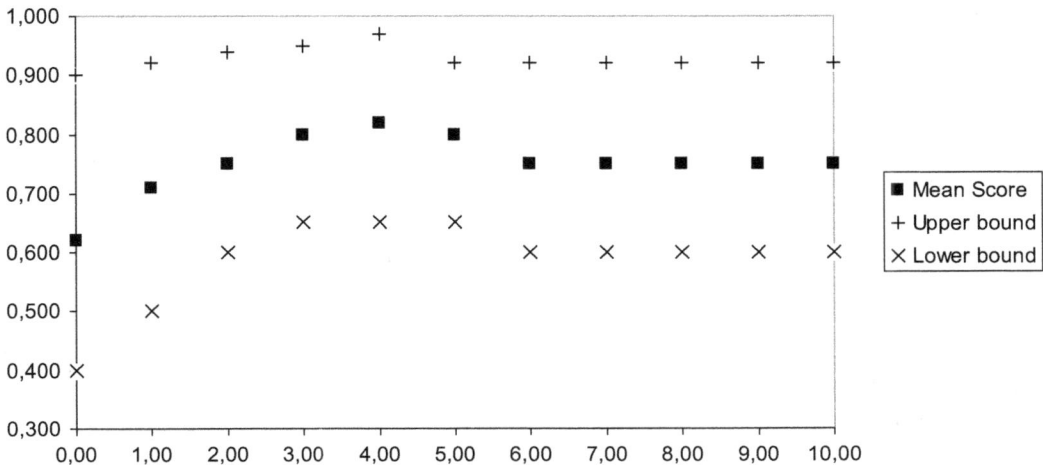

FIGURE 7.9 Depth fitting plot for the Decision Tree algorithm with the Gini splitting criterion, which is trained on the green channel data. The abscissa shows the values of the max depth parameter, and the ordinate shows the accuracy.

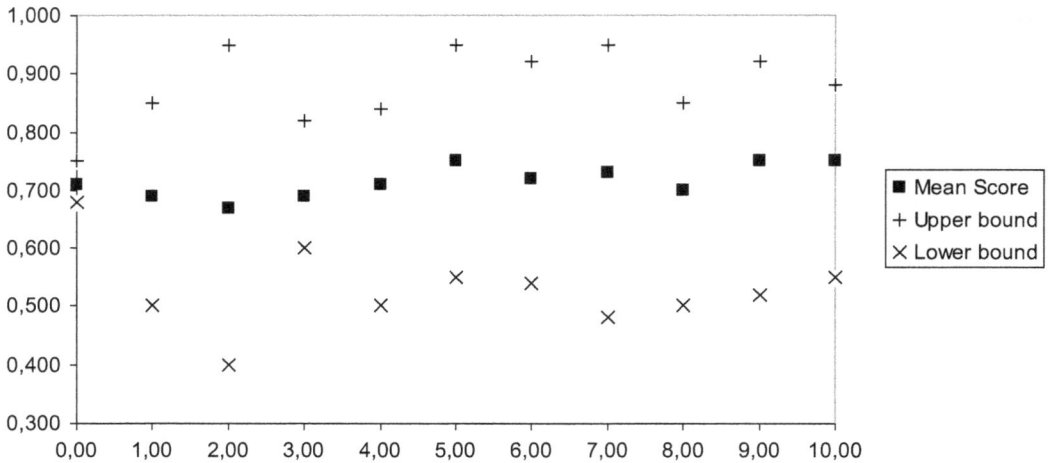

FIGURE 7.10 Depth fitting plot for a Decision Tree algorithm with a cross-entropy splitting criterion that trains on red channel data. The abscissa shows the values of the max depth parameter, and the ordinate shows the accuracy.

Sensitivity = 0.85
Specificity = 0.57

Decision Tree trained on data from the green channel.
Depth = 4.
Splitting criteria = Gini index.
Accuracy = 0.60
Sensitivity = 0.69
Specificity = 0.43

Decision Tree trained on data from the red channel.
Depth = 5.
Splitting criteria = cross entropy.
Accuracy = 0.50
Sensitivity = 0.77
Specificity = 0.0

The next issue for the aggregation of the Decision Tree algorithms is the use of the simple voting method (averaging the votes):

$$P(y = 1) = \sum_{i=1}^{3} T_i(x),$$

where $P(y = 1)$ is the probability that, given x, the result of the Random Forest will be class 1 (breast cancer patient), T_i are Decision Tree algorithms that produce a class 1 probability. When testing this version of the Random Forest algorithm, the following results were obtained:

- Accuracy = 0.70
- Sensitivity = 0.85
- Specificity = 0.42

Also, based on the previously obtained trees, logistic regression was applied. The input logistic regression algorithm takes class 1 (breast cancer patient) probabilities that were generated from each of the three decision trees. Training of logistic regression lasts as long as the maximum component of the loss function is greater than 10^{-4}. Therefore, the modification of the Random Forest algorithm gave the following results:

- Accuracy = 0.75
- Sensitivity = 0.69
- Specificity = 0.86

In addition, the Random Forest algorithm was tested with the bootstrap aggregation technique of distributing data into 100 subsamples to train the appropriate number of Decision Trees with the Gini splitting criterion. The trees are split until each letter contains training examples of only one class, or there are no more than two examples in the letter. This Random Forest variant gave the following results:

- Accuracy = 0.90
- Sensitivity = 0.92
- Specificity = 0.85

7.7.4 CONCLUSIONS ON RANDOM FOREST

The Random Forest algorithm was tested, and beautiful results were obtained. The best result was shown by the Random Forest algorithm from bootstrap aggregation and 100 decision trees: accuracy (90%), sensitivity (92%), and specificity (85%).

The idea of building a Random Forest based on three decision trees, each of which is trained on its own (blue, green, red) data channel, has not shown its effectiveness. The decision tree built on the data from the blue channel shows the same accuracy as the Random Forest built on these trees using logistic regression.

At the same time, the trees built on the green and red data channels show very low results. Considering that the logistic regression weights for the decision tree trained on the blue channel data are the largest, it can be concluded that the blue data channel is the most informative. However, other data channels should not be discarded from consideration, their importance is confirmed by the high accuracy of the Random Forest algorithm with 100 trees, which was studied on all data channels at once.

7.8 CONCLUSION

Machine-learning methods for diagnosing breast cancer based on the fractal dimension of buccal epithelium nuclei is proposed in the work. The cancer diagnosis method with 95% accuracy, 92% sensitivity, and 100% specificity is developed. The significance of the data from blue, green, red channels is checked using the Random Forest algorithm and logistic regression. The blue data channel is more important than the other two channels. However, the best results are obtained when using all data channels.

Future scope of the work consists in considering images with yellow and violet filters (only images without filters are used in this work), and in using other measures of fractal dimension.

REFERENCES

Adam, R., Silva, R., Pereira, F. et al. 2006. The fractal dimension of nuclear chromatin as a prognostic factor in acute precursor B lymphoblastic leukemia. *Cellular Oncology* 28: 55–59. doi: 10.1155/2006/409593

Adhraryn, S. G., Dave, B. J., and Trivedi, A. H. 1991. Cytogenetic surveillance of tobacco-arecaunt (mava) chewers, including patient with oral cancers and premalignant conditions. *Mutation Research* 261, no. 1: 41–49. doi: 10.1016/0165-1218(91)90096-5

Andreichuk, A. V., Boroday, N. V., Golubeva et al. 2021. Artificial Intelligence System for Breast Cancer Screening Based on Malignancy-Associated Changes in Buccal Epithelium. In: *Enabling AI Applications in Data Science*, ed. A. H. Hassanien, A. E. Taha, and N. E. M. Khalifa, 266–285. Cham: Springer.

Bedin, V. et al. 2010. Fractal dimension of chromatin is an independent prognostic factor for survival in melanoma. *BMC Cancer* 10: 260. https://bmccancer.biomedcentral.com/articles/10.1186/1471-2407-10-260. doi:10.1186/1471-2407-10-260

Bikou, O. et al. 2016. Fractal Dimension as a Diagnostic Tool of Complex Endometrial Hyperplasia and Well-differentiated Endometrioid Carcinoma. *In Vivo* 30: 681–690.

Boroday, N., Chekhun, V., Golubeva, E. et al. In Vitro and in Vivo Densitometric Analysis of DNA Content and Chromatin Texture in Nuclei of Tumor Cells under the Influence of a Nano Composite and Magnetic Field. *Advances in Cancer Research and Treatment*. 2016, 706183. doi: 10.5171/2016.706183

Breiman, L. 2021. Random Forests. *Machine Learning* 45, no. 1: 5–32.

Butakov, V. and Grakovskiy, A. 2005. Evaluation of arbitrary time series stochastic level by Hurst parameter. *Computer Modelling and New Technologies* 9, no. 2: 27–32.

D'Orsi, C. J. and Sickles, E. A. 2017. Breast Cancer Surveillance Consortium Reports on Interpretive Performance at Screening and Diagnostic Mammography: Welcome New Data, But Not as Benchmarks for Practice. *Radiology* 283, no. 1: 7–9.

Einstein, A., Wu, H., Sanchez, M., and Gil, J. 1998. Fractal characterization of chromatin appearance for diagnosis in breast cytology. *The Journal of Pathology* 185: 366–381. doi: 10.1002/(SICI)1096-9896 (199808)185:4<366::AID-PATH122>3.0.CO;2-C

Hastie, T., Tibshirani, R., and Friedman, J. 2009. *Elements of Statistical Learning*. Cham: Springer.

Ho, T. 1998. The Random Subspace Method for Constructing Decision Forests. *IEEE Transactions on Pattern Analysis and Machine Intelligence* 20, no. 8: 832–844. doi:10.1109/34.709601

Hu, Q., Whitney, H. M., and Giger, M. L. 2020. A deep learning methodology for improved breast cancer diagnosis using multiparametric MRI. *Scientific Reports* 10: 10536. 10.1038/s41598-020-67441-4

Kavitha, T., Mathai, P. P., Karthikeyan, C. et al. 2022. Deep Learning Based Capsule Neural Network Model for Breast Cancer Diagnosis Using Mammogram Images. *Interdisciplinary Sciences–Computational Life Sciences* 14: 113–129. 10.1007/s12539-021-00467-y

Khamparia, A., Bharati, S., Podder, P. et al. 2021. Diagnosis of breast cancer based on modern mammography using hybrid transfer learning. *Multidimensional Systems and Signal Processing* 32: 747–765. 10.1007/s11045-020-00756-7

Klyushin, D., Golubeva, K., Boroday, N. et al. 2021. Breast cancer diagnosis using machine learning and fractal analysis of malignancy-associated changes in buccal epithelium. Chapter: *Artificial Intelligence, Machine Learning, and Data Science Technologies Future Impact and Well-Being for Society 5.0*, ed. N. Mohan, R. Singla, P. Kaushal, and S. Kadry, 1–17. London: Taylor & Fransis.

Lieberman-Aiden, E. et al. 2009. Comprehensive mapping of long-range interactions reveals folding principles of the human Genome. *Science* 326, no. 5959: 289– 193. doi: 10.1126/science.1181369.

Losa, G. and Castelli, C. 2005. Nuclear patterns of human breast cancer cells during apoptosis: characterization by fractal dimension and (GLCM) co-occurrence matrix statistics. *Cell and Tissue Research* 322: 257–267. doi: 10.1007/s00441-005-0030-2

Losa, G. 2012. Fractals and their contribution to biology and medicine. *Medicographia* 34: 365–374.

Metze, K. 2010. Fractal dimension of chromatin and cancer prognosis. *Epigenomics* 2, no. 5: 601–604. doi: 10.2217/epi.10.50

Metze, K. 2013. Fractal dimension of chromatin: potential molecular diagnostic applications for cancer prognosis. *Expert Review of Molecular Diagnostics* 13, no. 7: 719–735. doi: 10.1586/14737159.2013.828889

Nair, U., Obe, G., Nair, J., and Maru, G. B. 1991. Evaluation of frequency of micronucleated oral mucosa cells as a marker for genotoxic damage in chewers of betel quid with or without tobacco. *Mutation Research* 261, no. 2: 163–168.

Nelson, H. D., Fu, R., Cantor, A., Pappas, M., Daeges, M., and Humphrey, L. 2016. Effectiveness of breast cancer screening: systematic review and meta-analysis to update the 2009 U.S. Preventive Services Task Force Recommendation. *Annals of Internal Medicine* 164, no. 4: 244–255. doi: 10.7326/M15-0969

Nieburgs, H. E. 1968. Recent progress in the interpretation of malignancy associated changes (MAC). *Acta Cytologica* 12: 445–453.

Nieburgs, H. F., Herman, B. E., and Reisman, H. 1962. Buccal cell changes in patients with malignant tumors. *Laboratory Investigation* 11, no. 1: 80–88.

Obrapalska, E., Cadel, Z., and Kostyrka, J. 1973. Ocena cytologic zna nablonka jamy ustney u chorych na nowotwory zlosliwe. *Nowotwory* 1973, 23, no. 1/2: 25–29 (in Polish).

Ogden, G. R., Cowpe, J. G., and Green, M. W. 1990. The effect of distant malignancy upon quantitative cytologic assessment of normal oral mucosa. *Cancer* 65: 477–480. doi:/10.1002/1097-0142(19900201) 65:3<477::AID-CNCR2820650317>3.0.CO;2-G

Ohri, S., Dey, P., and Nijhawan, R. 2004. Fractal dimension in aspiration cytology smears of breast and cervical lesions. *Analytical and Quantitative Cytology and Histology* 26: 109–112.

Palcic, B. 1994. Nuclear texture: can in be used as a suurrogate endpoind biomarker? *Journal of Cellular Biochemistry* 19, no. 1: 40–46.

Patil, A., Tamboli, D., Meena, S., Anand, D. et al. 2019. A. Breast Cancer Histopathology Image Classification and Localization using Multiple Instance Learning. In: *2019 IEEE International WIE Conference on Electrical and Computer Engineering (WIECON-ECE)*, 1–4. doi: 10.1109/WIECON-ECE48653.2019.9019916

Prasad, M. P., Mukundan, M. A., and Krishnaswamy, K. 1995. Micronuclei and carcinogen DNA adducts as intermediate end points in nutrient intervention trial of precancerous lesions in the oral cavity. *European Journal of Cancer* 31B(3): 155–160. doi: 10.1016/0964-1955(95)00013-8

Punitha, S., Al-Turjman, F., and Thompson, S. 2021. An automated breast cancer diagnosis using feature selection and parameter optimization. *ANN, Computers and Electrical Engineering* 90: 106958.

Rathbone, M. J., Drummond, B. K., and Tucker, I. G. 1994. The oral cavity as a site for systemic drug delivery. *Advanced Drug Delivery Reviews* 13, no. 1–2: 1–23.

Rosin, M. 1992. The use of the micronucleus test on exfoliated cells to identify anticlastogenic action in humans. *Mutation Research* 287, no. 2: 265–276. doi: 10.1016/0027-5107(92)90071-9

Sagan, H. 1994. *Space-filling curves*. New York–Berlin: Springer-Verlag.

Sarto, F., Tomanin, R., Giacomelli L. et al. 1990. The micronucleus assay in human exfoliated cell of the nose and mouth: application to occupational exposures to chromic acid and ethylene oxide. *Mutation Research* 244, no. 2: 345–351. doi: 10.1016/0165-7992(90)90083-V

Schonwetter, B., Stolzenberg, E., and Zasloff, M. Epithelial antibiotics induced at sites of inflammation. *Science* 257, no. 5204: 1645–1648. doi: 10.1111/j.1600-0757.2010.00373.x

Tolbert, P. E., Shy, C. M., and Allen, J. W. 1992. Micronuclei and other nuclear anomalies in buccal smears development. *Mutation Research* 271, no. 1: 69–77. doi: 10.1016/0165-1161(92)90033-i

Yan, R. et al. 2018. A Hybrid Convolutional and Recurrent Deep Neural Network for Breast Cancer Pathological Image Classification. In: *2018 IEEE International Conference on Bioinformatics and Biomedicine (BIBM)*, 957–962. doi: 10.1109/BIBM.2018.8621429

Yang, H., Kim, J. -Y., Kim, H., and Adhikari, S. P. 2019. Guided Soft Attention Network for Classification of Breast Cancer Histopathology Images. *IEEE Transactions on Medical Imaging* 39, no. 5: 1306–1315. doi: 10.1109/TMI.2019.2948026

Yifan, D., Jialin, L., and Boxi, F. 2021. Forecast Model of Breast Cancer Diagnosis Based on RF-AdaBoost. In: *2021 International Conference on Communications, Information System and Computer Engineering (CISCE)*, 716–719. doi: 10.1109/CISCE52179.2021.9445847

Zhu, J., Zou, H., Rosset, S., and Hastie, T. 2009. Multi-class AdaBoost. *Statistics and Its Interface* 2: 349–360.

8 Fractionalization of Early Lung Tumour Regions and Detection Using a Low Intricacy Approach

Thanushree Latha A.S., Pranav M., and Hemalatha Karnan
School of Chemical and Biotechnology, SASTRA, Thanjavur

CONTENTS

8.1 INTRODUCTION

Being among the major causes of death, cancer has attracted the attention of scientists from various interdisciplinary fields to try and fight the challenges it poses to the human healthcare industry. In

DOI: 10.1201/9781003333081-8

our attempt to join this battle against cancer, we have used various image-processing techniques to enhance the rate of successful diagnosis using medical images. This early detection will aid doctors in providing effective treatment plans to patients to save their lives [1].

8.1.1 SIGNIFICANCE OF LUNG TUMOURS

Globally, cancer is the leading cause of death, totaling nearly 10 million deaths in 2020 [2]. The most common cause of cancer death in 2020 is lung cancer Figure 8.1.

Detection of lung cancer usually is possible only in the advanced stages of cancer progression due to the late onset of noticeable physiological symptoms. Most of these symptoms are either slight or ignored. Even if cancer is suspected at earlier stages, the tumours are generally mistaken for small benign lung abscesses through the initial screening. A lung cancer diagnosis is initially done by analysing chest x-ray images of the patient [1]. These images show the tumour cluster as a white patch that is easily recognizable for large tumours. However, for the identification of smaller tumours in the initial stages of cancer progression, CT scan images are much more reliable [1,3].

8.1.2 ISSUES WITH LUNG TUMOUR DETECTION

Easy recognition of the small tumour clusters will reduce the occurrence of false negative cases/reports. Diagnoses using x-ray images had a rate of false negatives of 17.7% in 2021 [3]. More efficient diagnostic methods are urgently needed to improve the outlook on the survival rates of lung cancer patients. Early-stage detection of lung cancer enhances the chances of survival of the patient significantly [1]. This detection involves the identification of smaller tumours present within the chest or lung, which is much harder [4]. Automatic, fast, efficient, and reliable identification techniques can help improve the accuracy of identification and classification of tumours. Better detection strategies can help in the early recognition of cancer cells.

8.1.3 IMAGE PROCESSING FOR TUMOUR DETECTION

For automatic identification of tumours, various image-processing techniques have been used for different types of cancer diagnoses. For brain tumour detection, an automated system based on image segmentation was used to perfect the segmentation of the tumour region from brain MRI images [5]. Using OTSU segmentation, brain tumours were detected from medical images using MATLAB Software [6]. Based on various thresholding methods that could identify micro calcifications, early breast cancer was detected from mammogram images [7]. Lung tumours were detected from CT scan

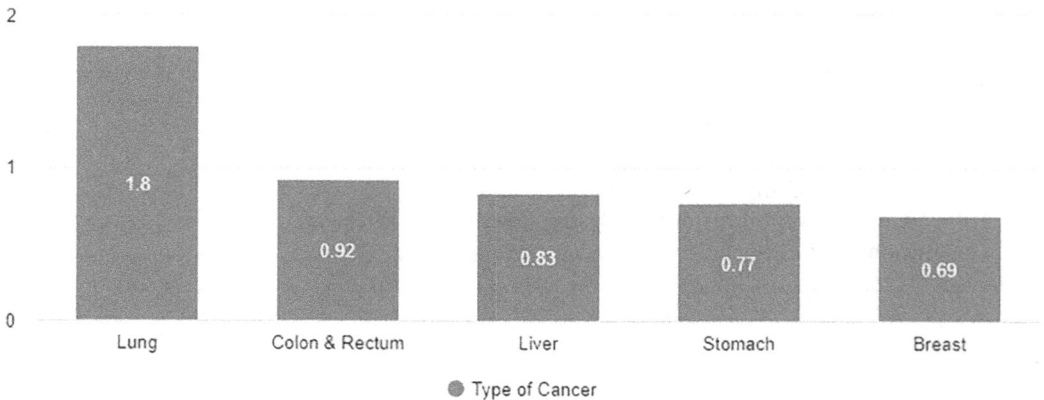

FIGURE 8.1 Most common causes of cancer death in 2020 (in millions).

images using feature extraction and contour modelling [8]. Detection of small metastatic lung cancer using direct 3D template-matching techniques [9] and detection of lung cancer in CT images using image-processing techniques based on mathematical morphological operations [10] are examples of image-processing applications for tumour detection, segmentation, and cancer diagnosis.

From these literature studies, it was considered apt to use OTSU segmentation and feature-extraction methodologies to segment the tumour region precisely. OTSU segmentation being a global adaptive binarization threshold image segmentation is a fast, straightforward method utilising mathematical morphological operations on the image. Its major advantage is that it is not affected by the contrast and brightness of images and hence yields the most precise results every time. However, being an iterative process, computational complexity increases with larger datasets, such as CT scan images. Feature extraction helps break down these large datasets (a large number of variables) into small relevant groups called features, therefore making processing easier. Even though these features are significantly small as compared to the original number of image variables, they represent the original dataset with accuracy and originality. To enhance the precision of outputs from these methods, various pre-processing techniques such as grayscale conversion, Top Hat filtering, histogram construction, distance transformation, and watershed transforms are performed on the original DICOM images derived from medical-image repositories. These methods are aimed to provide a process that accounts for high stability, precision, reliability, and efficiency. The process is then subjected to validation by performing Quad-tree decomposition and analysis through cumulative functional distribution and residual plots obtained from the histograms of the original and segmented image.

8.1.4 OBJECTIVES

To be able to automatically detect tumour regions from raw medical images, it will be possible to avoid the chances of tumour region nullification due to various image-processing techniques that are applied as default to make the medical image easily observable by the naked eye. Using pre-processing and segmentation techniques appropriate for the raw medical images, the tumour region can be retained and identified. The specific objectives of this project are:

1. To identify appropriate image pre-processing techniques to enhance the features of raw CT scan images of DICOM file format
2. To apply OTSU segmentation to detect tumour regions
3. To verify the segmented regions using Quadtree decomposition
4. To compare the histogram of the original image with the segmented image using distribution plots

8.2 LITERATURE SURVEY

To be able to perform efficient tumour fractionalisation and evaluation of the same, the following parameters should be satisfied in the most optimal way possible: (i) Initial image pre-processing and removal of noise to enhance the precision of the image segmentation technique employed in this project. (ii) Suitable segmentation techniques to distinguish the tumour regions accurately. This technique should be able to classify the pixels in the tumour region without committing to any errors that could produce false fractionalisation of tumour regions that cannot be accommodated. (iii) Analysis and evaluation for reliability of the employed segmentation techniques. This step should be able to examine if the proposed model is reliable without any bias. The results should be easily acceptable, interpretable, and understandable. This step is optional for fractionalisation of tumour regions. It only serves as a model evaluation technique.

Numerous literatures have been enumerated over lung cancer detections using CT images [8,11]. These studies also include various strategies for the selection of suitable pre-processing techniques to enhance the outcomes of diversified outputs obtained through the work.

8.2.1 REVIEW FOR IMAGE PREPROCESSING TECHNIQUES

By the inclusion of image processing and machine learning, a lung cancer detection system on CT images is framed by Rahane *et al.* (2018) [12]. The result of this project is a model that can classify lung CT images as regular and irregular. The abnormal images are then segmented to show emphasis on tumour regions. The various pre-processing techniques to improve contrast and clarity of images involved are grayscale conversion, noise reduction using median filter, image binarization techniques, and feature extraction.

To minimise lung cancer detection errors by humans, Kalaivani *et al.* (2017) [13] built an automated process for detection. This process for early-stage detection involves certain methods for image processing and also includes the concept of artificial neural networks. The image pre-processing techniques inculcated in this project are grayscale conversion, histogram equalization, image binarization, and feature extraction.

Using image-processing techniques, Kulkarni *et al.* (2014) [14] were able to classify lung cancers. A novel algorithm is developed with the help of image-clarifying techniques to identify cancer at naive stages by satisfying extensive accuracy. This process involves image pre-processing techniques and feature extraction. The pre-processing techniques include image smoothening using median filter and image enhancement using Gabor filter, which can perform texture analysis. The Gabor filter has an optimal localization in both the spatial and frequency domains.

Sujan *et al.* (2016) [5] used OTSU segmentation to perfectly segment the tumorous tissues from the human brain. The visual depiction is subjected to pre-processing techniques such as grayscale conversion, noise removal by median filtering, and image binarization. Morphological erosion is performed using a structural element shaped like a disc with an optimally required diameter. This element aids accurate tumor segmentation. Salt and pepper noises are removed using a median filter, and each pixel value is incremented by a value of 25 to enhance selection of optimal threshold.

In the paper by Saini *et al.* (2015) [6], image fractionalisation is performed to withdraw the numerous features of an image. Examination, observation, and interpretation can be easily done on these images. The work emphasises the identification of brain tumour and associated cells from MRI images using mathematical morphological alterations. Since ultrasound images consist of speckle noise and are of low contrast, pre-processing techniques become mandatory. These techniques include image restoration using level-set function, smoothening and edge sharpening using a Gabor filter, and contrast enrichment using histogram equalization. These are succeeded by OTSU's method for image segmentation and best suited global thresholding. The tumour regions are identified with the help of density-based clustering approach.

8.2.2 REVIEW FOR FEATURE EXTRACTION

Amutha *et al.* (2013) [8] used a level-set active contour model with a diminishing algorithm for lung tumour detection from CT scan images. For denoising, a kernel-based non-local neighbourhood algorithm is used. Feature extraction for image classification is executed with the aid of a second order histogram. Upon tumour detection, segmentation is performed through the use of level-set active contour modelling.

The work of Miah *et al.* (2015) [15] involves a series of processes such as image accession, pre-processing, image binarization, optimal thresholding technique, image segmentation, feature extraction, and a notion of neural network detection. After segmentation of the lung tumour from CT scan images, a robust feature extraction method is applied to take out information of selected lines. This information is used to tutor the neural network. The algorithm is tested on both tumorous and non-tumorous scans.

Katre *et al.* (2017) [16] aimed to classify lung tumour stages using familiar methods such as image processing and data classification. Image pre-processing techniques such as denoising using median filter, enhancement using a high boost operator, and image segmentation using marker-controlled watershed transforms are performed. Feature extraction helps identify the potential regions of tumour presence, which is the region of interest.

8.2.3 REVIEW FOR OTSU SEGMENTATION

A comparative analysis carried out by Gajanayake *et al.* (2009) [17] concludes that OTSU segmentation method is the best method to carry out segmentation of brain tumours from 2D brain MRI (magnetic resonance imaging) images. In this paper, all the familiar gray-level image-segmentation techniques such as OTSU segmentation, mean shift method, K-means, fuzzy c-means, and six other such methods, are compared to recognize the most satisfactory segmentation algorithm for the identification of tumours from 2D MRI images of the brain. The resultant images from each method are then compared by a panel of professional radiologists to conclude segmentation using OTSU method as the most reliable.

In the paper written by Huang *et al.* (2012) [18], the OTSU method was titled to be a simple and stable method widely applied for image segmentation as it has automatic control over threshold selection. However, they also found out that OTSU's method is highly sensitive to disturbances and target size. For images with more than a single peak, it is not as effective. When the contrast between two intra-class variances is high, threshold is more inclined toward the class with a larger intra-class variance. This outcome resulted in extra pixels of this class to be classified into an incorrect class. To improve the segmentation technique, the paper proposed two approaches. One, large parts of the gray values can be avoided, therefore limiting the threshold-selecting range. Two, removing gray values on both extremes of intensities, therefore reducing noises and false selection of threshold.

Xu *et al.* (2011) [19] through their work discovered a property of OTSU method that the optimal threshold of an image is equal to the average of the mean levels of the two classes separated by this threshold value. This was done through mathematical modelling. Therefore, they concluded that there will be a bias in favour of threshold for the class with the biggest variance when the intra-class variances of the two classes are different. To overcome this bias, a range-constrained OTSU segmentation method is proposed. Experiments revealed that this method yields satisfactory results and hence is a suitable improvement method for segmentation. The range-constrained OTSU method relied on an iterative process for the selection of an optimal threshold.

A paper published in The International Arab Journal of Information Technology [20] proposed a fast OTSU segmentation method to reduce computational complexity. The method involves creating checkpoints to drastically reduce the number of iterative cycles. Upon comparison of threshold values obtained from the classical OTSU method and the OTSU-checkpoints method on the same set of images, there is no deviation of the value of the optimal threshold. The checkpoints are framed using mathematical relations.

8.2.4 REVIEW FOR QUADTREE DECOMPOSITION

In the work framed by Dua *et al.* (2010) [21], they use an advanced edge-detection technique based on regional recursive hierarchical decomposition of an image called Quadtree decomposition. The validation and comparison studies were performed on diabetic retinopathy images obtained as a result of CT scanning. These tests rendered the method efficient and accurate. Successful segmentation of the image occurred using the Quadtree technique.

Subramaniam *et al.* (2013) [22] used the Quadtree decomposition method to estimate the variations between young and elderly healthy lungs from CT images. Here, the Quadtree method illustrated the changes in heterogeneity of the density of soft tissues between different subjects. The technique is sensitive enough to differentiate between heterogenous and homogenous regions and hence will be useful for tumour detection.

8.3 EXPERIMENTAL WORK/METHODOLOGY

The methodology of this project includes two major steps for image processing: image pre-processing techniques and OTSU segmentation. Image pre-processing is necessary to enhance the various features of the raw images such as brightness, contrast, etc. to ensure that during segmentation, no data is left unprocessed. All image-processing techniques are performed using MATLAB Software.

8.3.1 PRE-PROCESSING METHODOLOGIES

Pre-processing of the raw CT scan images of the chest involve the following steps: Figure 8.2

8.3.1.1 Selection of CT Scan Images

CT scans have the advantage of recording the structures of minute details, such as early tumours, because the imaging process involves scanning across various directions and in multiple planes that are reconstructed to ensure high accuracy in replicating internal body structures. All medical images, such as CT scans, MRIs, and ultrasounds, are suggested to be stored in the DICOM file format because it enables all of the metadata to remain attached to the file instead of being lost. DICOM files are compatible with various software and hence can be easily transferred and read without any incompatibility issues. The chest CT scans of patients with lung cancer have been obtained from the open-source medical image repositories. The source for the images used for processing in this project is acknowledged by the following citations [23,24], a publicly available

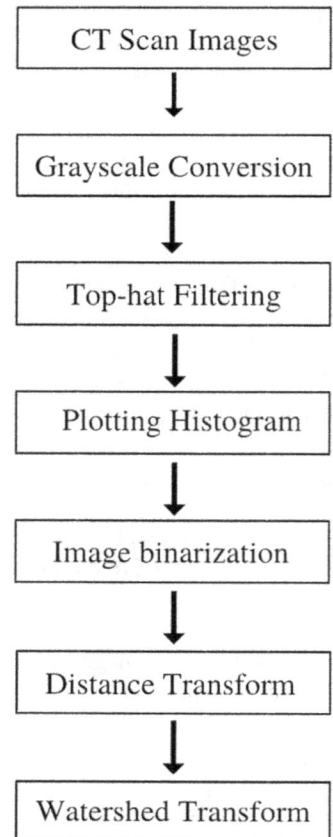

FIGURE 8.2 Image pre-processing methodologies.

archive of numerous medical CT images for lung cancer. The images are read using the syntax *I=dicomread("File_name")*.

8.3.1.2 Grayscale Conversion

The DICOM images are converted into a grayscale image using the syntax *J = im2gray(I)*. This technique involves the conversion of 24-bit values (RGB values) into 8-bit values (grayscale values). This process allows for feature extraction by reducing the number of large data for easier processing. The value of each pixel will only represent information on the intensity of light and will remove characteristics of saturation and color. This will reduce the computational complexity of data processing.

8.3.1.3 Top-Hat Filtering

The syntax used to achieve Top Hat filtering is *J = imtophat(I,strel('disk',10))* where the diameter of the structural element (strel) is chosen to be 10 units as it yields appropriate results. This filtering technique removes noises. The noises are identified as the minimal pixel-valued elements in the image. This principle of Top Hat filtering ensures that minute tumours are not identified as noises and removed during pre-processing. The algorithm of this technique involves the subtraction of morphological closing operations on the input image from the original input image. Here, closing operations help smoothen the contours of deformed images and therefore help remove small noises.

8.3.1.4 Plotting Histogram and Image Binarization

A histogram is plotted using the syntax *histogram(I)*. This plot shows the frequency distribution of grayscale-level intensities. It is in the form of a bar graph with the grayscale values of pixels plotted against the horizontal axis and the intensity values of the pixels plotted against the vertical axis. This graphical representation of an image is useful to obtain an optimal threshold to perform image binarization. The pixel values above the optimal threshold are assigned a value of 1, being completely white, and the pixel values below the optimal threshold are assigned a value of 0, being completely black. This assignment generates a binary (black and white) image. Binary images are required for other pre-processing techniques to enhance the precision of processing algorithms. The syntax used to find the optimal threshold is *level = graythresh(I)*.

8.3.1.5 Distance Transformation

The distance of a non-featured element from a featured element is measured using the syntax *D = bwdist(C)*. Here, the featured elements refer to the edges, points, or objects and the non-featured elements refer to the blank spaces. The blank spaces are generally set to 0 and the featured elements are set to 1 of the binarized image. Therefore, in simpler terms, the distance between the zero and the non-zero pixels of a binary image is calculated. Finding the Euclidean distance between the various elements helps to understand the spatial distribution of various elements of the image by giving us knowledge of the background and object features.

8.3.1.6 Watershed Transform

Watershed transform is applied to an image to examine it for high and low-level areas using the syntax *J = watershed(I)*. The low-level regions are compared to catchment basins and are correlated to the dark (0) pixels. The high-level regions are compared to the ridges and are correlated to light (1) pixels. Therefore, by treating the image as a topographical map, the brightness of each pixel is used to identify lines/ridges in the image. This allows for the segmentation of various regions of the image. The region consisting of the tumour is approximately identified using this methodology.

8.3.2   OTSU Segmentation

OTSU's method of segmentation involves the grouping of pixels into foreground and background classes to achieve automatic image thresholding. To achieve this classification, pixels are plotted into a histogram after which an optimal threshold value is obtained. This optimal threshold value is found using an iterative process that compares all the possible threshold values and the spread of the pixels on each side of the threshold value. The optimal threshold value is set when the sum of the foreground and background spreads is minimal, i.e., the intra-class spread should be minimal, whereas the inter-class spread should be maximal. This algorithm yields a single peak value that clearly distinguishes between the foreground and background pixels of the image. Based on this output, the tumour region which is made up of light pixels and correlates to the foreground pixels is precisely distinguished.

8.3.3   Analysis Using Quadtree Decomposition

The syntax used to perform Quadtree decomposition is $J = qtdecomp(I, minimum size of block)$. This technique yields information about the structure of an image. The method results in a subdivided image into homogenous regions. These subdivided regions are represented as blocks. The function initially divides the entire image into four equal-sized square blocks that are tested to meet a particular criterion of homogeneity by comparing them using a specific dynamic range. If the criterion is met by the block, it is not divided further, but if it fails to meet the criterion, it is in turn subdivided into four blocks and tested with the specified criterion again. This process occurs iteratively until each block meets the specified criterion. This process will result in homogenous square blocks of various sizes. This method is used to crosscheck the obtained OTSU segmented image by comparing the segmented regions to the homogenous blocks of wide spatial concentration.

8.3.4   Comparison Using Distribution Plots

The histograms of the original, segmented, and threshold images are obtained and compared with the aid of a distribution plotter available in MATLAB R2022 Online. The cumulative function distribution of the data of the original, segmented, and threshold images are then plotted in a graphical representation. The normal distribution and residual distribution of the original and segmented image are considered for a comparative study.

8.4   RESULTS AND DISCUSSION

Upon subjecting the CT scan images of the lungs to the various pre-processing techniques mentioned above and OTSU segmentation, the following results were obtained. Output images after each pre-processing methodology are displayed to compare, observe, and study its effects on enhancing the segmentation process.

8.4.1   Pre-processing Outputs

The first output image (Figure 8.3) is the raw CT scans DICOM image. The original image is displayed to make it possible to compare the effects of the various pre-processing and OTSU segmentation methods. A medical practitioner can identify the irregular white patches as potential tumour clusters. With our code, we will check if these tumour regions are being successfully detected by segmentation; see Figure 8.4.

The histogram is a graphical representation of an original image's pixel intensity distribution. The number of pixels found at each pixel value is plotted in a histogram. The lower signal values are typically represented on the left side of the graph, while the higher signal values are typically represented on the right side. It represents data points that are organized into ranges that the user specifies.

Original Image

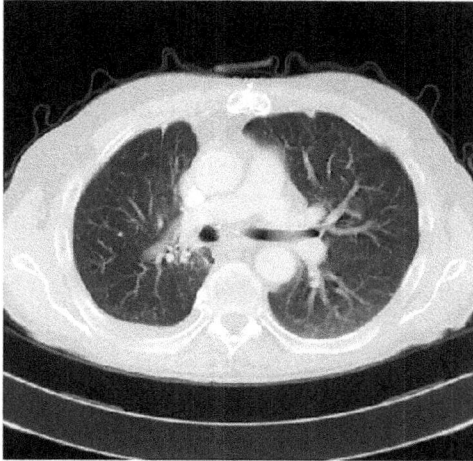

FIGURE 8.3 Original image.

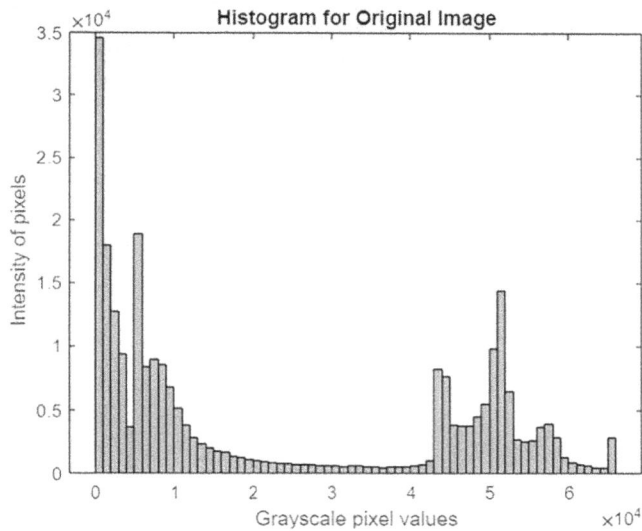

FIGURE 8.4 Histogram for original image.

Upon applying a Top Hat filter to the original image, within a radius of 10 units, the contrast between different structures are retained, whereas the bright regions of the chest wall are filtered out (Figure 8.5). This filtering ensures that the chest walls do not get wrongly diagnosed as a tumour since they both share the characteristic feature of reflecting as a white patch on CT scans. Minimal noise present in the original image (Figure 8.3) is eliminated in the resulting image upon Top Hat filtering (Figure 8.5).

The plotted histogram (Figure 8.6) depicts the frequency distribution of various grayscale levels of the filtered image (Figure 8.5). Though it does not provide any spatial information and inter-relation of the gray pixels, the pixels give information on the general shape and size of the gray value spread [25]. The x-axis represents the grayscale values of pixels, and the y-axis represents the intensity values of the pixels. It is noticeable that the frequency of 0-valued (black) pixels is much higher than the frequency of low-valued pixels. The frequency of high-valued pixels is significantly higher than the pixel values lying around its range; this makes it possible to correlate

Top-hat Filtering

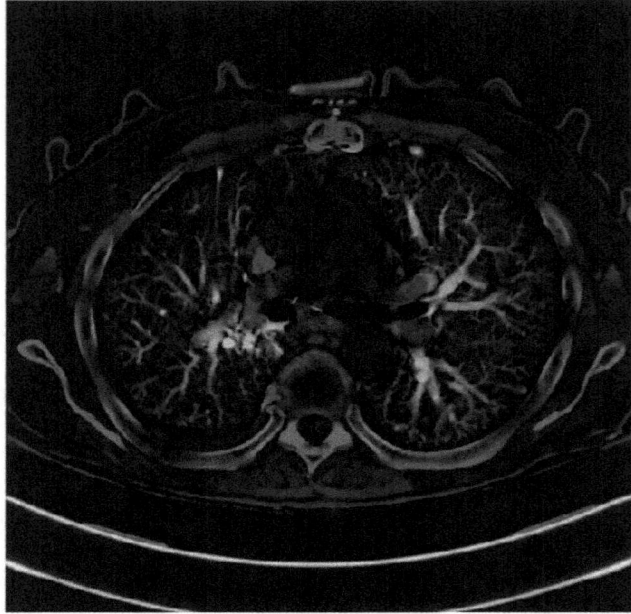

FIGURE 8.5 Top Hat filtering.

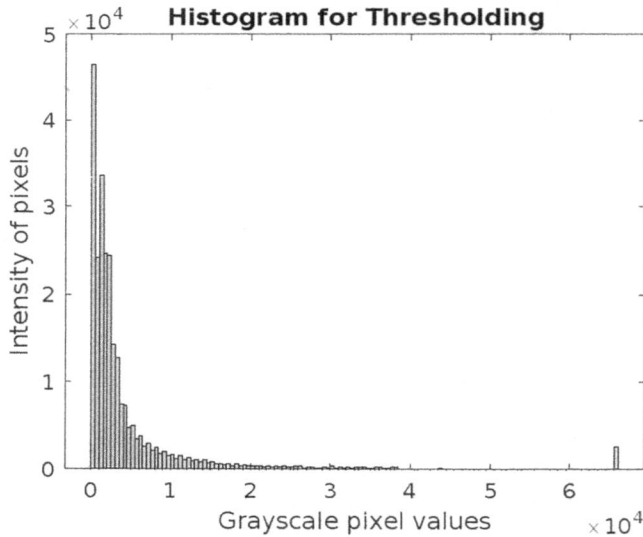

FIGURE 8.6 Histogram for thresholding.

the histogram (Figure 8.6) with the filtered image (Figure 8.5). Because there are more background pixels than foreground pixels in the filtered image, the majority of pixels are concentrated on the darker side of the grayscale in the histogram plot. The pixels toward the rightmost end of the histogram belong to the tumour.

  Upon image binarization using the optimal threshold derived from the histogram (Figure 8.6), the image (Figure 8.7) is seen to be depicted only by pixels with values strictly either 0 or 1. The

Binary Image

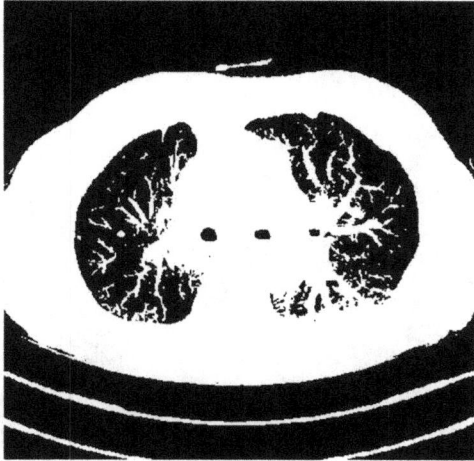

FIGURE 8.7 Binarization.

originally lighter regions are completely white, and the originally darker regions are completely dark. This outcome is achieved using thresholding techniques, as discussed prior.

The watershed transform (Figure 8.7) clearly depicts the various regions of the CT scan image. Upon comparison with Figure 8.3, it can be seen that the specific regions depict the following regions of the human chest anatomy (Table 8.1).

8.4.2 OTSU Segmentation Outputs

The histogram used for OTSU segmentation is displayed in Figure 8.8. The two characteristic peaks denote the intensity values of the pixels. The x-axis represents the grayscale values of pixels, and the y-axis represents the intensity values of the pixels. The peaks depict the lighter regions, and the valleys represent the darker regions of the CT scan. Upon finding optimal threshold values and processing the image, the OTSU segmentation technique yields the final output (Figure 8.9) of the project.

A defined outline of the high-intensity regions shows the potential regions of the tumour. Upon comparing Figure 8.9 with Figure 8.3, the segmented regions that represent bone can be voluntarily eliminated from evaluation. This step yields the expected outcome of the project by segmenting regions of tumour clusters. This output can also be observed in an inverse format, i.e., in the white and black format (Figure 8.10), based on the observer's preference. The inverse format is obtained by inverting the values of individual pixels. Pixels initially with a value of 1 now become 0 and vice versa.

TABLE 8.1
Regions of Watershed Transform

Colour of Region	Anatomical Region
Yellow	Right lung
Orange	External to body
Dark Blue	External to body
Light Blue	Left lung
Aqua Blue	Vertebral column
Green	Major tumour cluster

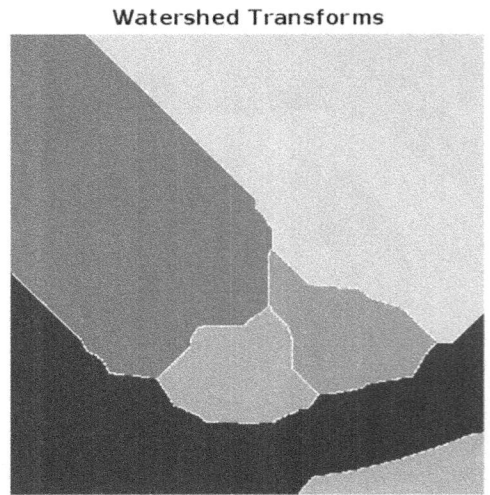

FIGURE 8.8 Watershed transforms.

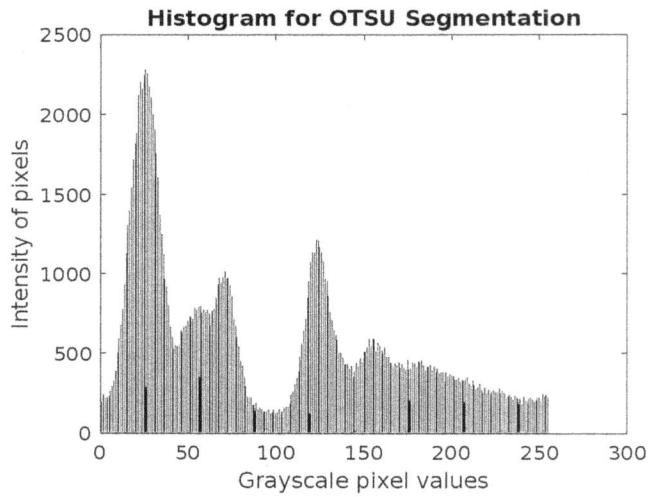

FIGURE 8.9 Histogram for OTSU Segmentation.

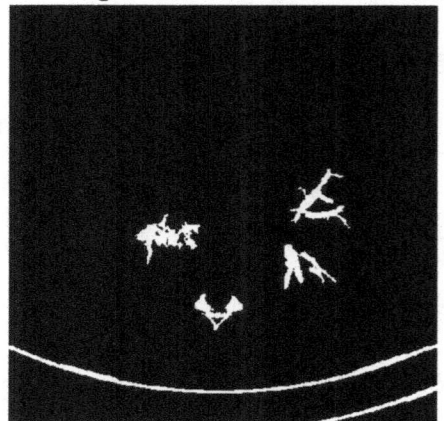

FIGURE 8.10 OTSU segmentation: black and white.

OTSU Segmentation-White and Black

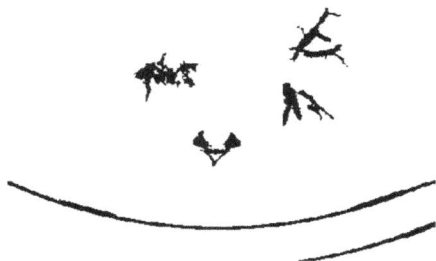

FIGURE 8.11   OTSU segmentation: white and black.

8.4.3   ANALYSIS USING QUADTREE DECOMPOSITION

From the subdivided/decomposed image (Figure 8.11), the tumour regions can be identified as the larger homogeneous blocks after eliminating the consideration of completely low pixel valued blocks. The subdivided blocks with majorly high valued pixels can be correlated to the segmented tumour regions obtained in Figure 8.9. This serves as a verification for the OTSU segmentation derived output.

8.4.4   COMPARISON OF HISTOGRAMS USING DISTRIBUTION PLOTS

The data of the cumulative function distribution is seen to converge within the data range zero to one data points. This distribution significantly shows the interpolation of tumorous regions with respect to the original and segmented pixel distribution. The confidence interval allowed for the data is 99%. The normal distribution and residual distribution along the mean have a concurrent residual distribution between 3.5 to 5.5 raised to the fourth power, which matches with the fit plot. Figure 8.12 and Figure 8.13 emphasize more upon the fractionalization of regions restricted to tumour occurrences, thereby helping the observer look into the region-specific region of the tumour Figure 8.14.

Quadtree Decompositon

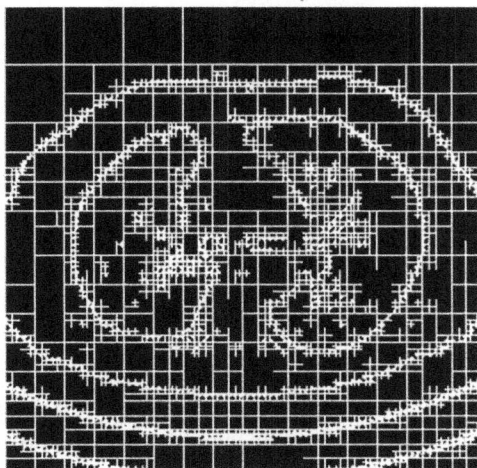

FIGURE 8.12   Quadtree decomposition.

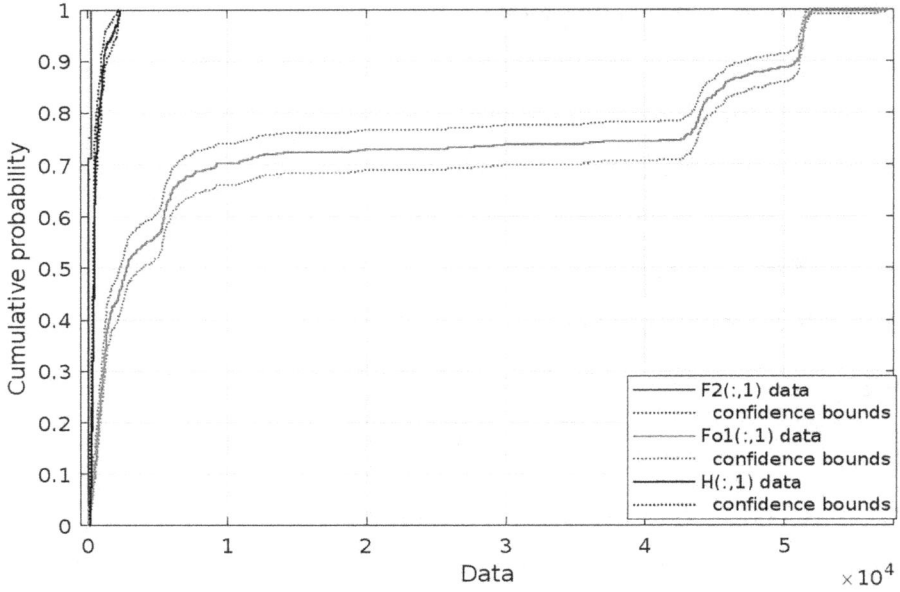

FIGURE 8.13 Cumulative function distribution.

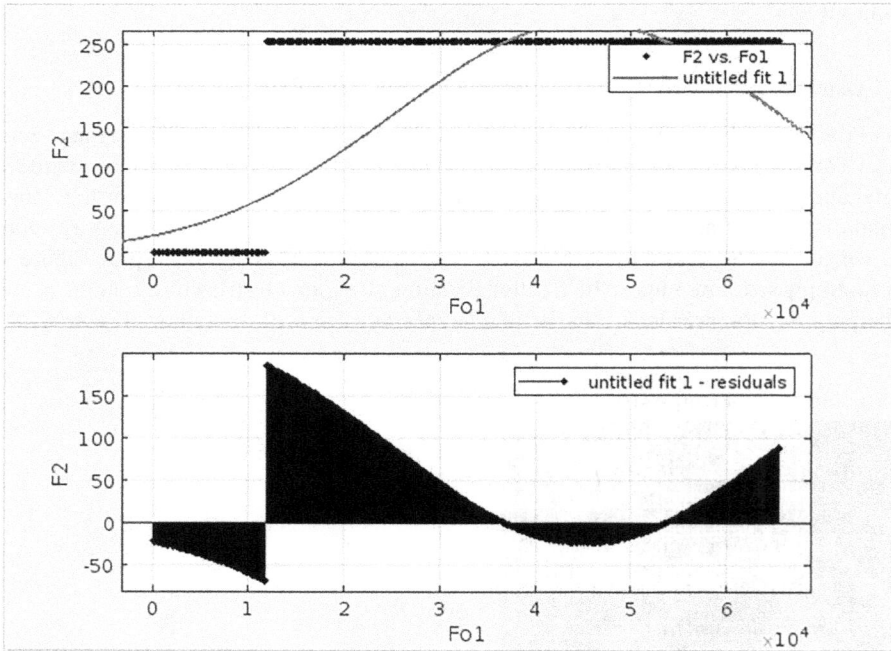

FIGURE 8.14 Residual plots.

8.5 CONCLUSIONS AND FURTHER WORK

The final result of the project mainly focuses on the segmented tumour regions from raw CT scan images of the chest. This model was reliable due to the individual advantages of the various processing techniques, such as Top Hat filtering, watershed transforms, thresholding, and OTSU segmentation. An appropriate and effective pre-processing methodology was developed for CT scan images. OTSU segmentation derived the most reliable outputs by accurately segmenting the tumour regions upon validation tests. The algorithm is tested using a DICOM image to ensure that the model will be usable with any medical equipment or accessory equipment, such as scanners, transmitters, printers, etc., since all medical images are stored in DICOM file format. The developed algorithm is reliable for automatic segmentation of lung cancer from CT scans. To automatically eliminate the bony structures that are mistaken for tumour regions, direct 3D template-matching methods can be implemented. This will allow only the tumour regions to be visible on the final output image result. Quadtree decomposition verifies the segmented tumour regions. Distribution plots allow for efficient comparison between the original image and segmented image.

The algorithm can be improved to be adaptable for other medical images, such as MRIs and ultrasound images. This improvement will need less specific pre-processing methodologies or more adaptable pre-processing techniques since different medical imaging will need enhancement of different features of the raw DICOM image. OTSU segmentation can be used advantageously for the automatic segmentation of tumours of the different organs of the body.

REFERENCES

[1] Purandare, N. C., & Rangarajan, V. (2015). Imaging of lung cancer: Implications on staging and management. *The Indian Journal of Radiology & Imaging*, *25*(2), 109–120. 10.4103/0971-3026.155831

[2] Ferlay, J., Ervik, M., Lam, F., Colombet, M., Mery, L., Piñeros, M., et al. (2020). *Global Cancer Observatory: Cancer Today*. Lyon: International Agency for Research on Cancer. (https://gco.iarc.fr/today, accessed February 2021.

[3] Whelan, C. (2022). Can CT Scans Accurately Detect Lung Cancer?

[4] Palcic, B., Lam, S., Hung, J., & MacAulay, C. (1991). Detection and localization of early lung cancer by imaging techniques. *Chest*, *99*(3), 742+. https://link.gale.com/apps/doc/A10656613/AONE?u=anon~2d8283b6&sid=googleScholar&xid=1fd01168

[5] Sujan, M., Alam, N., Noman, S. A., & Islam, M. J. (2016). A segmentation based automated system for brain tumor detection. *International Journal of Computer Applications*, *153*(10), 41–49.

[6] Saini, P. K., & Singh, M. (2015). Brain tumor detection in medical imaging using MATLAB. *International Research Journal of Engineering and Technology*, *2*(02), 191–196.

[7] Al-Bayati, M., & El-Zaart, A. (2013). Mammogram images thresholding for breast cancer detection using different thresholding methods.

[8] Amutha, A., & Wahidabanu, R. S. D. (2013, April). Lung tumor detection and diagnosis in CT scan images. In *2013 International Conference on Communication and Signal Processing* (pp. 1108–1112). IEEE.

[9] Wang, P., DeNunzio, A., Okunieff, P., & O'Dell, W. G. (2007). Lung metastases detection in CT images using 3D template matching. *Medical Physics*, *34*(3), 915–922.

[10] Nadkarni, N. S., & Borkar, S. (2019, April). Detection of lung cancer in CT images using image processing. In *2019 3rd International Conference on Trends in Electronics and Informatics (ICOEI)* (pp. 863–866). IEEE.

[11] Sammouda, R. (2016). Segmentation and analysis of CT chest images for early lung cancer detection. In: Global Summit on Computer & Information Technology.

[12] Rahane, W., Dalvi, H., Magar, Y., & Kalane, A. (2018). Lung cancer detection using image processing and machine learning healthcare. In: IEEE International Conference on Current Trends toward Converging Technologies (ICCTCT).

[13] Kalaivani, S., Chatterjee, P., Juyal, S., & Gupta, R. (2017). Lung cancer detection using digital image processing and artificial neural networks. In: International Conference on Electronics, Communication and Aerospace Technology (ICECA).

[14] Kulkarni, A., & Panditrao, A. (2014). Classification of lung cancer stages on CT scan images using image processing. In: International Conference on Advanced Communication Control and Computing Technology (ICACCCT).

[15] Miah, M. B. A., & Yousuf, M. A. (2015, May). Detection of lung cancer from CT image using image processing and neural network. In *2015 International Conference on Electrical Engineering and Information Communication Technology (ICEEICT)* (pp. 1–6). IEEE.

[16] Katre, P. R., & Thakare, A. (2017, April). Detection of lung cancer stages using image processing and data classification techniques. In *2017 2nd International Conference for Convergence in Technology (I2CT)* (pp. 402–404). IEEE.

[17] Gajanayake, G. M. N. R., Yapa, R. D., & Hewawithana, B. (2009, December). Comparison of standard image segmentation methods for segmentation of brain tumors from 2D MR images. In *2009 International Conference on Industrial and Information Systems (ICIIS)* (pp. 301–305). IEEE.

[18] Huang, M., Yu, W., & Zhu, D. (2012, August). An improved image segmentation algorithm based on the Otsu method. In *2012 13th ACIS International Conference on Software Engineering, Artificial Intelligence, Networking and Parallel/Distributed Computing* (pp. 135–139). IEEE.

[19] Xu, X., Xu, S., Jin, L., & Song, E. (2011). Characteristic analysis of Otsu threshold and its applications. *Pattern Recognition Letters, 32*(7), 956–961.

[20] AlSaeed, D. H., Bouridane, A., & El-Zaart, A. (2016). A novel fast otsu digital image segmentation method. *International Arab Journal of Information Technology, 13*(4), 427–434.

[21] Dua, S., Kandiraju, N., & Chowriappa, P. (2010). Region quad-tree decomposition based edge detection for medical images. *The Open Medical Informatics Journal, 4*, 50.

[22] Subramaniam, K., Hoffman, E. A., & Tawhai, M. H. (2013, March). Using CT imaging to quantify differences between young and elderly healthy lungs. In *Medical Imaging 2013: Biomedical Applications in Molecular, Structural, and Functional Imaging* (Vol. 8672, pp. 236–241). SPIE.

[23] Albertina, B., Watson, M., Holback, C., Jarosz, R., Kirk, S., Lee, Y., … Lemmerman, J. (2016). Radiology Data from The Cancer Genome Atlas Lung Adenocarcinoma [TCGA-LUAD] collection. *The Cancer Imaging Archive*. 10.7937/K9/TCIA.2016.JGNIHEP5

[24] Clark, K., Vendt, B., Smith, K., Freymann, J., Kirby, J., Koppel, P., Moore, S., Phillips, S., Maffitt, D., Pringle, M., Tarbox, L., & Prior, F. (December, 2013). The Cancer Imaging Archive (TCIA): Maintaining and Operating a Public Information Repository. *Journal of Digital Imaging, 26*(6), 1045–1057. (paper)

[25] Bashir, U., Siddique, M. M., Mclean, E., Goh, V., & Gary, J. (2016). Imaging Heterogeneity in Lung Cancer: Techniques, Applications, and Challenges. *Cook American Journal of Roentgenology, 207*(3), 534–543.

9 Reshaping the Pathology

An AI Perspective

Juhi Dwivedi, Bramah Hazela, Shikha Singh, Pallavi Asthana, and Vineet Singh
Amity University, Uttar Pradesh, India

CONTENTS

9.1 INTRODUCTION: BACKGROUND AND DRIVING FORCES

The stimulation of human intelligence by machines is artificial intelligence. The theory and creation of computer programs can carry out tasks and resolve issues that call for the human intellect.

9.1.1 How Does AI Operate?

With large volumes of labeled training data, AI systems analyze the data for connections and patterns. They forecast future conditions based on these patterns. Additionally, by studying millions of instances, an image-recognition program can learn to recognize and characterize things in photos.

Reverse engineering human traits and abilities into a machine and exploiting its computing prowess to outperform us is the process of creating an AI system. Numerous sub-domains of artificial intelligence are applied to the various fields of the industry to better understand how AI functions [1–3].

- Machine learning (ML): ML teaches a computer to draw conclusions and make decisions based on prior knowledge. Without relying on human experience, it recognizes patterns and examines historical data to deduce the significance of these data points and reach a potential conclusion.
- Deep learning: Deep learning is a machine-learning (ML) technique that trains a computer to process inputs through layers to categorize, infer, and predict the outcome.
- Neural networks: These algorithms simulate how the human brain processes data by capturing the link between several underlying variables.
- Natural language processing (NLP): NLP is the process through which a machine reads, comprehends, and interprets a language.
- Computer vision: Computer-vision algorithms attempt to comprehend a picture by dissecting the image and examining various aspects of the object. The machine may then classify and learn from a collection of images to get superior results based on earlier findings.
- Cognitive computing: By analysing text, audio, images, and other input the way a human would, cognitive computing algorithms seek to simulate the functioning of the human brain and attempt to produce the intended results.

9.1.2 The Three Cognitive Skills of AI

- Learning processes: This area of AI programming is concerned with gathering data and formulating the rules that will transform the data into meaningful knowledge. The algorithms give computing devices detailed instructions on how to carry out a specific task.
- Reasoning processes: This area of AI programming is concerned with selecting the best algorithm to produce the desired result.
- Self-correction processes: This feature of AI programming is to optimize algorithms and make sure they deliver the best outcomes [3].

9.2 AI ADVANCEMENT IN PATHOLOGY: AN INTRODUCTION

Artificial intelligence has made its remarkable way into the field of pathology. AI has proved to be an asset in a wide variety of markets. Some examples include its applications in healthcare, business, education, reinforcement, finance, law, manufacturing, banking, transportation, and security.

AI refers to educating a computer to solve a problem without giving explicit instructions on each step. It is common to draw a contrast between traditional machine learning and more contemporary methods like deep learning. AI applications have multiplied exponentially due to several developments during the past 10 years. Among the advancements are better hardware, better algorithms, and an increasing quantity of available data. These developments were in line with the pathology field's growing digitization trend [4,5]. Algorithms using AI and ML are beneficial for solving simple problems. Analysis of tissue samples from significant screening initiatives, such as colorectal cancer screening, and situations when numerous slides with identical content are submitted (such as with sections of prostate specimens) are included in routine pathological diagnosis.

One of the most promising areas of diagnostic medicine is digital pathology. It is a popular area of primary study. Digital pathology encompasses more than merely converting histopathology slides into digital images. Combining many data sources with recent developments in artificial intelligence and machine learning makes novel knowledge measurable by a human expert available. An integrated strategy is needed to build a solid foundation for an "augmented pathologist."

9.3 LITERATURE REVIEW

Artificial intelligence can detect specific features within that image (characterizing an image in terms of classification labels) that contribute to understanding its clinical behavior. The image analysis may be robust and provide more information than the unaided morphological interpretation by the human mind. However, the capability may get compromised by the vast annotated datasets required for supervised deep-learning training as currently implemented. The unsupervised experiential training that occurs in the case of humans is not currently helpful. However, multiple weakly supervised strategies substantially reduce the amount of specific annotation mandatory for training.

9.3.1 ARTIFICIAL INTELLIGENCE IN PATHOLOGY

The use of AI-assisted methods in medical contexts has recently increased. They might be used more widely, especially in the field of imaging. For instance, numerous businesses now provide solutions for radiology that address regular diagnostic issues, yet none of these services are used nationally. This trend occurs cautiously in pathology because full-slide scanners are still infrequently employed for formal diagnosis due to many complicated causes, such as high investment costs, security concerns, or pathologists' objections. Specific academic and commercial institutions are conducting ground-breaking research in this field [6].

9.3.1.1 Applications in Medical Imaging

The ability to identify pulmonary nodules with CT, detect polyps in CT colonography, screen for breast cancer, find microcalcification clusters (early signs of breast cancer) in mammography, and detect masses for benign or malignant in mammography. AI with computer-aided detection methods in mammography increase the diagnostic precision for the classification of breast cancer.

The diagnosis of stroke utilizing neuroimaging with CT and MRI with deep-learning technologies automates the extraction and classification of imaging information with speed and power. Radiomics, picture segmentation, and multimodal prognostication are significant research fields. On the CT front, a decision-support tool automating the Alberta Stroke Program Early CT Score (ASPECTS) assessment tool for early ischemia alterations is now under development. This tool is comparable to one recently approved by the FDA. Additionally, AI is combined with CT angiography to distinguish between carotid plaque and free-floating intraluminal thrombus and to accurately assess the level of cerebral edema to predict recovery following stroke. It might help in the early triage of stroke patients who would benefit from craniectomy.

By enabling doctors in isolated and rural areas to contact and consult with specialized pathologists, AI, in conjunction with digital pathology, may even advance telepathology (the practice of pathology over the internet). These two technologies have the potential to reduce inter-reader variability among pathologists by making it simple to transmit photos so that a second reader may validate findings. AI will be used in digital pathology methods to identify information in images not visible to the human eye, such as molecular markers in cancers. Such findings might support early diagnosis and result in new illness micro classifications [7].

9.3.1.2 Addressing Bio-disaster X Threats with Artificial Intelligence and 6G Technologies

According to studies, bio-disaster X could ruin economies and upend people's lives and livelihoods. In essence, it represents a growing threat to civilizations everywhere. In detail, effective AI and 6G-enabled strategies were observed to shed light on bio-disaster X threats. These strategies ranged from natural language processing to deep-learning-based image analysis to address problems like early bio-disaster X detection (like identification of suspicious behaviors), remote design and development of pharmaceuticals (like treatment development), and public health interventions (like reactive shelter-at-home mandate enforcement), as well as disaster resiliency.

Due to the possible adverse effects bio-disaster X could have on people and the economy, it is an impending but preventable catastrophe. Deploying technology-based solutions to avoid and contain bio-disaster X risks may be more realistic and cost-effective than relying on the professional attention of overworked medical professionals and government officials. More research could investigate how the fusion of AI and 6G systems could improve high-impact readiness even more [8].

9.3.1.3 Prostate Cancer Risk Stratification via Light Sheet Microscopy

Most prostate cancer diagnosis depends on pathologists' interpretation of thin 2D sections of prostate biopsies. With the aid of these 2D sections, it is possible to deduce the 3D structure of cancer and grade it using the ISUP grading system, which positively correlates with patient outcomes and aids in formulating crucial clinical judgments.

The findings demonstrate that 3D pathology with AI outperforms AI approaches utilizing conventional 2D sections and accurately stratifies high-risk versus lower-risk patients. The study is noteworthy for its use of artificial intelligence to 3D digital pathology datasets from clinical biopsies and an ex-vivo microscopy approach (light-sheet microscopy), which allows for 3D imaging of the complete prostate core needle biopsies. The method offers a promising novel prostate cancer diagnosis that can be utilized in conjunction with pathologist interpretation of conventional 2D sections if proven in more significant patient cohorts [9].

9.3.1.4 The Applications of Artificial Intelligence in Chest Imaging of COVID-19 Patients

Worldwide healthcare and economic crisis occurred during the outbreak of COVID-19 (coronavirus disease 2019) infection, often known as the SARS-CoV-2 [Severe Acute Respiratory Syndrome Coronavirus 2 (SARS-CoV-2)]. The clinical evaluation of patients with suspected or confirmed COVID-19 infection required diagnostic imaging for disease identification, screening, and stratification. However, imaging aids in the differentiation of COVID-19 from other lung infections and illnesses. Imaging helps distinguish COVID-19 from other lung infections and diseases.

AI-based COVID-19 classification and segmentation models are developed by first training them on various image sources, often normal and abnormal (COVID-19, non-COVID-19) chest pictures. Thus, gathering data is considered mandatory. The system's working is portrayed in the flowchart in Figure 9.1.

After ethical approval, patient data must be retrieved, queried, accurately de-identified, and securely kept. Pseudonymization is the best method for de-identification; when the DICOM pictures are pseudonymized, the subject's identity is replaced with "pseudonyms" or identifiers [10].

9.3.1.5 A Narrative Review of Digital Pathology and Artificial Intelligence Focusing on Lung Cancer

With the development of whole-slide imaging (WSI) technologies, pathology diagnosis is also possible online. The uses of digital pathology are constantly growing, from helping rural institutions with a pathologist shortage to everyday use in diagnoses like lung cancer.

The use of whole-slide images (WSIs), also virtual slides, has substantially increased thanks to improvements in the speed of glass slide digitization technology and the decline in storage costs. Users of WSIs can view digital slides on electronic displays at various magnifications, just like in the Google Maps app. The adoption of digital pathology has been more gradual for a variety of reasons, such as the difficulty in determining the return on investment. Adoption still presents difficulties, despite the regulatory approval of numerous commercial systems. Pathology lab procedures, such as slide preparation, quality control, labeling, and bespoke integration with current laboratory information systems, must be changed significantly to digitalize a pathology practice (LIS).

Hiring someone to look after storage systems and the systems themselves is expensive [11].

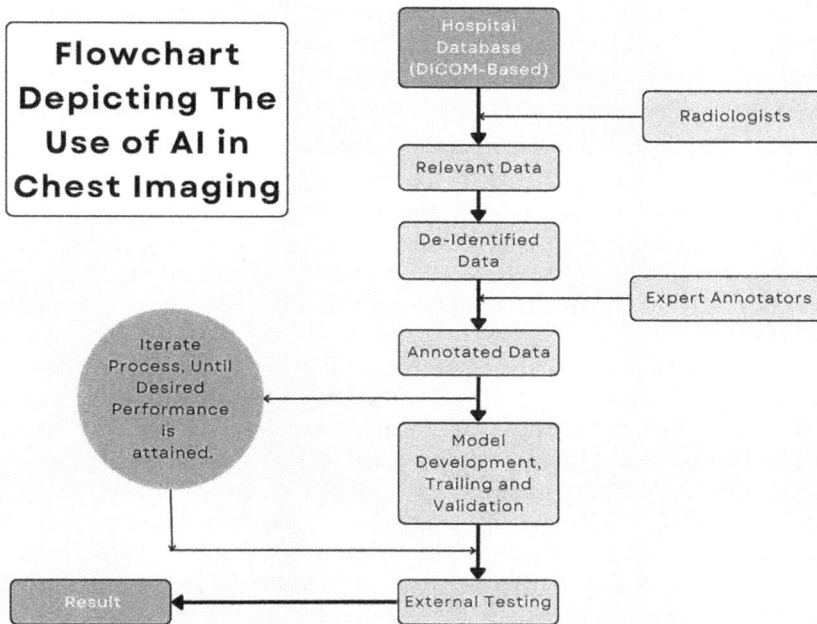

Flowchart Depicting The Use of AI in Chest Imaging

Hospital Database (DICOM-Based)

Radiologists

Relevant Data

De-Identified Data

Expert Annotators

Annotated Data

Iterate Process, Until Desired Performance is attained.

Model Development, Trailing and Validation

Result

External Testing

FIGURE 9.1 Flowchart depicting the use of AI in chest imaging.

9.3.1.6 Artificial Intelligence-based Analysis of Genetic Data

The concept of genotype-phenotype coupling implicates that it is highly likely that changes in morphology in tumor tissue—for example, with a mutation in a critical gene—are also identified. Besides the ability to anticipate molecular or clinical factors based on histo-morphological data, AI applications will play an increasingly essential role in interpreting molecular pathological data. As an illustration, deep-learning categorizes the deoxyribonucleic acid (DNA) methylation profiles of lung squamous cell carcinomas to separate metastatic head and neck cancer from primary lung cancer.

9.3.1.7 First FDA-cleared AI Product in Digital Pathology

On September 21st, 2021, the FDA granted Paige the first marketing authorization for an AI product in digital pathology for its prostate cancer diagnosis system: Paige Prostate. In addition to data analysis of digitally scanned whole-slide images (WSIs) produced from prostate biopsies, the software is designed to help pathologists identify areas suspected of malignancy. The FDA gave their product a brand-new classification: "Software algorithm device to aid users in digital pathology." A software algorithm device to aid pathologists in digital pathology is an *in vitro* diagnostic device meant to analyze acquired scanned pathology entire slide images, according to this general type of equipment description.

It uses computer algorithms to provide details on picture elements' presence, position, and properties that have therapeutic consequences. The user is supposed to use the information collected from this gadget to make a pathological diagnosis [12].

9.4 METHODOLOGY

H&E-stained slides are used for scanning the majority of the digital pathology images for AI. Tissue sectioning, staining, paraffin embedding, grossing, and formalin fixing are just a few processes pathology samples undergo. Each step in the process and the different hardware and software used with the digital image scanners can impact the quality of the digital photographs, including their color, brightness, contrast, and scale. It is strongly encouraged to reduce the influence of these variances before using the images in automated analysis activities for the best outcomes.

One method used to lessen such discrepancies is normalization. $\left[V(new) = \frac{\{V(old) - a\}}{\{f(scale) + b\}} \right]$ It is used for the values of each channel in color images or the pixels in grayscale images. Since images taken from separate devices can have varying pixel sizes, even at the same magnification level, scale normalization is a concern when numerous image acquisition devices are employed. Since they all used the same image acquisition method, such as a specific microscopic camera or digital slide scanner, scale normalization has not been mentioned in related research [13–16].

Many researchers favored CNN as a base algorithm for their deep-learning models. Deep-learning-based models, particularly CNNs, have recently gained considerable attention.

Transfer learning and data augmentation should be employed to get better results. While later layers, such as fully connected layers or deconvolutional layers, are initialized randomly in transfer learning, the convolutional layer parameters of a CNN are imported into the target CNN as layer initialization. A well-known dataset like ImageNet is used to pre-train a CNN's convolutional layer parameters. Different training stages can update only the imported layer parameters or all of the layer parameters, including the ones that were randomly initialized for the layers. The development of a model without transfer learning is supposed to produce superior outcomes when there is adequate data.

An efficient way to improve image data is to apply multiple transformations to the provided image while maintaining its core elements. These transformations include rotation (90, 180, and 270 degrees), flipping (horizontal/vertical), scaling, random translations, blurring, and sharpening, as well as introducing jitters to the color and brightness and adjusting the contrast histogram, among others [17,18].

Since applying large medical images directly to CNN is challenging, another type of augmentation uses the patch construction method. From a sizeable problematic image with a size between 1024×1024 (camera) and $> 104 \times 104$ (scanner) pixels, smaller patches with sizes between 32×32 and 512×512 pixels are recovered for use in training and inference of CNNs.

Instead of using the pre-generated image patches throughout the training phase, resampling patches throughout each training epoch can increase the variance in training data and decrease the likelihood of overfitting. Once the patch-level CNN is trained, a different ML model is usually made for the decision at the complete picture level. A patch-level decision is taken for each patch in the training images to produce heatmap-like output, from which many features are retrieved using traditional image-analysis methods. The gathered feature values from the training images are then supplied into the target picture-level ML model [16].

Figure 9.2 shows the framework of a CNN Model.

Machine learning (ML) uses data to develop predictive models to find patterns or carry out operations like regression or classification. ML techniques fall into two categories: supervised learning and unsupervised learning. In various implementations, WSIs are normalized for quick processing, annotated by a skilled user, and divided into image patches after being aligned using a multiresolution registration technique. To uncover properties that are useful for recognizing and classifying ROIs in images, an ML model may be trained using the image patches [19].

In CAD methodology, the image's general qualities are the foundation for the optimization. A typical image index is built utilizing these global image features after each image in a database of images with a known ROI has evaluated its global image characteristics. Based on their image characteristic index, the database's photos are divided into several image groups, with the CAD scheme for each group. The global image features of the digitized picture are established when the

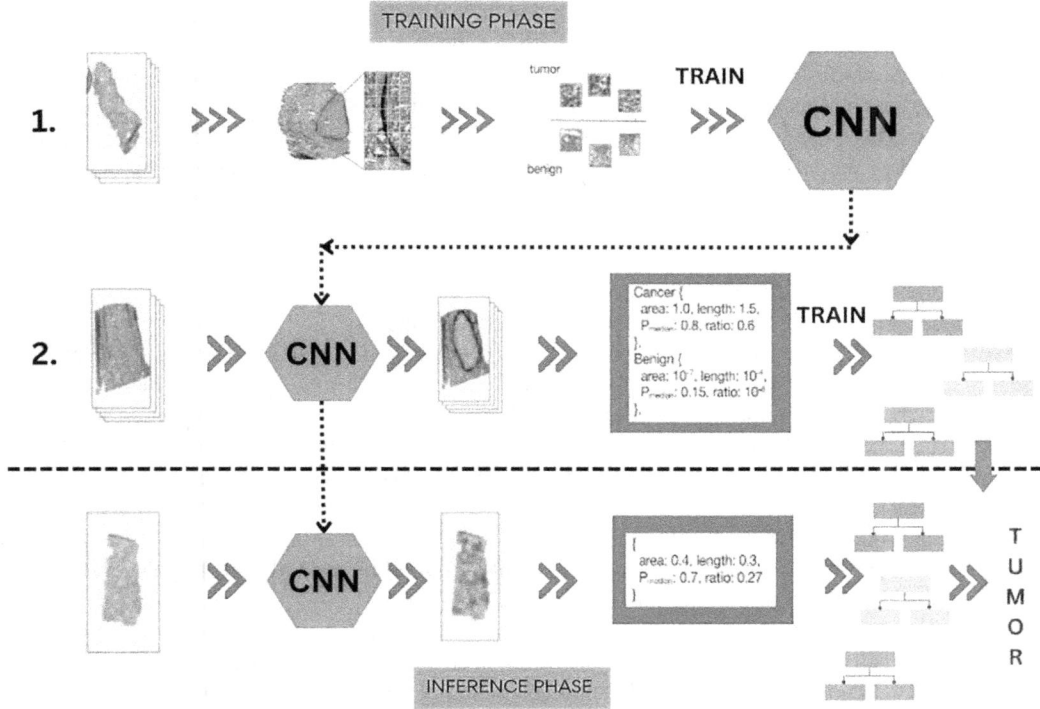

FIGURE 9.2 CNN deep-learning based model.

construction of classification criteria optimizes the CAD system for processing a digital image based on that image's characteristics. The digitized image is given an image rating once the global image attributes are detected, and the image is then assigned to an image group based on the image rating. A detection method adapted to the designated image group is used to determine the ROI shown in the image [20–23].

9.5 DISCUSSION

Pathologists often annotate structures, train, and evaluate algorithms to detect and classify these structures, and then validate the algorithms. In this scenario, the taught AI platform will absorb all the biases of the pathologists who developed the ground truth. A competent pathologist who signs off on the case would study the results produced by AI, determine whether they should be used, and evaluate the accuracy of the predictions made by the technology.

The ground truth, for instance, might differ between an algorithm created under the direction of a top expert pathologist and a platform developed using a solid and convincing correlation to clinical data such as prognosis and therapy effectiveness. Therefore, explaining how ground truth was established for each algorithm is crucial in developing AI algorithms [24,25].

The paucity of prospective, randomized, multi-center trials evaluating the benefit for pathologists and patients is now the most significant obstacle to using AI-based methods. Studies are necessary to identify AI solutions that improve outcomes. For research, high-quality clinical data are just as important as photographic data. Considering these issues, the use of digital pathology and AI has the potential to revolutionize the industry and help pathologists complete their work more efficiently and adequately.

In this review study, we gathered data on prior developments, assessed the industry's position now, and speculated on potential future trends of AI in DP.

However, the studies mentioned above, and reviews did not demonstrate sufficient robustness and reproducibility to be incorporated into routine clinical practice because of biases in datasets, either too small or too heterogeneous, poor data integration, or insufficient validation. Additionally, specific machine-learning models could exhibit bias due to overfitting and underfitting. A specific criterion was set for including and excluding the chosen research to overcome the constraints associated with selection bias [26].

To minimize existing prejudices and further widening health disparities, many healthcare workers believe in decoding the present and restructuring current practices before involving AI. This mindset has proved to be a hindrance in AI advancement [27].

Artificial intelligence has come a long way in the previous 65 years. Healthcare-related AI research has advanced over the preceding two decades and is now applied in many different medical subspecialties, including pathology, radiology, and dermatology. A national or worldwide plan is needed for AI and digital pathology (DP) to be used for automated diagnosis, case triaging for improved workflow, or providing pathologists with new insights. The DP system will provide a second opinion and the advantages of time and cost savings over the traditional microscope-based pathology approach. It will also lessen the inter- observer variation problem if the system's requirements—appropriate slide image management software, integrated reporting systems, faster scanning, and high-quality images—are met.

However, AI methods, including deep learning, are subject to legitimate criticism because it is unknown how they function internally to make decisions by design. As a result, it will be necessary to resolve any legal and regulatory difficulties before realizing any benefits. Despite the few setbacks, precision image processing at a faster rate is one of AI's most significant advantages in pathology. Additionally, it aids in the early detection of biomarkers during testing, saving pathologists time studying samples. The development of brightfield and fluorescent slide scanners has also made it possible for pathologists to detect concealed problems. In their daily work, medical personnel is helped by procedures like immunohistochemistry and digital histopathology. A cloud-based data management system can be used to store digital data, enabling remote access to other pathology centers located in various locations [28].

The multidimensional applications of AI in the field of pathology and its future objectives have been graphically represented in Figure 9.3.

9.6   FUTURE SCOPE

Several models have been proposed in various research, as stated in this study; hence, these models must be further validated and applied in other domains to ensure that these models can be implemented in various locations efficiently. Due to the primary concerns in healthcare systems late diagnosis, incorrect treatment, and misinterpretation—appropriate systems must be created with the incorporation of cutting-edge software, tools, and technology.

To successfully utilize artificial intelligence in the creation of smart cities, it is required to analyze and save the available data so that it can be used to produce effective AI and deep learning algorithms for the advancement of pathologies [29,30].

It is promising that the automated morphological analysis has become more accurate thanks to DL technology. The pathology definition in AI is increasing to encompass prognosis prediction and assessment of illness severity. A pathological diagnosis is more than just a morphological diagnosis; it involves a nuanced process of analyzing and making decisions based on clinical information about various organs and illnesses. A large amount of data, including genetic data, clinical data, and digital images, is necessary to construct AI that can manage a variety of clinical circumstances.

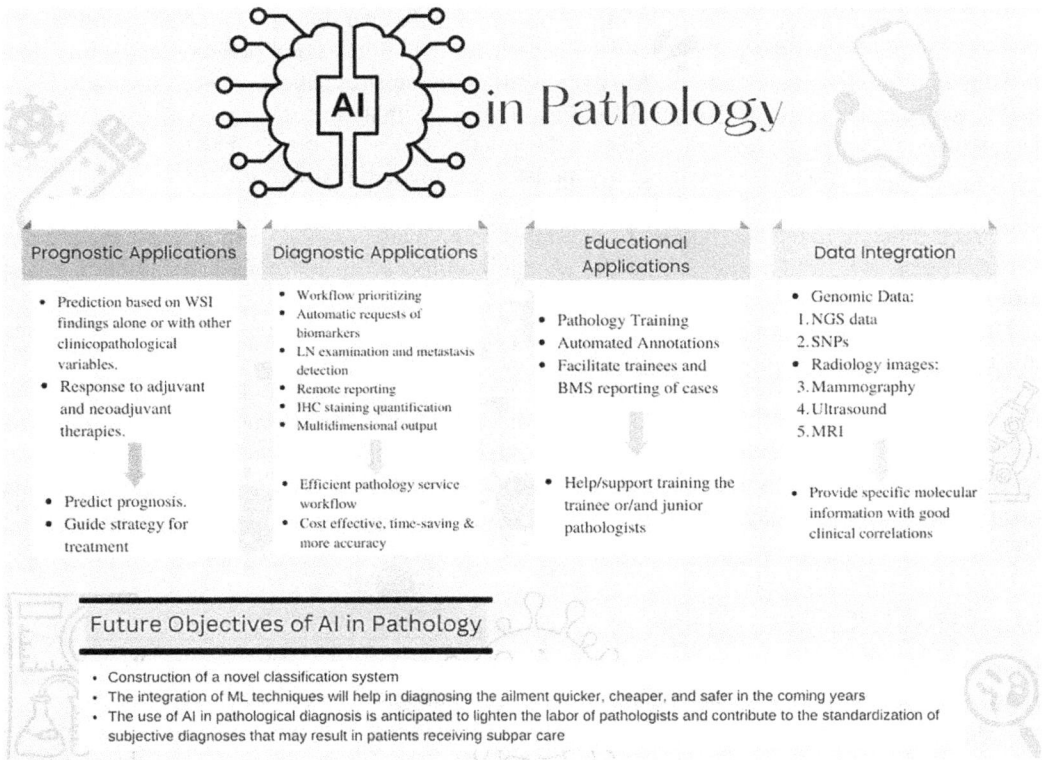

FIGURE 9.3 AI applications in the field of pathology.

Various types of research have been done using public medical databases, like TCGA. They are an excellent place to start when researching and developing medical AI, but much more high-quality data is required. For instance, to develop an AI that can analyze pathology images and human pathologists, it is necessary to create and validate detailed annotations on many pathology images.

9.6.1 Challenges in the Implementation of Artificial Intelligence-based Diagnosis

Although artificial intelligence and machine learning have the potential to revolutionize the area of pathology, their translational use confronts several significant challenges. The amount of data consumed, and an AI system's accuracy are closely related. In the study by Campanella et al., the validation error decreased by around 10 when 100 times more occurrences were analyzed. However, a dearth of histopathological specimens is available in digital form for computer analysis. Additionally, digitalization always requires high up-front costs.

Even though there will be a significant increase in the volume of digital data over the medium term, or at the latest, within the next 10 years, a complete study and detailed description of these data by experienced pathologists are still lacking.

Another factor that substantially influences the accuracy of an AI model is the data quality, which has significant implications for it (garbage in, garbage out problem). The guide "Digital Pathology," published by the professional association of German pathologists (Berufsverband Deutscher Pathologen e. V.), offers aid with the digitization of pathology. It notably encourages the use of digital technology while highlighting the freedom of method choice and the pathologist's responsibility for the selected diagnosis route [31].

The most significant obstacle to using AI-based methods now is the lack of prospective, randomized, multicentered trials evaluating the benefit for pathologists and patients separately. Such investigations are crucial to discover AI solutions that can improve patient-related outcomes. High-quality clinical data are equally crucial for this research as imaging data. Essentially, this is about the possible predictive application of AI-based methods. If these problems are fixed, AI and digital pathology have the potential to change the industry and make it possible for pathologists to finish their tasks more swiftly and precisely.

Privacy protection, the utilization of proprietary techniques, a lack of funding, and the absence of pathologists who can participate in the annotation process are difficulties in producing such high-quality data.

The ultimate solution to such challenges is collaborating with numerous hospitals and medical labs to create a sizable amount of meticulously labeled and annotated medical data.

A medical AI prognostic prediction model that combines clinical data, genetic data, and morphology will eventually exist. Additionally, an AI model learned from the patient's prognosis mixed with several characteristics such as tumor markers, morphology, and treatment options can develop a new grading system relevant to other tumor types. This system will overcome the inconsistent current grading and staging results across pathologists and help to improve patient clinical outcomes [32–34].

9.7 CONCLUSION

By automating processes like finding metastases, recognizing tumor cells, and counting mitoses shortly, AI has the potential to change the quality completely, precision, and effectiveness of pathology. The use of AI in pathological diagnosis is anticipated to lighten the labor of pathologists and contribute to the standardization of subjective diagnoses that may result in patients receiving subpar care.

Pathologists interested in AI/ML envision various tools that may provide better efficiency and accuracy in the regular diagnostic workflow. These tools could scan slides to count elements such as lymph node metastases, mitoses, inflammatory cells, or pathologic organisms, presenting results at sign-out and flagging examples for review. AI/ML tools could even flag regions on a slide and prioritize cases based on slide content. Future systems may be able to correlate patterns across multiple inputs from the medical record, including genomics, allowing a more comprehensive prognostic statement in the pathology report.

Integrating ML techniques will help diagnose the ailment quicker, cheaper, and safer in the coming years. However, various biases stand as a hurdle. They must be overcome to develop other ML-based algorithms to guarantee sufficient robustness and reproducibility for their integration into clinical practice. Many proposed ML models could not be proven fit for translation in clinical practice. Higher-quality datasets, articles with sufficient documentation, and external validation are required to give the currently developed ML models sufficient robustness and reproducibility to integrate them into the existing clinical practice.

It is perhaps sufficient to say that AI advancements in pathology hold the potential to revolutionize the healthcare industry. However, the journey to make our expectations a reality is not an easy one. It would require a breakthrough that will gain the trust of pathologists across the globe. The results so far are accurate to a certain extent but not enough to be independent of human intelligence.

To conclude, despite the many challenges posed by society, funding departments, and lack of appropriate technology, AI advancements are gradually advancing in the field of pathology. Many pathologists have their hopes tied to the progress of AI/ML to assist them in their workload and give patients a better healthcare environment Table 9.1.

TABLE 9.1

Key Terms Used

S.No.	Term	Description
1	Artificial intelligence	Computer behavior resembles intelligent or human behavior. Methods like machine learning are employed to assist with this intelligence.
2	Machine learning	Computer algorithms improve with experience and generate artificial knowledge.
3	Deep learning	A subfield of machine learning is mainly concerned with using artificial neural networks.
4	Artificial neural network	Ths network consists of artificial neurons arranged in layers or planes, or one after the other. They are used in deep-learning applications.
5	Convolutional network	A subtype of artificial neural networks reduces the input of presumably relevant features by using specific folding matrices. They are used in automated image-recognition applications.
6	Recurrent neural network	In recurrent neural networks, weighted connections exist not only in the direction of the output layer but also in preceding layers or levels, creating a kind of memory that is useful in recognizing sequences.
7	Support vector machine	The support-vector machine, a popularly used illustration of traditional mechanical science, illustrates a mathematical pattern-recognition model. The goal of classification is to create as much space between each subject as possible by classifying objects.
8	Transfer learning	Artificial neural networks employ transfer learning. This learning explains how a network is initially trained on a dataset before being applied to further data.
9	Graphical processing unit	This unit is frequently used hardware components for artificial neural network training.
10	Multiple instance learning	A technique wherein, not every training example is annotated. Instead, some situations—like all picture tiles—are assigned to a slide. The annotating procedure is made more accessible.

REFERENCES

[1] McCarthy, J. (2004). What is artificial intelligence. *URL*: http://www-formal.stanford.edu/jmc/whatisai.html

[2] Dick, S. (2019). Artificial intelligence.

[3] Davenport, T. H., & Ronanki, R. (2018). Artificial intelligence for the real world. *Harvard Business Review*, 96(1), 108–116.

[4] Jiang, Y., Yang, M., Wang, S., Li, X., & Sun, Y. (2020). Emerging role of deep learning-based artificial intelligence in tumor pathology. *Cancer Communications*, 40(4), 154–166.

[5] Niazi, M. K. K., Parwani, A. V., & Gurcan, M. N. (2019). Digital pathology and artificial intelligence. *The Lancet Oncology*, 20(5), e253–e261.

[6] Cui, M., & Zhang, D. Y. (2021). Artificial intelligence and computational pathology. *Laboratory Investigation*, 101(4), 412–422.

[7] Mason, J., Morrison, A., & Visintini, S. (2018). *An Overview of Clinical Applications of Artificial Intelligence*. Ottawa: CADTH.

[8] Su, Z., McDonnell, D., Bentley, B. L., He, J., Shi, F., Cheshmehzangi, A., ... & Jia, P. (2021). Addressing Biodisaster X threats with artificial intelligence and 6G technologies: literature review and critical insights. *Journal of Medical Internet Research*, 23(5), e26109.

[9] Xie, W., Reder, N. P., Koyuncu, C., Leo, P., Hawley, S., Huang, H., Mao, C., Postupna, N., Kang, S., Serafin, R., Gao, G., Han, Q., Bishop, K. W., Barner, L. A., Fu, P., Wright, J. L., Keene, C. D., Vaughan, J. C., Janowczyk, A., Glaser, A. K., Madabhushi, A., True, L. D., & Liu, J. T. C.. (2022 Jan 15). Prostate Cancer Risk Stratification via Nondestructive 3D Pathology with Deep Learning-Assisted Gland Analysis. *Cancer Research*, 82(2), 334–345. doi: 10.1158/0008-5472.CAN-21-2843. Epub 2021 Dec 1. PMID: 34853071; PMCID: PMC8803395.

[10] Laino, M. E., Ammirabile, A., Posa, A., Cancian, P., Shalaby, S., Savevski, V., & Neri, E. (2021). The applications of artificial intelligence in chest imaging of COVID-19 patients: a literature review. *Diagnostics, 11*(8), 1317.

[11] Sakamoto, T., Furukawa, T., Lami, K., Pham, H. H. N., Uegami, W., Kuroda, K., ... & Fukuoka, J. (2020). A narrative review of digital pathology and artificial intelligence: focusing on lung cancer. *Translational Lung Cancer Research, 9*(5), 2255.

[12] Jurmeister, P., Bockmayr, M., Seegerer, P., et al. (2019). Machine learning analysis of DNA methylation profiles distinguishes primary lung squamous cell carcinomas from head and neck metastases. *Science Translational Medicine, 11*, eaaw8513.

[13] Chang, H. Y., Jung, C. K., Woo, J. I., Lee, S., Cho, J., Kim, S. W., & Kwak, T. Y. (2019). Artificial intelligence in pathology. *Journal of Pathology and Translational Medicine, 53*(1), 1–12.

[14] Komura, D., & Ishikawa, S. (2018). Machine learning methods for histopathological image analysis. *Computational and Structural Biotechnology Journal, 16*, 34–42.

[15] Li, Y., & Ping, W. (2018). Cancer metastasis detection with neural conditional random field. *arXiv preprint arXiv:1806.07064.*

[16] Mobadersany, P., Yousefi, S., Amgad, M., Gutman, D. A., Barnholtz-Sloan, J. S., Velázquez Vega, J. E., ... & Cooper, L. A. (2018). Predicting cancer outcomes from histology and genomics using convolutional networks. *Proceedings of the National Academy of Sciences, 115*(13), E2970–E2979.

[17] Zhang, L., Sonka, M., Lu, L., Summers, R. M., & Yao, J. (2017, April). Combining fully convolutional networks and graph-based approach for automated segmentation of cervical cell nuclei. In *2017 IEEE 14th International Symposium on Biomedical Imaging (ISBI 2017)* (pp. 406–409). IEEE.

[18] Ailia, M. J., Thakur, N., Abdul-Ghafar, J., Jung, C. K., Yim, K., & Chong, Y. (2022). Current Trend of Artificial Intelligence Patents in Digital Pathology: A Systematic Evaluation of the Patent Landscape. *Cancers, 14*(10), 2400.

[19] Sakamoto, T., Furukawa, T., Lami, K., Pham, H. H. N., Uegami, W., Kuroda, K., Kawai, M., Sakanashi, H., Cooper, L. A. D., Bychkov, A., et al. (2020). A narrative review of digital pathology and artificial intelligence: Focusing on lung cancer. *Translational Lung Cancer Research, 9*, 2255–2276.

[20] Gur, D., & Zheng, B. (21 August 2001). Image Quality Based Adaptive Optimization of Computer Aided Detection Schemes. *U.S. Patent, 6*(278), 793.

[21] Lange, H., Krueger, J., Young, G. D., Johnson, T., Voelker, F., & Potts, S. (8 November 2016). Cell-Based Tissue Analysis. *U.S. Patent, 9*(488), 639.

[22] Bachelet, I., Pollak, J. J., Levner, D., Bilu, Y., & Yorav-Raphael, N. (24 November 2020). Apparatus and Method for Analyzing a Bodily Sample. *U.S. Patent, 10*(843), 190.

[23] Eshel, Y. S., Lezmy, N., Gluck, D., Houri Yafin, A., & Pollak, J. J. (26 May 2020). Methods and Apparatus for Detecting an Entity in a Bodily Sample. *U.S. Patent, 10*(663), 712.

[24] Marble, H. D., Huang, R., Dudgeon, S. N., Lowe, A., Herrmann, M. D., Blakely, S., ... & Lennerz, J. K. (2020). A regulatory science initiative to harmonize and standardize digital pathology and machine learning processes to speed up clinical innovation to patients. *Journal of Pathology Informatics, 11*(1), 22.

[25] Serag, A., Ion-Margineanu, A., Qureshi, H., McMillan, R., Saint Martin, M. J., Diamond, J., ... & Hamilton, P. (2019). Translational AI and deep learning in diagnostic pathology. *Frontiers in Medicine, 6*, 185.

[26] Davenport, T., & Kalakota, R. (2019). The potential for artificial intelligence in healthcare. *Future Healthcare Journal, 6*(2), 94.

[27] Tizhoosh, H. R., & Pantanowitz, L. (2018). Artificial intelligence and digital pathology: challenges and opportunities. *Journal of Pathology Informatics, 9*(1), 38.

[28] Hosny, A., Parmar, C., Quackenbush, J., Schwartz, L. H., & Aerts, H. J. (2018). Artificial intelligence in radiology. *Nature Reviews Cancer, 18*(8), 500–510.

[29] Osamura, R. Y., Matsui, N., Kawashima, M., Saiga, H., Ogura, M., & Kiyuna, T. (2021). Digital/Computational Technology for Molecular Cytology Testing: A Short Technical Note with Literature Review. *Acta Cytologica, 65*(4), 342–347.

[30] Barisoni, L., Gimpel, C., Kain, R., Laurinavicius, A., Bueno, G., Zeng, C., ... & Hewitt, S. M. (2017). Digital pathology imaging as a novel platform for standardization and globalization of quantitative nephropathology. *Clinical Kidney Journal, 10*(2), 176–187.

[31] Rashidi, H. H., Tran, N. K., Betts, E. V., Howell, L. P., & Green, R. (2019). Artificial intelligence and machine learning in pathology: the present landscape of supervised methods. *Academic Pathology, 6*, 2374289519873088.

[32] Dash, R. C., Robb, J. A., Booker, D. L., Foo, W. C., Witte, D. L., & Bry, L. (2012). Biospecimens and biorepositories for the community pathologist. *Archives of Pathology & Laboratory Medicine*, *136*(6), 668–678.

[33] Willemink, M. J., Koszek, W. A., Hardell, C., Wu, J., Fleischmann, D., Harvey, H., ... & Lungren, M. P. (2020). Preparing medical imaging data for machine learning. *Radiology*, *295*(1), 4–15.

[34] Rakha, E. A., Toss, M., Shiino, S., Gamble, P., Jaroensri, R., Mermel, C. H., & Chen, P. H. C. (2021). Current and future applications of artificial intelligence in pathology: a clinical perspective. *Journal of Clinical Pathology*, *74*(7), 409–414.

10 Influence of Community Mobility Habits on the COVID-19 Pandemic
A Case Study on India

Vikas Thada
Department of CSE, Poornima University Jaipur, Rajasthan, India

Shweta Sinha
Department of CSE, Amity University, Gurgaon, Haryana, India

Utpal Shrivastava
Chitkara University School of Engineering and Technology, Badi, Solan, Himachal Pradesh, India

CONTENTS

10.1 INTRODUCTION

The rapid spread of COVID-19 urged WHO to declare it an epidemic of international concern and, soon after, on March 12, 2020, WHO announced it as a global pandemic [1]. COVID-19 is spread by severe acute respiratory syndrome coronavirus 2 (SARS-CoV-2), which are enveloped RNA viruses and have a crown-like appearance. Over the years, seven strains of these viruses have spread, having mild to fatal impacts on the human race [2]. With the second-highest population globally, India is having a hard time dealing with the COVID-9 disease. The early COVID-19 cases in India were due to people coming from abroad. By March 7, around one lakh people in the country had been infected with the disease. Owing to its fast transmission rate, the ministry of home and family welfare, the government of India, issued several advisories related to travel, including quarantine rules for 14 days, a social distance of one meter, and compulsory mask wearing to avoid disease transmission. However, even after these steps, the disease spread across the country at a very rapid pace. On May 18, 2020, the total number of confirmed cases reached one lakh, and by July 18, 2020, it crossed the mark of 8.5 lakhs. During this period, the government imposed the first phase of lockdown for 21 days. This closing was a complete lockdown, which reduced social, retail, park visits, grocery, and pharmacy mobility by −73.4%, −46.3%,−51.2%, respectively [3]. It also influenced the transit to outstations and parks along with workplaces. But, as the number of positive cases was still growing, India's government extended this lockdown until May 3, 2020, in the second phase, and it was further extended until May 31 in the third phase. The Indian Council of Medical Research (ICMR) projection highlighted that social distancing and quarantine interventions might reduce the growth rate by 62% [4]. To increase the effects of measures the Indian government was taking, the GOI levied the quarantine law under the Epidemic Disease Act, 1897. This law allowed inspecting people traveling by rail/ship (extended to cover flight) and make the suspects stay in separate places in the hospital.

Even though several measures were used and the lockdown was extended phase by phase, by the end of all of these measures, India had experienced 1,90,648 confirmed cases along with 5407 deaths [1]. Undoubtedly, with the country's huge population, the statistics highlight the government's success to no small extent. The earnest efforts of all the front-line workers, especially the doctors, nurses, and paramedics, are noteworthy. The lockdown simultaneously had a destructive impact on society, mainly on the small, medium, and large enterprises. The suddenly imposed lockdown forced millions of migrants to move to their place with no money to pay for shelter and food. This total shutdown increased the unemployment rate to 19% after one month of lockdown [5]. In general, the coronavirus disease took life through virus incursion. It badly influenced the economic and mental health of the people, in both developed and developing countries.

In the last few months, scientists have worked extensively to develop vaccines to combat the disease. After the successful trial, the vaccine has been administered to people in different countries. In India, at present, only front-line workers are being vaccinated against the virus. Until the entire population is covered, people must follow the guidelines and restrict their mobility. Previous studies have mainly focussed on the detection and forecasting of positive cases [5,6]. Few studies have highlighted the challenges the Indian government faces in tackling the situation of rural and urban India [7,8]. Apart from this challenge, the global scientific community has also addressed the environmental and social factors [9]. From the start of the spread of COVID-19 until the present, the lockdown of cities/regions and mobility restriction is the most common norm followed across the world.

In contrast to this issue, the effect of humans' mobility on the spread of COVID-19 is rarely investigated [10]. The Indian government took a very early decision to open the lockdown in a phased manner to minimize the adverse effect on the economy while considering the health challenges ahead. With the revocation of the lockdown, with several precautionary measures, people's mobility to places like parks, grocery stores, pharmacy, recreation, and transit to stations started. Google produced a dataset of these mobility patterns named Google COVID-19 Community Mobility Reports [11]. The purpose of this data was to show movement trends compared to the baseline dates that are based on the regular days.

This research aims to discuss the transmission of COVID-19 and relate it with the population mobility, with India as a case study. The purpose is to forecast the disease growth based on the current mobility pattern. The research focuses on analyzing how the number of confirmed cases is related to mobility habits a few days ago. The present analysis will also help us understand how population mobility interventions can help us fight the epidemic. To analyze the mobility influence, it is deemed suitable to first look into the COVID-19 challenges and their consequences for Indian citizens. The information will help understand the mobility pattern and also clarify its necessity. The paper is organized as follows: Section 10.2 discusses the COVID-19 in the Indian scenario. Section 10.3 reports the material and methods used for the analysis. Section 10.4 describes the main findings, and the conclusion is documented in section 10.5.

10.2 COVID-19 AND INDIA

The very first case of COVID-19 was reported in India on January 30, 2020, in Kerala. The patient was a student of Wuhan University, China [12]. Within one month, more patients were reported from the patients having travel history to Italy. During a brief span, the number of cases increased across the world and also in India. To date (February 7, 2021), in India, a total of 10,904,940 COVID-19 positive patients have been reported, and the total death count has reached 155,673, with around 200 positive cases being reported on average every day. As the number of cases has sharply declined, we look back to the approaches and efforts of the Indian government to tackle COVID-19 and its impact on society. The overall discussion can be summarized into two phases: the lockdown phase and the post-lockdown India.

10.2.1   India During Lockdowns of COVID-19

In India, inside the country boundary, the first step to control the spread was taken on March 16, 2020, when the ministry of home and family welfare (MOHFW) of India proposed to implement social distancing [13] to control the spread rate of the disease. Then, on March 22, a Janta curfew of 14h was implemented in India [14], and soon after, on March 24, 2020, a 21-day lockdown was announced. Consecutively, India's government prioritized individuals' health and extended this lockdown in phases until May 31, 2020. This sudden lockdown negatively influenced the Indian economy and Indian lifestyle in terms of education: financial, recreational, and social activities. The GDP growth rate was the worst in history and was recorded as −23.9% [15] for April-June 2020. But, simultaneously, this lockdown came as a boon for the environment. Reduced vehicle and electric equipment due to several service sectors and offices' closures positively impacted the environment. Rivers became clearer, and air quality improved due to industry closure.

10.2.2   COVID-19 Post-Lockdown Scenario in India

Partial unlocking occurred on June 1, 2021, when the reopening's primary focus was the economy. With several government guidelines, the country moved toward opening all the financial sectors in phases. The healthcare sector's key constraints were identified at the early stage to contain the epidemic within these critical constraints. The Indian economy sustained during this challenging time as compared to other countries, even when around 14 crore people lost their job and many more saw a salary cut. Unemployment rose to 26%, and it was predicted that India would witness the worst recession since independence. The government decided to work on it, and the life vs. livelihood debate played out. The government announcement of prioritizing life over livelihood changed to equal priority to both. The Indian government made an early decision to resume economic activities. The country's medical facilities were strengthened, and strict norms were followed during mobility, quarantine, and moving around public places.

As soon as the lockdown was revoked, traffic at grocery stores, pharmacies, parks, etc. has increased. The rise in mobility influences the spread of disease. Despite attempts to permanently unlock all the services, the lockdown has been enforced by different state governments time and again. To date, many benefits have not yet started to their full capacity. It can be hypothesized that people's mobility trend directly influences the number of positive cases, and these trends can also forecast the direction of disease. The aim is also to study the influence of the COVID-19 positivity rate on the mobility habits of people. The next section presents this relation and utilizes it for predicting the direction. Today, when vaccines are in the market, we see the mobility to different places and social gatherings are increasing. But, as the vaccine has not reached the mass population, we ignore its impact on the trend.

10.3   METHOD AND MATERIAL

As stated in section one of this research paper, one of this study's aims was to investigate how citizens' mobility impacts the coronavirus pandemic's spread. The data considered for this estimation was taken from Google community mobility data [11].

This data was collected to analyze how the visits to places like grocery stores, pharmacies, and parks are changing in a different geographic region. Out of all the information available for other parts of the world, the present study uses only data for India. This data highlights the mobility trends to workplaces, residential areas, restaurants, cafes, public transport hubs, and parks. Google's data shows the changing trend of visits and length of stay at different places concerning a baseline. Each day's changes are obtained by comparing with a baseline value that is fixed for each day of a week. In general, the baseline is the median value obtained over five weeks for each day before the spread of COVID-19. Since the baseline value calculation period is between January 3, 2020, and February 6, 2020, the median value is selected to represent the data's central tendency compared to the average. During this period, the mobility on a few days may be influenced by extreme weather conditions and festivals in several regions of the country, giving rise to skewed data. The selection of the median was only to reduce the impact of skewed data. Further, to make this data usable, some places with similar characteristics due to social-distancing guidelines were grouped. Combining grocery and pharmacy into a single group, using the park as the representative of national forests, castle, etc., are few examples.

To study the influence of mobility on COVID-19, the need is to investigate citizens' mobility patterns during COVID-19. Figure 10.1 represents the mobility of people to different places in the pre-lockdown and the lockdown period. Both the transition statistics are based on the mobility for essential goods like grocery and pharmacy, and the data has been taken randomly for only the two most significant states of India. The demand for essential items has increased during the lockdown, as is visible in the plot. Also, it can be seen that the median values in both the states have increased during the lockdown. Also, the values seem to be influenced by the outliers that may represent instances when people stocked up the essentials as much as possible during the lockdown period due to panic due to total shutdown and other constraints.

After extending the lockdown in phases, when the government announced unlocking different sectors in several stages, the collected mobility data highlights the trend in places like parks, recreational activities, grocery and pharmacy, transit stations, and workplaces. Figure 10.2 presents the trend of mobility in these places throughout the lockdown and unlock period. The plot of mobility trends directly poses a question "Are we ready to open?". To answer this question, it would be better to analyze these trends concerning the change in COVID-19 cases during this duration. This analysis will also prove our hypothesis that the transition in mobility, mainly the positive growth, influences the positivity rate of COVID-19 in the country.

To find the relation between the mobility and COVID-19 cases in India, the statistics for COVID-19 in India have been extracted from [16]. For this study, only the daily cases and the total number of positive cases have been considered each day. Apart from these, the databases also

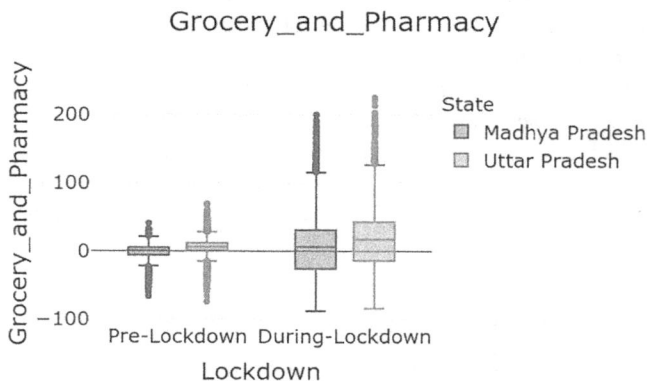

FIGURE 10.1   Mobility trend for essential services in pre-lockdown and lockdown period.

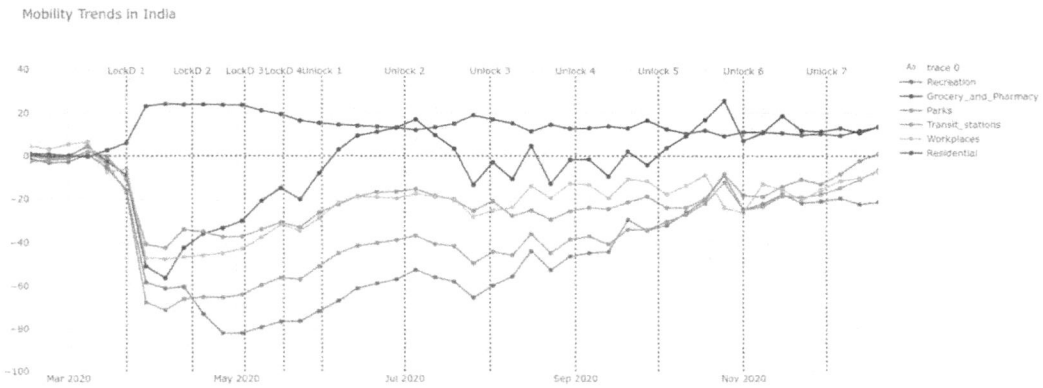

(a) Mar 2020 to Nov 2020

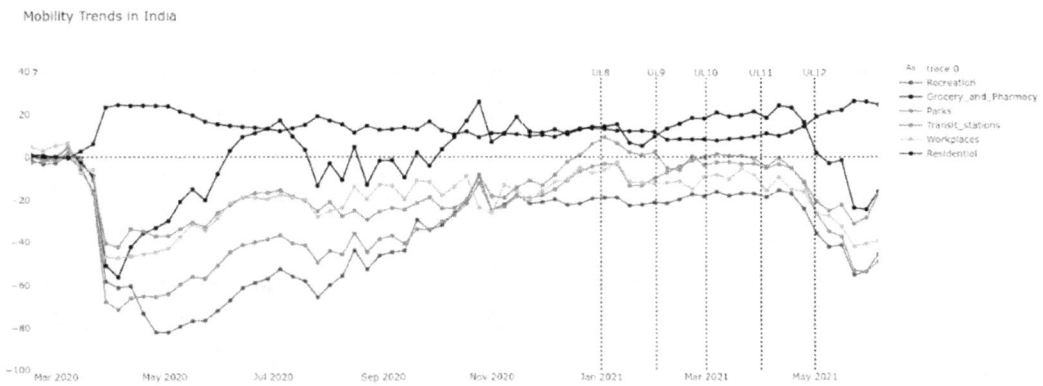

(b) Mar 2020 to May 2021

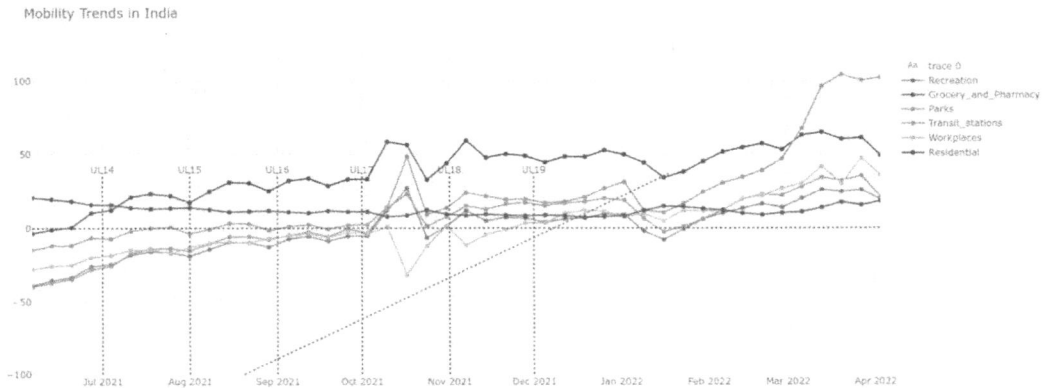

(c) Jul 2021 to Apr 2022

FIGURE 10.2 (a),(b) and (c) Mobility trends for different places during lockdown and post lockdown periods.

consist of information such as the number of recovered and deceased on a per-day basis, which has been ignored at this stage. Blank records of missing entries were discarded. We have selected places like grocery and pharmacy, recreation, transit stations, and parks to analyze the influence. The residential and workplaces have been intentionally ignored for obvious reasons. Figure 10.3

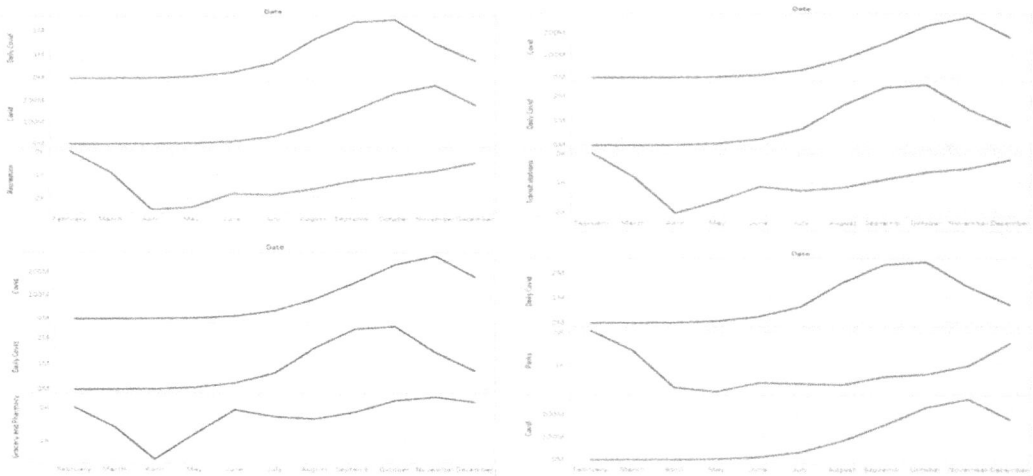

FIGURE 10.3 Trend analysis of COVID-19 and citizen mobility data in different places (a) mobility trend in recreation (b) transit station (c) grocery and pharmacy (d) park.

presents the trend plot for community mobility in different places and the COVID-19 disease progression during the same time. We discuss and analyze these plots in the next section.

This study's second objective was to predict and forecast the disease progression based upon the citizen mobility data. To meet our objective, we used an ARIMA (auto-regressive integrated moving average) model. ARIMA includes the auto-regressive(AR) model, a moving average (MA) model, and is integrated to make the moving stationary. It is a time-series forecasting model that uses historical data to predict the future. In simple words, ARIMA uses its own lags along with the lagged forecast errors [17] to formulate an equation that can be used to forecast future values. In general, ARIMA uses three terms during forecasting. The first is the order of the AR term (p). This p refers to the number of past observations and is used to represent predictors. The second term is the moving-average order (q), and it represents the number of past errors in the forecast that should be included in the ARIMA model. The third term is the differencing number and is needed for stationary time series. The stationary time series is obtained by subtracting the previous value from the current one. This difference may be computed several times depending on the series complexity. For any stationary time series, $d = 0$. The autocorrelation function (ACF) and partial autocorrelations (PACF) [18] are used to find these ARIMA model parameters. Figure 10.4 represents the process followed by ARIMA for forecasting.

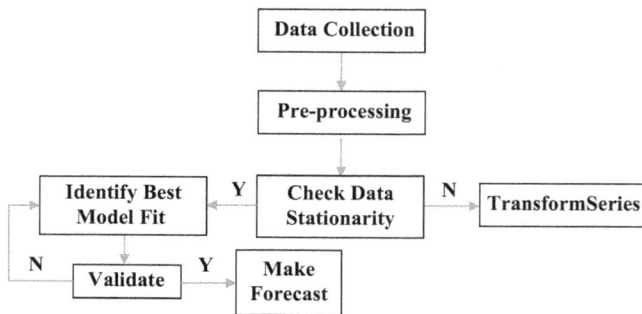

FIGURE 10.4 Processing ARIMA model for the forecast.

10.4   RESULTS AND DISCUSSIONS

As the number of positive COVID-19 cases reported started to decline, the government took decisions regarding the opening of different service sectors in a phased manner. Advocates have said that owing to the economic strengthening of the country, these decisions for the opening were essential. The opening was allowed with moderation in the stringent rules regarding traveling, social distancing, organizing social events, etc. Even though the unlock phases have started, it is important to evaluate that we are ready for opening. The plot of Figure 10.2 represents the mobility trends of the population in different sectors. Until March 2020, the baseline's mobility trend is considered an average trend in these sectors. As the news of disease spread reached every individual, there was a sudden dip in mobility toward the lockdown phases. Even though there were fluctuations in the mobility trend, they were far away from normal mobility. It is clear that apart from the residential sector, grocery and pharmacy is the other sector that observed mobility that was more than the ordinary phenomena. This result was because these are essential commodities and need to be reserved as stock. During the initial lockdown, the shortage of these items in the market influenced people's behaviours. The trend graph also points out that by the seventh lockdown phase, most of the sectors observe mobility toward the normal, pointing to the return of normalcy in society.

Although the number of cases is declining and most of the sectors have started working, it is crucial to determine the impact of this mobility transition on the COVID-19 cases. Figure 10.3 presents the mapping of COVID-19 cases on the citizen mobility data in different places like recreation, transit station, grocery and pharmacy, and park. It is observed that during March-April, the mobility in the recreation sector was negative, and rarely was any case of COVID-19 reported in the country during that time. But, around June 2020, when the first phase of unlocking started, the mobility of citizens increased, and the number of cases being positive also started to rise. After a steep dip in the movement at transit stations until April 2020, people began moving from one place to another. With the availability of public transport, this movement further increased. The impact of the increase is visible as a surge in the number of positive cases during June-July. Undoubtedly, the pandemic constraints have minimally affected the movements in places associated with grocery and pharmacy. By October 2020, the movements in these places have reached normal, and the number of positive cases reached a peak during this time. An interesting phenomenon was observed at places falling in the park category. The plot shows that people rarely visited these places during this time. Even though a few people may have visited, the open area and other environmental factors may have worked positively to avoid the spread. The increasing trend cannot be attributed to mobility in parks.

The paper's second objective was to forecast the disease progression in the country based on these citizen mobility trends. The ARIMA model is used to predict disease progression. To implement this model, the most important aspect is identifying the most suitable model for identifying the parameters. With the help of ACF and PACF, the best model was determined, and the parameters of the ARIMA model were set to (5,1,0) for (p,q,d) triplet. To train the system, the mobility data from February 2, 2020, to October 17, 2020, is taken for different sectors. The train test ratio for the model is 80:20. Based on the data for the above-mentioned duration, the ARIMA (5,1,0) model is used to predict the disease status for the period October 18, 2020, to December 2020. Figure 10.5 represents the forecasted mobility pattern and the actual data obtained by Google for the next 60 days in the three major places: grocery and pharmacy, recreation centers, and transit stations. The forecast's performance evaluation based on each sector is estimated in terms of root mean square error (RMSE). The RMSE statistics for datasets are considerably useful as RMSE is below 10% for the mean of the test data for every data sector.

Since we have already observed that citizen mobility influences the positivity rate, we discuss the prediction in reverse order. Based on the COVID-19 data for the total number of positive cases taken from [16], predictions are made regarding the disease spread for the next 60 days, starting from October 18, 2020. These predictions are then mapped on the citizen mobility trend, and, for each of these sectors, it is visible that as the COVID-19 cases are decreasing, mobility is increasing (Figure 10.6).

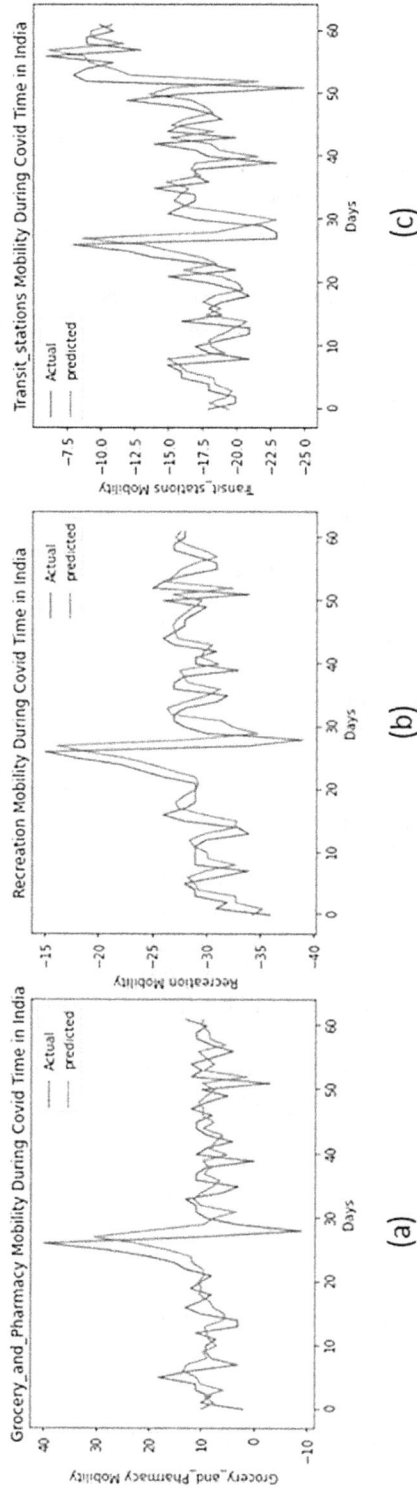

FIGURE 10.5 Mobility trend forecast using ARIMA (5,1,0) model for (a) grocery and pharmacy, (b) recreation, (c) transit stations.

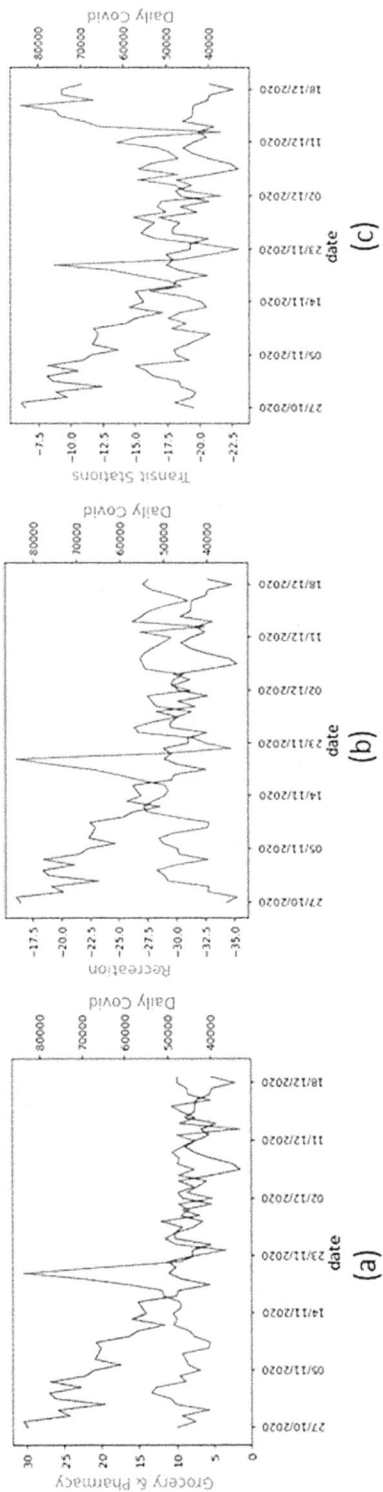

FIGURE 10.6 COVID-19 cases and mobility trend forecast using the ARIMA model for (a) grocery and pharmacy, (b) recreation, (c) transit stations.

The prediction of mobility trends and the trend of COVID-19 in the country may help the government prepare for the future. In general, we can sum up to say that COVID-19 positivity and the mobility trend both reciprocally influence each other.

Proper care and precautions must be followed while opening up to avoid the next surge of disease spread.

10.5 CONCLUSION

The matter this paper discusses concerns the topics of the Indian government's efforts toward dealing with the devastating disease of COVID-19 and the relationship between the citizen mobility trend and the spread of COVID-19. The paper investigates the influence of mobility trends on the COVID-19 disease propagation and tries to predict the mobility transition and the disease propagation in society based on the historical data. The case study is based on India, a country with the second-highest population in the world. The work examines the conjecture that mobility habits influence the spread of COVID-19 and that the positivity rate impacts people's mobility habits. The places of visits have been divided into categories to investigate the influence of mobility habits on the disease spread. It also highlights the fact that not all areas have a similar effect on the disease spread.

To pursue the research aims, quantitative estimates are made through the ARIMA model. The prediction results showed that mobility habits represent the variables that mainly affect the number of COVID-19 infections. Furthermore, the presence of other variables on the spread of disease can't be ignored. Also, the other side of the analysis highlights that as the disease propagation slows down, the mobility transition increases and more people start coming out. This transition generates the highs and lows in the number of daily COVID cases being reported. The results presented here are original, and further analysis may lay the groundwork for handling health-related emergencies and controlling the further spread.

Authors Contributions
Data Collection, analysis, interpretation, methodology and implementation work has been done by Vikas Thada. Literature survey, writing original draft has been done by Shweta Sinha. Review, editing has been done by all authors. Complete formatting and final editing has been done by Utpal Shrivastava.

Conflicts of Interests
None

Role of funding source
The work is not funded by any source.

REFERENCES

[1] Ghosh, Aritra, Srijita Nundy, and Tapas K. Mallick. "How India is dealing with COVID-19 pandemic." *Sensors International* 1 (2020): 100021.

[2] Tang, Xiaolu, et al. "On the origin and continuing evolution of SARS-CoV-2." *National Science Review* 7.6 (2020): 1012–1023.

[3] Saha, Jay et al. "Lockdown for COVID-19 and its impact on community mobility in India: An analysis of the COVID-19 Community Mobility Reports, 2020." *Children and Youth Services Review* 116 (2020): 105160. 10.1016/j.childyouth.2020.105160

[4] Sahu, Kamal Kant, et al. "India fights back: COVID-19 pandemic." *Heart & Lung: The Journal of Cardiopulmonary and Acute Care* 49.5 (2020): 446–448.

[5] Sarkar, Kankan, Subhas Khajanchi, and Juan J. Nieto. "Modeling and forecasting the COVID-19 pandemic in India." *Chaos, Solitons & Fractals* 139 (2020): 110049.

[6] Bastos, Saulo B., and Daniel O. Cajueiro. "Modeling and forecasting the Covid-19 pandemic in Brazil." *arXiv preprint arXiv:2003.14288* (2020).

[7] Dutta, Anwesha, and Harry W. Fischer. "The local governance of COVID-19: Disease prevention and social security in rural India." *World Development* 138 (2021): 105234.

[8] Kumar, Anant, K. Rajasekharan Nayar, and Shaffi Fazaludeen Koya. "COVID-19: Challenges and its consequences for rural health care in India." *Public Health in Practice* 1 (2020): 100009.

[9] Nakada, Liane Yuri Kondo, and Rodrigo Custodio Urban. "COVID-19 pandemic: environmental and social factors influencing the spread of SARS-CoV-2 in São Paulo, Brazil." *Environmental Science and Pollution Research* (2020): 1–7.

[10] Cartenì, Armando, Luigi Di Francesco, and Maria Martino. "How mobility habits influenced the spread of the COVID-19 pandemic: Results from the Italian case study." *Science of the Total Environment* 741 (2020): 140489.

[11] Google LLC. "Google COVID-19 Community Mobility Reports." https://www.google.com/covid19/mobility/ Accessed: 22-12-2020

[12] Singhal, Tanu. "A review of coronavirus disease-2019 (COVID-19)." *The Indian Journal of Pediatrics* 87.4 (2020): 281–286.

[13] Kaushik, S., S. Kaushik, Y. Sharma et al. "The Indian perspective of COVID-19 outbreak." *VirusDis* 31 (2020): 146–153 .

[14] "What Is Janata Curfew: Self Isolation by the People, for the People to Prevent Coronavirus, The Times of India." 2020. https://timesofindia.indiatimes.com/india/janata-curfew-march-22-all you-need-to-know/articleshow/74716032.cms. Accessed 14-12-2020.

[15] "GDP growth at −23.9% in Q1; first contraction in more than 40 years, The Economic Times." 2020. https://economictimes.indiatimes.com/news/economy/indicators/gdp-growth-at-23-9-in-q1-worst-economic-contraction-on-record/articleshow/77851891.cms Accessed on 10-12-2020.

[16] COVID19 India. https://www.covid19india.org/ Accessed on 25-12-2020.

[17] Khan, Farhan Mohammad, and Rajiv Gupta. "Arima and nar based prediction model for time series analysis of covid-19 cases in india." *Journal of Safety Science and Resilience* 1.1 (2020): 12–18.

[18] Alsharif, Mohammed H., Mohammad K. Younes, and Jeong Kim. "Time series ARIMA model for prediction of daily and monthly average global solar radiation: The case study of Seoul, South Korea." *Symmetry* 11.2 (2019): 240.

11 Impact of Social Media Platforms on Vaccination Drive during COVID-19 Pandemic in India

Prince Nagpal, Kartikey Gupta, Unnati Rastogi, and
Jyoti Singh Kirar

Banaras Hindu University, Varanasi, Uttar Pradesh, India

CONTENTS

11.1 INTRODUCTION

Coronavirus disease (COVID-19) is an infectious disease caused by a newly discovered coronavirus. 'CO' stands for corona, 'VI' for virus, and 'D' for disease. Formerly, this disease was referred to as '2019 novel coronavirus' or '2019-nCoV'. The COVID-19 virus is a new virus linked to the same family of viruses as Severe Acute Respiratory Syndrome (SARS) and some types of common cold.

The symptoms of COVID-19 can include fever, cough, and shortness of breath. In more severe cases, infection can cause pneumonia or breathing difficulties. More rarely, the disease can be fatal. These symptoms are similar to the flu or the common cold, which are a lot more common than COVID-19. This similarity is why testing is required to confirm if someone has COVID-19.

Most people infected with the COVID-19 virus will experience mild to moderate respiratory illness and recover without requiring special treatment. Older people, and those with underlying medical problems, like cardiovascular disease, diabetes, chronic respiratory disease, and cancer, are more likely to develop serious illness.

11.1.1 How Does COVID-19 Spread?

The virus is transmitted through direct contact with respiratory droplets of saliva or discharge from the nose when an infected person coughs or sneezes, so it's important that people also practice

DOI: 10.1201/9781003333081-11

respiratory etiquette (for example, by coughing into a flexed elbow). Individuals can also be infected from touching surfaces contaminated with the virus and touching their face (e.g., eyes, nose, mouth). The COVID-19 virus may survive on surfaces for several hours, but simple disinfectants can kill it.

The best way to prevent and slow down transmission is to be well informed about the COVID-19 virus, the disease it causes, and how it spreads. Protect yourself and others from infection by washing your hands or using an alcohol-based rub frequently and not touching your face.

11.1.2 WHO IS MOST AT RISK?

We are learning more about how COVID-19 affects people every day. Older people, and people with chronic medical conditions, such as diabetes and heart disease, appear to be more at risk of developing severe symptoms. As this is a new virus, we are still learning about how it affects children. We know it is possible for people of any age to be infected with the virus, but so far, there are relatively few cases of COVID-19 reported among children. This is a new virus, and we need to learn more about how it affects children. The virus can be fatal in rare cases, so far, mainly among older people with pre-existing medical conditions.

According to the WHO, in India, from 3 January 2020 to 5 June 2021, there have been 28,694,879 confirmed cases of COVID-19 with 344,082 deaths. Indicating that around 2.88Cr number of persons were affected by COVID-19 with around 3.47L persons losing the war against COVID-19 to date.

Currently, COVID-19 vaccines are one of the most important achievements of modern medicine. However, their acceptance is only partial, with vaccine hesitancy and refusal representing a major health threat. As of 31 May 2021, a total of 218,358,591 vaccine doses have been administered. COVID-19 vaccines stimulate discussions both in the real world and online. Social media is currently a significant source of health and medical information. Elucidating the association between social media engagement and COVID-19 vaccination is important and may be applicable to other vaccines.

Vaccination against COVID-19 is a significant and cost-effective protective mechanism for reducing the disease burden related to its morbidity and mortality. Nevertheless, at the population level, its coverage is insufficient due to factors influencing vaccination decisions and hesitancy, such as risk-benefit misperception or accessibility to the healthcare system. A major contribution to these factors is communication, involving both social and mass media, family, friends, and healthcare professionals. More specifically, social media and Simple Notification Service (SNS) have been used to improve vaccine response worldwide. However, they are also a forum for vaccine opponents and spreading of fake news. Understanding social media engagement, influence, and reliability is a critical point for improving the efficacy of advertising and publicity policies on social media. Our primary aim is to support the design and the implementation of future eHealth strategies and interventions on social media to increase the quality of targeted communication campaigns and the COVID-19 vaccination rates. Our main objective is to describe and characterize profiles regarding the COVID-19 vaccination affect the compliance of the population to vaccination guidelines. For example, those who advocate against vaccines use social media to disseminate their messages on a large scale, increasing vaccine hesitancy or refusal in the population.

Concerning the new COVID-19 vaccines, evaluating the relationship between the population's perception and compliance with the vaccine against COVID-19 is important. Therefore, this will contribute to creating effective means of online communication to improve vaccine acceptance. Social media platforms have been used to improve COVID-19 vaccine responses worldwide. However, they are also a forum for vaccine opponents and spreading of fake news. Understanding social media engagement, influence, and reliability is a critical point for improving the efficiency of advertising and publicity policies on social media. Our primary aim is to support the design and the implementation of future eHealth strategies and interventions on social media to increase the quality of targeted communication campaigns and the COVID-19 vaccination rates. Our main objective is to describe and characterize profiles regarding COVID-19 vaccination and their association with social media engagement, influence, and reliability. We specifically focus on the Indian population in this study. The findings of this research may then support vaccination campaigns against COVID-19 in the future. Our goal is to identify socio-demographic and social media engagement attributes affecting COVID-19 vaccination compliance. This research characterizes the differences between individuals vaccinated or not vaccinated against coronavirus during the 2021 season. We attempt to understand whether there is a link between vaccination against COVID-19 and social media engagement, influence, and perception of reliability during the COVID-19 pandemic.

- To study the extent of influence of social media (if any) on the vaccination drive, public health awareness, and prevention against this COVID-19 pandemic.
- To understand the role of social media so that the results can help the government in strategizing and implementation of future vaccination drive to increase the quality of targeted communication campaigns and the COVID-19 vaccination rates.
- To help improve the social media posts through early detection and monitoring the quality of post posted by users on social media.

11.2   PROPOSED APPROACH

In this work, we aim at determining the impact of social media on general public as a classification approach. In this work, we collected the data using a survey. The collected data is then pre-processed. Finally, the processed data is used for classification as positive and negative impact with various classifiers. Each step of this model is described in detail, below. (Figure 11.1)

11.2.1   Dataset Description

[1]A quantitative approach and several social media platforms namely WhatsApp, Facebook, LinkedIn, Telegram, Instagram, etc. were used to collect data via Google Forms questionnaires shared among social media users. This survey was conducted with the target population as the residents of India. With a structured questionnaire of 24 questions in total, 590 responses in all were collected. The responses of this survey were collected during the months May and June of 2021. Mainly, the data collected is divided into three categories: youths, adults, and senior citizens. Respondents answered 24 questions related to social media activities, COVID-19 vaccination, social media usage, COVID-19 and vaccination-related information and behaviour, health-related information and some related to the nature of the respondent toward these social media platforms. Convenience sampling, which is one of the non-probability sampling methods, has been used in this research because of the ease of accessibility of the sample [1,2]. (Table 11.1)

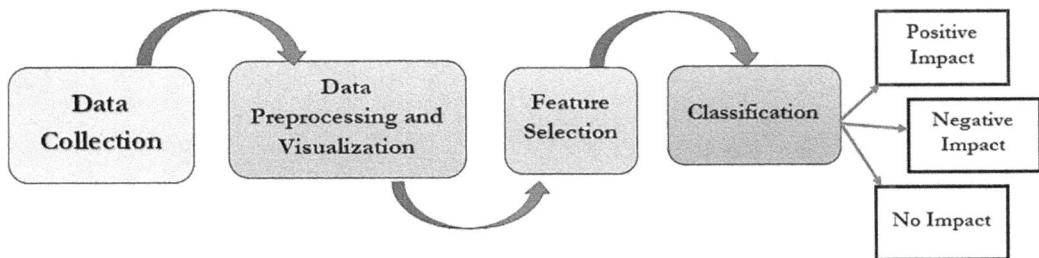

FIGURE 11.1   Flow diagram of proposed model.

TABLE 11.1

Showing Dataset Used in the Survey

Dataset of the survey

S.No.	Questionnaire	Responses
F1	Gender	Male, Female, prefer not to say
F2	State / UT	All states of India
F3	Age	18–24, 25–64, Above 65 years
F4	Educational Qualification	Bachelors, Masters, PhD, Associate
F5	Which Social Media platform's you mostly prefer?	Facebook, WhatsApp, Instagram, LinkedIn, Twitter, Telegram, YouTube
F6	Which Social Media platform do you think give more reliable information?	Facebook, WhatsApp, Instagram, LinkedIn, Twitter, Telegram, YouTube
F7	What are your usual activities on social media platforms?	Messaging, Writes post, Responds to posts, Just Scrolling, Not an Active User
F8	How long do you browse social media?	Less than half hour, In between $1/2$ hour to 2 hours, In between 2 hour to 3 hour, More than 3 hours
F9	Do you see any Health related post on social media?	No, Yes,Sometimes
F10	If yes, then What impression does that post create of the vaccination drive?	Fear and Anxiety, Hope and Encouragement
F11	Have you posted anything related to COVID and vaccination drive on social media?	Yes, No
F12	If yes, then What impression does that create of the vaccination drive?	Fear and Anxiety, Hope and Encouragement
F13	How many posts you had posted related to it?	No posts, 1–2 Times, 2–5 times, 6–10 times, More than 10 times
F14	Has someone in your family got covid positive?	No, Yes
F15	Have you got vaccinated?	Yes, No
F16	If no, then Why not?	Not Interested, Heard bad rumours on social media, Unsure about the efficacy of vaccines, Confused between the vaccines, Not able to book slot online
F17	If yes, then from where you have taken your vaccine?	Government Hospital, Private Hospital
F18	Which Vaccine did you take?	Covishield, Sputnik-V, Covaxin
F19	After taking vaccine, Have you posted it on social media?	Yes, No
F20	Do you verify the information on social media with the attending physician/family physician?	No, Yes,Sometimes
F21	How do you determine that the information on social media is reliable?	Published by Government/Health Organization, Provided by Healthcare professionals, Browsing in Scientific Publications, Shared by someone I know, It seems convincing to me
F22	Have you searched vaccine related information on WHO site?	Yes, No
F23	Please rate the level of information reliability about vaccine information on social media?	1,2,3, … .10

11.2.2 Dataset Pre-Processing [3] and Visualisation

Data pre-processing is a data-mining technique that transforms raw data into a useful and efficient format. This process has four main stages: data cleaning, data integration, data transformation, and data reduction.

- **Data cleaning** will fill in missing values, smooth noisy data, identify or remove outliers and resolve inconsistencies.
- **Data integration** is integration of multiple databases, data cubes or files.
- **Data transformation** is done to transform the data in appropriate forms suitable for mining process.
- **Data Reduction** is done to handle high volume of data when analysis becomes harder.

After the collection of responses, first, we had transformed the raw data into an understandable format, which in this case, was stored in a comma-separated values (CSV) format. Here, all irrelevant and duplicate values and the missing variables were taken out of the dataset to get high quality of data for good results. Also, normalization was performed on the dataset to improve its integrity. Features of the dataset collected are gender, state, age, educational qualification and other similar features.

Data visualization is the graphical representation of information, patterns, and trends in the processed dataset. For data visualisation, we used some descriptive statistics methods, i.e. pie charts and bar graphs to extract the simple summary of our collected dataset. (Figure 11.2a) to (Figure 11.2p) shows the visualization of different responses of the survey's questionnaire. First, we observed gender distribution data where around 55% of the respondents were male and around 44% were female. Further, we observed that majority of the respondents were holding at least a bachelor's degree, which represents a good sign of analysis [(Figure 11.2a) and (Figure 11.2b)]. In (Figure 11.2c), the blue bar represents "How many users prefer these Social Media Platforms" and orange bar represents "Which Social Media platform give more reliable information?" where in majority of the respondents uses WhatsApp, but they do agree it spreads fake news. On the other hand, the bar representing LinkedIn users showed that the numbers of respondents using it and thinking it gives reliable information were almost equal, while for Twitter, even respondents who don't use it think that it gives more reliable information. (Figure 11.2d) represents a majority of the users who use social media platforms for messaging and scrolling, while (Figure 11.2e) represents a large number of users who spend around 30 minutes to 2 hours on social media. While scrolling the newsfeed, they do encounter health-related posts, which can be pictorially represented by (Figure 11.2f). From (Figure 11.2g), we can see that viral posts on social media give hope and encourage other users to get vaccinated. Social media posts are encouraging other users to get vaccinated, but still, the majority of users have not been vaccinated, as depicted in (Figure 11.2h); the reason is that they were not able to book a slot online, as shown in (Figure 11.2m), and the reason for it may be due to a limited supply of the vaccines or the negative posts creating rumours against vaccination. So, the government may use these social media platforms for encouraging users as a reliable source to share information, which may remove confusions regarding vaccination.

Our analysis shows that even social media users are using these platforms to encourage other users to get vaccinated (Figure 11.2j) and for that, they are posting many posts on their newsfeed [(Figure 11.2h)] because of which many users took Covishield vaccine [(Figure 11.2l)] and that too from government hospital [(Figure 11.2k)].

Even though 90% of our questionnaire was filled by respondents who were holding at least a bachelor's and master's degree, when it comes to verification of information on social media, only 50% do it; see (Figure 11.2n), (Figure 11.2o) and (Figure 11.2p).

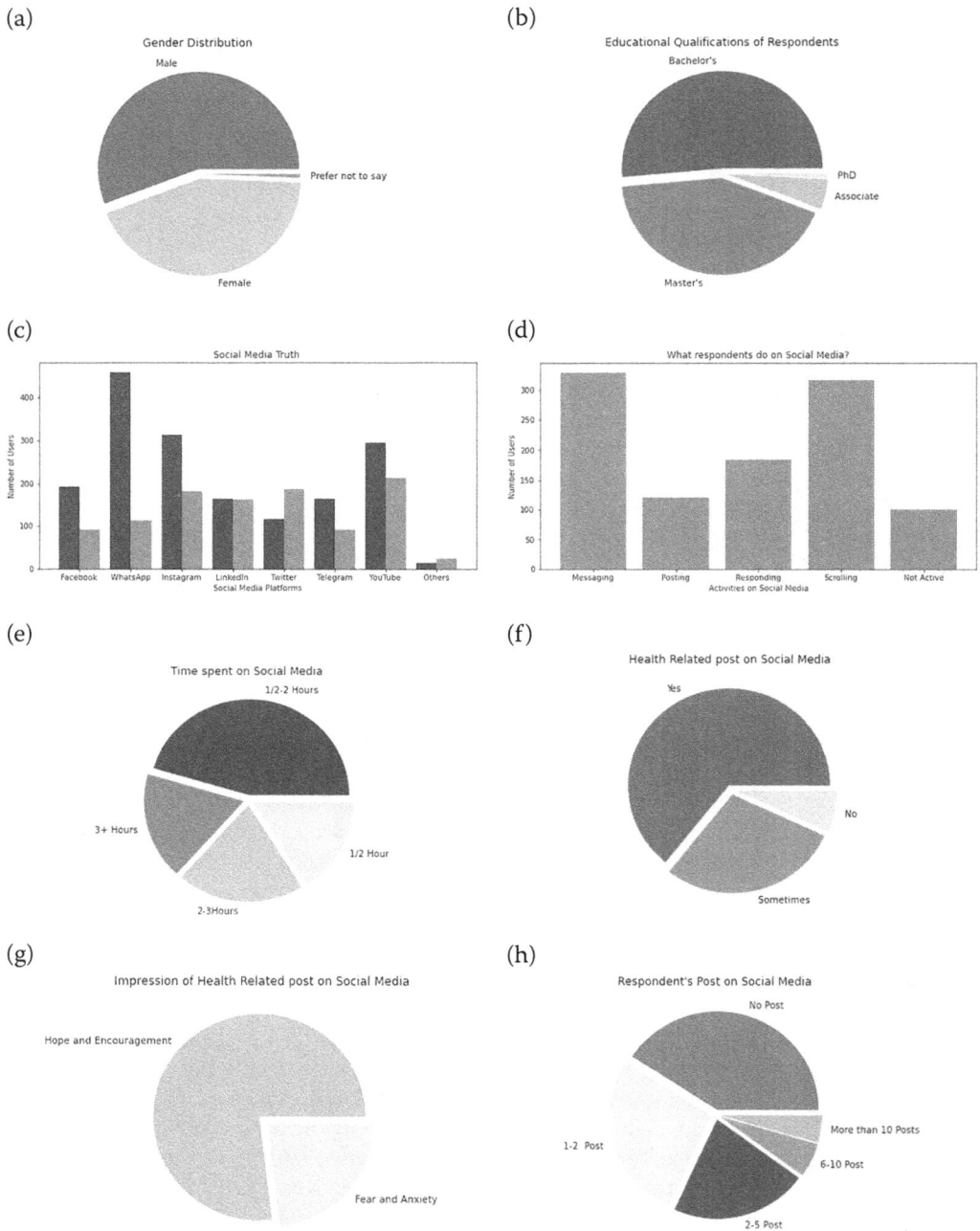

FIGURE 11.2 (a). Gender distribution, (b). Educational qualification, (c). Social media reliability, (d). Activity on social media, (e). Time duration on social media, (f). Visibility of health-related posts on social media, (g). Effect of health-related posts, (h). Count of posting health-related posts, (i). Number of respondents vaccinated, (j). Vaccinated respondent posts on social media, (k). Type of vaccination centre, (l). Preference of vaccine, (m). Causes of no vaccination, (n). Credibility of vaccine-related information on social media, (o). Number of respondents who verify information on social media with physician, (p). Verification of social media posts with WHO website.

(i)

Number of Respondent's got Vaccinated

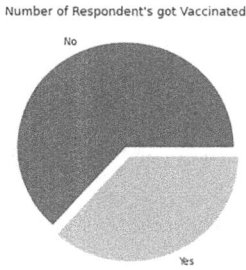

(j)

Has Respondent Posted on Social Media related to Vaccination

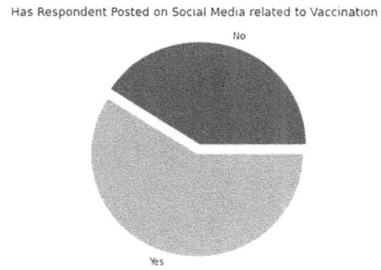

(k)

Respondent took vaccines from

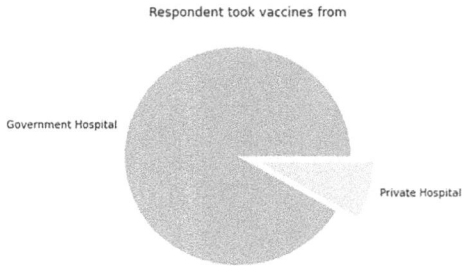

(l)

Respondent's Choice on Vaccine

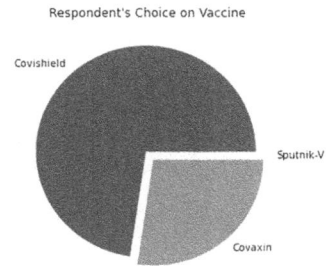

(m)

Why respondents have not got vaccinated?

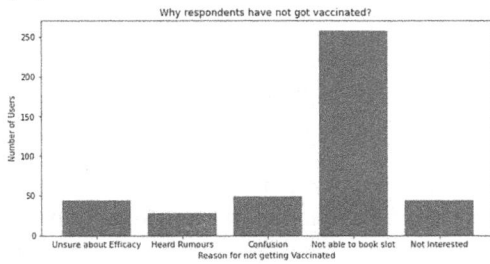

(n)

Respondent's verification of Information on Social Media

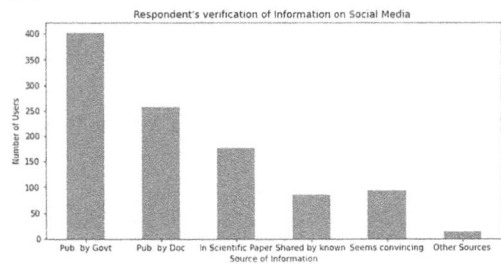

(o)

Verification of information on Social Media with physician

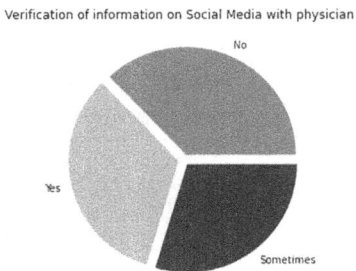

(p)

Verification related information on WHO

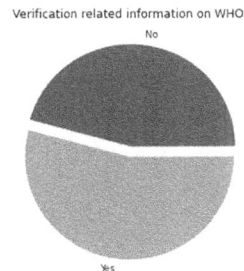

FIGURE 11.2 (*continued*)

11.2.3 FEATURE SELECTION

SEQUENTIAL BACKWARD SELECTION (SBS) [4] ALGORITHM

Step1 Start with a subset of features which are relevant to our problem of study and calculate its entropy i.e.

$$Y_0 = X \tag{11.1}$$

Step2. Each feature is deleted one at a time, and then its entropy is computed and the worst feature is discarded, i.e.

$$x^- = arg\ max\ J\,(Y_k - x)\ where\ x \epsilon Y_k \tag{11.2}$$

Step3. Again, each feature from remaining features is deleted one at a time, and the worst feature is discarded, i.e.

$$Y_{k+1} = Y_k - x^-;\ \ k = k + 1 \tag{11.3}$$

Step4. This procedure continued until a predefined number of features are left.

The feature selection is used to reduce the number of input variables to those that are believed to be most useful to a model to predict the target variable. Initially in our decision tree classifier, we took 14 features out of 23 that we found were the best fit, and to select the best out of these 14 features, we have used backward feature elimination.

Sequential backward selection (SBS) [4] is a search method that starts with all the features (an empty set of features) and removes a single feature at each step with a view to improving the cost function. This algorithm aims to reduce the dimensionality of the initial feature subspace from N to K-features with a minimum reduction in the model performance to improve upon computational efficiency and reduce generalization error.

Here, we started with 14 features and removed the least significant feature at each iteration, one that no longer improved the performance of the model and change in entropy. We repeated this iteration until no improvement is observed on removal of features and change in entropy. At the removal of the 11th feature, there was an increase in entropy. So, we stopped at feature 11 and found our model performance is at the peak. (Table 11.2), (Figure 11.3)

TABLE 11.2
Showing Observations from Features Selection

Features	Accuracy	Entropy
{F1,F4,F8,F9,F10,F11,F12,F13,F14,F15,F19,F20,F22}	0.991(0.009)	0
{F4,F8,F9,F10,F11,F12,F13,F14,F15,F19,F20,F22}	0.986(0.010)	0
{F8,F9,F10,F11,F12,F13,F14,F15,F19,F20,F22}	0.993(0.008)	0
{F8,F9,F10,F11,F12,F13,F14,F15,F19,F20}	0.992(0.008)	0

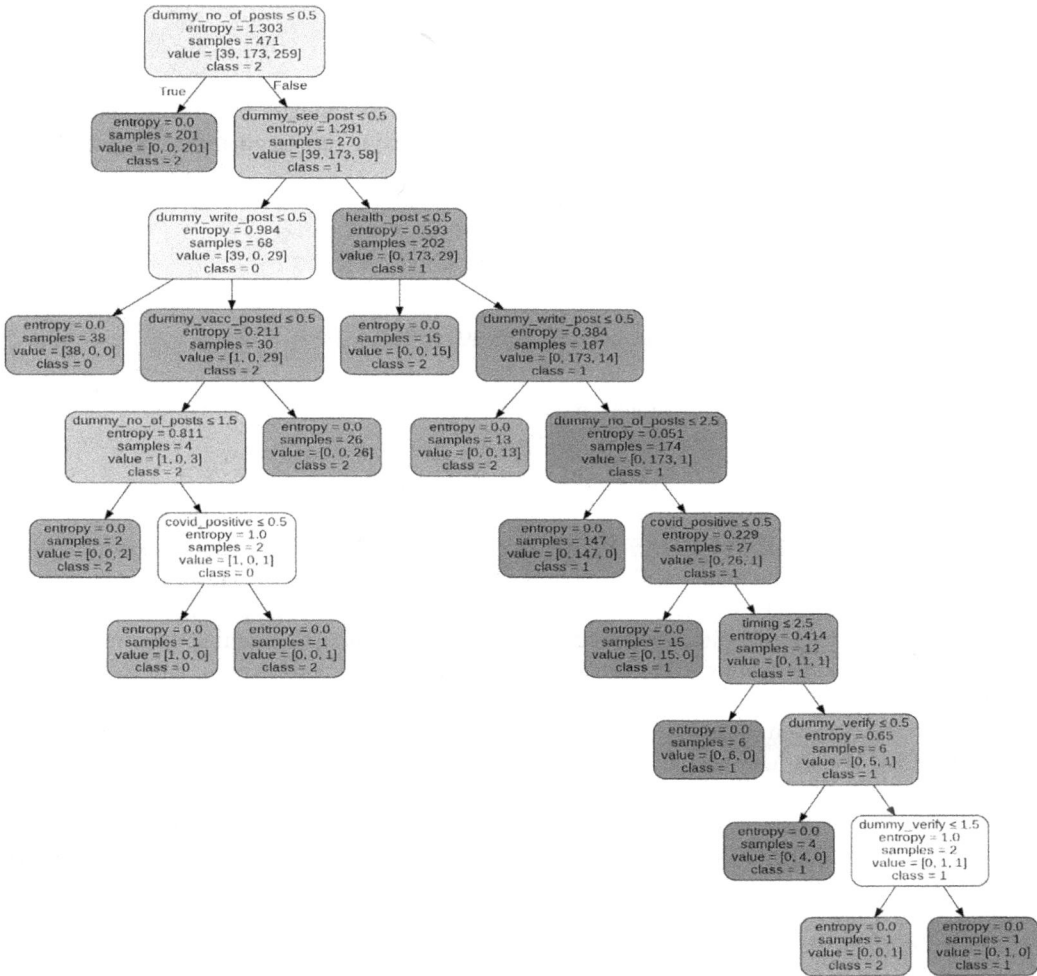

FIGURE 11.3 Decision tree obtained using backward feature selection.

11.2.4 CLASSIFICATION [3,5–7]

On analysing our survey data, we brought down our results to three classes: positive impact, negative impact, and no impact. This is a problem of multiclass classification. The algorithm will be given training data with populations that have positive, negative, and no impact on social media users. The model will find the features within the data that correlate to either class and create the mapping function: Y = f(x). Then, when provided with an unknown observation, the model will use this function to determine whether or not the respondent is impacted by these posts. Classification problems can be solved with numerous algorithms.

In this research work, we have used different classifications of supervised data-mining and machine-learning techniques. With the implementation and help of these methods, we tried to get the most accurate results. The techniques used in our research work are listed below:

- Decision Tree Classification Algorithm (DT) [5]
- Random Forest Classifier (RFC) [5]
- Support Vector Classifier (SVC) [5]

- K-Nearest Neighbour (K-NN) [5,8]
- Logistic Regression (LR) [5]

Following parameters have been used in this research work to compare the performance of different classifiers in determining 'The impact of social media on vaccination drive in India'. (Figure 11.4)

And Model Performance is given as follows

$$\text{Accuracy} = (TN + TP)/(TN + FP + FN + TP) \tag{11.4}$$

$$\text{Precision} = TP/(FP + TP) \tag{11.5}$$

$$\text{Sensitivity} = TP/(TP + FN) \tag{11.6}$$

$$\text{Specificity} = TN/(TN + FP) \tag{11.7}$$

We have used **the K FOLD CROSS VERIFICATION METHOD** [9–12], a resampling procedure used to evaluate machine-learning models on a limited data sample. This approach involves randomly dividing the set of observations into k groups, or folds, of approximately equal size. The first fold is treated as a validation set, and the method is fit on the remaining k − 1 folds. Here, we have discussed the results we get after implementing the above-discussed classification. (Figure 11.5)

The accuracy achieved with Decision Tree using k fold cross validation is 0.995(0.008), representing 99.5% of the time our classifier will be able to correctly identify users on whom social media has created positive, negative, or no impact on vaccination drive. The accuracy achieved with Random Forest using k fold cross validation is 0.997(0.007) representing 99.7% of the time our classifier will be able to correctly identify users on whom social media has created positive, negative, or no impact on vaccination drive. The accuracy achieved with the support vector classifier using k fold cross validation is 0.937(0.007), representing 93.7% of the time our classifier

		PREDICTED CLASS	
		NO	YES
OBSERVED CLASS	NO	TN	FP
	YES	FN	TP

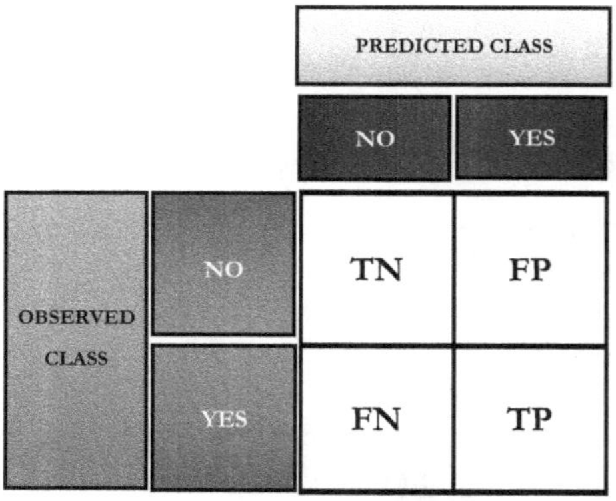

CONFUSION MATRIX AND ROC CURVE

where

TN	True Negative
FP	False Positive
FN	False Negative
TP	True Positive

FIGURE 11.4 Showing the formulas used to calculate the above quantitative observations.

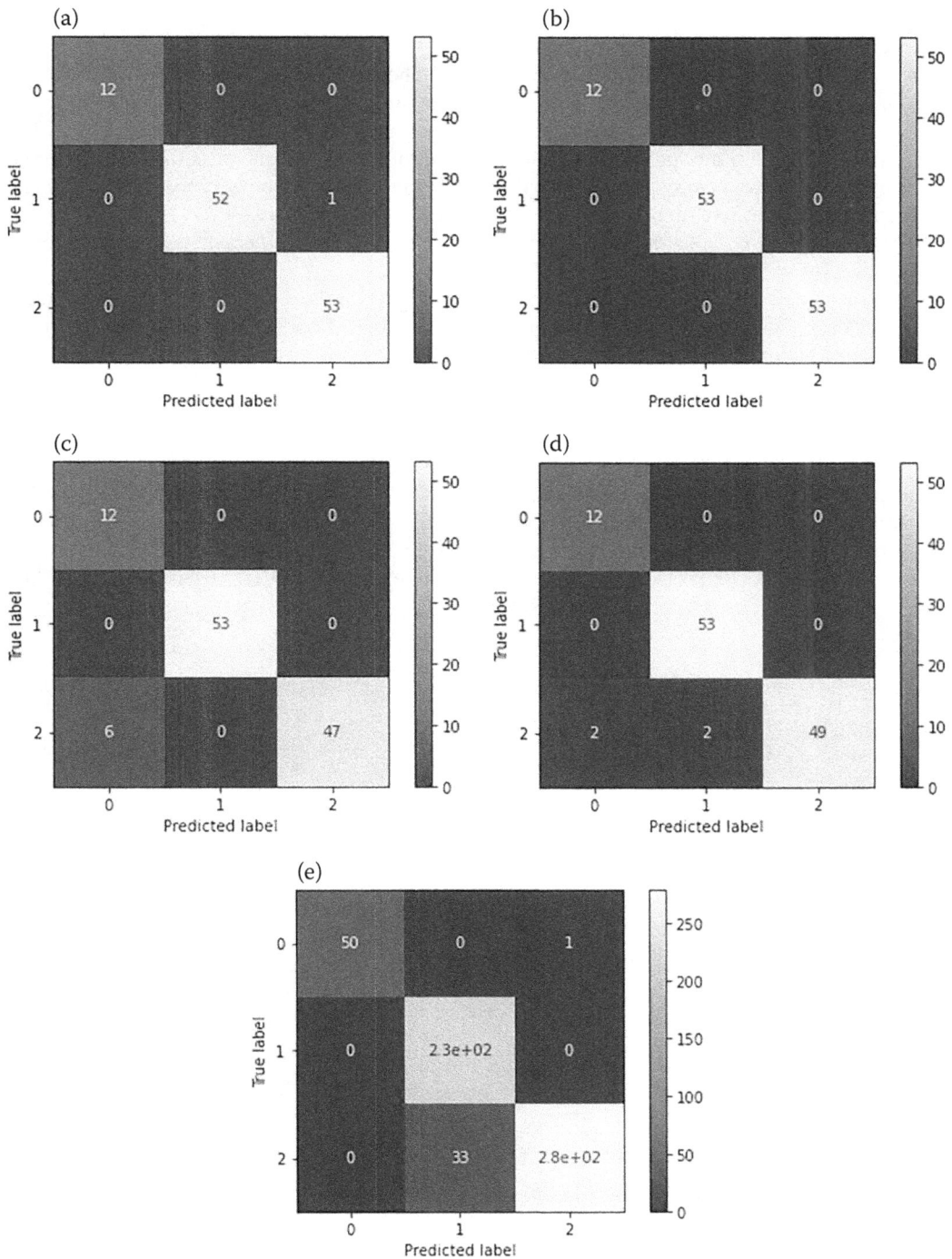

FIGURE 11.5 (a). Confusion matrix obtained from Decision Tree Classifier, (b). Confusion matrix obtained from Random Forest Classifier, (c). Confusion matrix obtained from SVM Classifier, (d). Confusion matrix obtained from KNN Classifier, (e). Confusion matrix obtained from Logistic Regression Classifier.

will be able to correctly identify users on whom social media has created positive, negative, or no impact on vaccination drive. (Figure 11.6)

The accuracy achieved with the k-nearest neighbors using k fold cross validation is 0.952(0.018), representing 95.2% of the time our classifier will be able to correctly identify users on whom social media has created positive, negative, or no impact on vaccination drive. The accuracy achieved with the logistic regression using k fold cross validation is 0.924(0.030), representing 92.4% of the time our classifier will be able to correctly identify users on whom social media has created positive, negative, or no impact on vaccination drive.

Following results demonstrates the comparison of different classifiers in terms of different parameters. (Table 11.3)

The goal behind selecting this topic for the research work is to check the influence of social media platforms on COVID-19 vaccination by using various classification techniques of supervised machine learning so that the common people can get the essence of Artificial Intelligence at an affordable cost in less time [9, 10] . K-Nearest Neighbor, Logistic Regression, Support-Vector Classifier, Decision Tree, and Random Forest Classifier are the classification algorithms used on the dataset to build the best predictive model with the highest accuracy among all [6,7,11].

From the analysis done, we found that Decision Tree and Random Forest give the best accuracy, precision (What percent of your predictions were correct?), recall (What percent of the positive cases did you catch?), and f1-SCORE (What percent of positive predictions were correct?) [12].

The main findings revealed that the use of social media platforms had a significant positive influence on public health protection and vaccination drive against COVID-19 as a pandemic. And

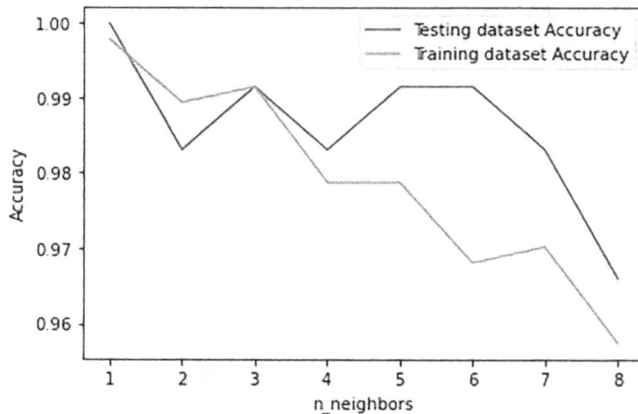

FIGURE 11.6   Training-testing accuracy using KNN classifier.

TABLE 11.3
Showing Comparison of Different Classifiers

Model	ACCURACY	PRECISION	RECALL	f1-SCORE
Logistic Regression	0.934	1.00	1.00	1.00
Decision Tree	0.990	1.00	0.98	0.99
Random Forest	0.997	1.00	1.00	1.00
SVM	0.952	1.00	1.00	1.00
KNN	0.952	1.00	1.00	1.00

also, the posts shared in these platforms regarding vaccination encourage the other users to get vaccinated, which predicts that in the future, the probability of vaccinated people will increase and reach nearly to 100 percent, i.e., every single person may get vaccinated in the future.

11.3   CONCLUSION AND FUTURE WORK

Today, social media has become an important part of everyone's life. Now everyone directly or indirectly depends on social media platforms. These platforms have become a mirror of all activities done in our country. During this COVID-19 pandemic period, the vaccination drive also became a part of it. But it is quite unknown how much social media has influenced public health awareness and prevention against this COVID-19 pandemic and its vaccination in a developing country like India.

The main purpose of this research work was to find out the impact of the social media platforms on the COVID-19 pandemic using various data-mining techniques and machine-learning algorithms, including K-Nearest Neighbour, Logistic Regression, Support-Vector Classifier, Decision Tree, and Random Forest Classifier, which are used on the dataset to build the best predictive model with the highest accuracy. The data was taken from a survey that was later cleaned to improve the overall quality and increase the productivity [11]. Besides this, data pre-processing and data-analysis methods were used, which helped us improve the data visualization and overall accuracy of our machine-learning algorithm. Data standardization procedures kept all the features in the same scale and helped us in predicting the impact of social media on vaccination drive.

The main finding revealed that social media platforms have a significant positive influence on the vaccination drive. Moreover, the government can use Twitter as a reliable source to spread required information in the future and inform the public about possible preventions and cures of other COVID-19 mutations. Therefore, a better understanding of the effects of using social media platforms is required, as well as a specificaiton of the profiles of social media engagement regarding vaccine and their association with knowledge and compliance to support improvement of future vaccination campaigns.

Public health authorities may use social media platforms as an effective tool to increase public health awareness through dissemination of brief messages to targeted populations. However, more research is needed to validate how social media channels can be used to improve health knowledge and adoption of healthy behaviours in a cross-cultural context.

The study was confined to residents of India only, but it can be extended to residents of all over the world. The method of sampling used was convenience sampling, which being a non-probability sampling method may have introduced some bias, which can be eliminated by taking a large sample. Many different adaptations, tests, and experiments have been left for the future due to lack of time (i.e., the experiments with real data are usually very time consuming). Future work concerns deeper analysis of particular mechanisms, new proposals to try different methods, or simply curiosity. More research is needed to validate how social media channels can be used to improve health knowledge and adopt healthy behaviours in a cross-cultural context.

Conflicts of Interest
The authors report no conflicts of interest

NOTE

1 https://colab.research.google.com/drive/1h5PsDvr5QjR1iK7Ln4FUThrGBo21tjpE?usp=sharing#scrollTo= 6RZ4Ig6sSgdt- **link for the dataset**

REFERENCES

[1] S. Shabnoor, S. Tajinder. "Social Media its Impact with Positive and NegativeAspects", *IJCATR*, 5(2), 71–75, 2016.

[2] P. Viswanath, T. H. Sarma, "An improvement to k-nearest neighbor classifier", *Recent Advances in Intelligent Computational Systems (RAICS)*, 2011 IEEE, Sept. 2011.

[3] S. García, S. Ramírez-Gallego, J. Luengo, J. M. Benítez, F. Herrera, "Big data preprocessing: methods and prospects".

[4] M. Karnan, P. Kalyani, "Attribute reduction using backward elimination algorithm", 2010 IEEE.

[5] P. -N. Tan, M. Steinbach, V. Kumar, "Introduction to DATA MINING".

[6] *Wes Mckinney,* "Python For Data Analysis", *the first specialized Python book on Data Analysis and Data Science.*

[7] F. A. Farris, "The Gini Index and Measures of Inequality" December 2010.

[8] J. Han, M. Kambar, J. Pei, "Data Mining Concepts and Techniques", Elsevier Second Edition.

[9] J. D. Rodríguez, A. Pérez, J. A. Lozano, "Sensitivity Analysis of k-Fold Cross Validation in Prediction Error Estimation", *IEEE Transactions on Pattern Analysis and Machine Intelligence*, 32(3), 569–575, April 2010, Source, IEEE Xplore.

[10] WHO coronavirus (COVID-19) Dashboard, https://covid19.who.int/,daily report on covid cases.

[11] M. J. Berry, G. S. Linoff, *Data Mining Techniques For Marketing, Sales And Customer Support.* Wiley, New York, 1997.

[12] H. Huang, X. Wu, R. Relue, "Association analysis with one scan of databases", In: Proceedings of the 2002 IEEE international conference on data mining (ICDM'02), 629–632, 2002.

12 Pneumonia Detection Using Chest X-Ray with the Help of Deep Learning

Milind Udbhav and Robin Kumar Attri
Department of Computer Science, School of Engineering and
Technology, K.R. Mangalam University, Gurugram, India

Meenu Vijarania and Swati Gupta
Centre of Excellence, Department of Computer Science, School of
Engineering and Technology, K.R. Mangalam University, Gurugram, India

Khushboo Tripathi
Department of Computer Science & Engineering, Amity University
Haryana, India

CONTENTS

12.1 INTRODUCTION

As previously stated, pneumonia affects a wide range of people, especially children, particularly in developing and impoverished countries, which are defined by risk factors like overcrowding, sanitation, and hygiene. Bad fitness and malnutrition are associated with a lack of suitable medical

DOI: 10.1201/9781003333081-12

facilities. This acute lung infection can be brought on by viruses, fungi, or microorganisms. It affects the lungs, infecting the air sacs and leading to pleural effusion, which causes the lungs to fill with fluid. Germs, which are responsible for pneumonia, are contagious. Both viral and bacterial pneumonia are communicable and spread to others. By coming in contact with contaminated surfaces or objects, people can also get infected. Inhalation of airborne droplets from sneezing and coughing may also result in pneumonia infection. Symptoms of pneumonia are: coughing, mucus production, excessive sweating or chills, feeling of tiredness or stress, vomiting or nausea, and loss of appetite, etc. As mentioned in [1]. Physical examinations such as x-rays of the chest, blood cultures, pulse oximetry, CT scans, fluid samples, and bronchoscopies can be used to identify pneumonia disease. The disease is more prevalent in underdeveloped and developing nations, where medical resources are limited and environmental factors like congestion, pollution, and unhygienic environments make the disease worse. Therefore, preventing death from the illness can be greatly helped by early identification and management. More than 15% of all deaths in children under the age of five are attributable to it. As mentioned in [2], diagnosis is frequently done using a chest x-ray, radiography, commonly known as x-rays, computed tomography (CT), as well as magnetic-resonance imaging (MRI). A vital artificial intelligence technology called "deep mastering" plays a key role in resolving a variety of challenging computer vision issues. For many picture-categorization problems, deep-learning models—especially cumulative neural networks (CNNs)—are often used. However, those models perform best when given a large amount of data. For the trouble biomedical photograph category, it is far hard to achieve a big amount of labelled data as it requires scientific professionals to categorise each photo, which is a high-priced and time-consuming assignment. Transition learning is one way to overcome this barrier. In this approach, to remedy trouble involving a small facts set, a version trained on a big dataset is reused, and the lattice weights defined in this model are carried out. CNN models are skilled on a large dataset like ImageNet, inclusive of more than 14 million photos, usually used for biomedical photograph-classification responsibilities. As mentioned in [3], the optimum treatment for pneumonia must be determined as soon as possible to avoid risking the patient's life. The most common method for diagnosing pneumonia is a chest radiograph, although this method is difficult to use because of inter-magnification variability, and the prognosis depends on how well clinicians can recognise early pneumonia lines. Chest x-ray imaging is the method that is most usually used to diagnose pneumonia. Examining chest x-rays, however, is a difficult undertaking that is subject to subjectivity. To diagnose contamination, the radiologist will search for white spots inside the lungs (known as infiltrates) when interpreting the x-ray. According to [4], this examination will even help determine whether you have any headaches connected to pneumonia, such as pleural effusions or abscesses (fluid surrounding the lungs). The overall radiographic clearance rate in patients with mild to moderately severe pneumonia is 30% after 10 days and 70% after 1 month, in conclusion. The degree of pneumonia at the time of admission was associated with delayed radiological clearance. A chest x-ray is typically used to diagnose pneumonia. Blood tests, such as a complete blood count (CBC), can help find out how well a person's immune system is working to help avoid contamination. Pulse oximetry calculates how much oxygen is present in the blood. Pneumonia can prevent the lungs from supplying blood with enough oxygen. ResNet, a crucial component of a deep convolutional neural network that excels at image recognition-related tasks, is used in the study presented here. The project helps to talk about the working of Google Collab and its resources and how it can be implemented to solve high-level problems of deep learning and its various methodologies where the dataset is in the form of images, text, and videos. As mentioned in [5], TensorFlow plays a major role in building convolutional neural networks. The identification and detection of pneumonia are done using the ResNet architecture and perform well. The model can be deployed to get real-time responses using APIs. The major key takeaway from the project is to utilize the data and should be made balanced; resampling techniques should be applied for the proper working of the deep-learning model. Other things to try, such as medical problem statements, are complex, and there's a high chance to miss some important points before solving the issue for proper implementation. Different companies make different x-ray scanners, and processing and working methods are different. As mentioned in [6], to improve the existing dataset, collection of x-rays from multiple hospitals and different machines can be implemented. Using a deep-learning model, the project gives confidence to users to perform more classification tasks and image-processing tasks. For pneumonia detection, the basics of Python and machine-learning algorithms like logistic regression and linear regression play a major role in the real-life implementation and help to fulfill the basics need of the image-processing environment. The project focuses on proper classification, causes detection, and helps people to avoid pneumonia infection by the use of ANN (artificial neural network) and CNN (convolutional neural network) systems and their working methodologies. The main benefit of the project highlights how Resnets work better than plain networks and help in improving the model accuracy as well show its implementation. Using deep learning, many lives can be saved from pneumonia infection, helping people to live a healthy and prosperous life.

12.2 LITERATURE REVIEW

Detection of pneumonia from chest radiographs has been difficult for many years; the primary problem is the lack of posted information. Conventional systems are gaining knowledge of strategies and have been studied. A maximum of the deep getting-to-know techniques are required for detection of pneumonia awareness on the usage of a single CNN model. However, an organization gaining knowledge permits the consolidation of picks made via more than one CNN method. This efficiently incorporates the essential information, collecting additional facts from distinctive classifiers and considering more efficient choice making. This pattern is not often explored in the quest to diagnose pneumonia. (Nayak, [1]) mined common devices and kind strategies. (Rautaray, [7]) describes a transfer getting-to-know method within the global mag of new generation and engineering. (Germany, D.S. et al., [5]) identified a clinical diagnosis and a treatable sickness with the assistance of images, primarily based on deep learning. Variable generalization performance of a deep-mastering version helped find pneumonia in chest radiographs and thus itchanged into a move-sectional test which was performed by the authors in their research paper (Zech, [8]). In the assessment of device-learning algorithms, for which handcrafted capabilities need to be extracted and decided on for class or segmentation, deep gaining knowledge of based totally techniques perform give up-to-end kind, wherein the applicable and informative features are mechanically extracted from the input statistics and categorized. CNNs are desired for picture facts class because they automatically extract translationally invariant functions through the convolution of the entered picture and filters. CNNs are translationally invariant and conduct better than device mastering or traditional photograph-processing methods in photo category obligations and, as a result, are widely utilized by researchers [9]. The radio-logistic stage of pneumonia detection with x-ray via the help of deep analysis was conducted by (Rajpurkar, [2]). (Xu et al., 2019) helped through using the making of the deep studying gadget to screen coronavirus disease and pneumonia. (Simonyan, [3]) made a deep convolutional community for the large scale of the images for their popularity. Rahman et al. 2014, Liang et al. 2014, Ibrahim et al. 2014, and Zubair et al. 2014 implemented without a doubt transfer mastering strategies wherein first-rate CNN fashions pre-educated on ImageNet records are used for pneumonia elegance. To categorise the lung regions from chest x-ray images, Chandra et al. (2015) segmented the lung sections and extracted eight statistical features from these regions [10]. Multi-layer perceptron (MLP), random wooded area (RWA), sequential minimum optimization (SMO), type through regression, and logistic regression are the five conventional classifiers they successfully implemented. They tested their method on 412 images and found that the MLP classifier had an accuracy rate of 95.39%. 2019s Kuo et al. used 11 methods to identify pneumonia in 185 schizophrenia patients. They used those skills in a wide range of regression and type patterns, including logistic regression, decision trees, and support-vector machines, and they compared the results of those models. They used a decision tree classifier and achieved an accuracy rate of 94.5%; the other models failed due to the use of huge margins. In addition, Yue et al. 2021 employed six functions to identify pneumonia in 52 patients' chest CT scan pictures; the astounding AUC value they achieved was 97%. When compared to the requirements for in-depth analysis, the information provided in the challenge we created only had 5,800 images [11,12]. A branch of machine learning called deep learning employs mathematical formulas to translate the input to output. The available functions can build a courtship-like relationship between the input and the output by extracting non-redundant information or patterns from the data. In many conditions, the count may even be up to hundreds or thousands of images, which is a little difficult for the processing to be finished using local machines [13]. The version that is used within the project is quite heavy and could eat a lot of time for running on a normal CPU. Resolving this following difficulty, the project was utilized in Google Collaborator, which helped it plenty in the deep-learning model. Google Collab is a part of Google research projects, which is a lot beneficial in machine-learning education and its research and is likewise hosted on Google Cloud example, which all can use without cost and with less difficulty than others [14].

12.3   TECHNOLOGIES USED IN PNEUMONIA DETECTION

12.3.1   DEEP LEARNING AND NLP THE TECHNOLOGIES PLAYING A MAJOR ROLE IN REAL-LIFE IMPLEMENTATION

Deep learning is a form of technology that makes it simple to solve extremely difficult computational problems. Image processing, picture classification, image segmentation, image tagging, sound classification, video analysis, and other practical issues are examples [15]. Deep learning comes under the ideology of neural networks. A collection of algorithms makes up the neural network. That helps in recognizing relationships with the help of a dataset through which it mimics a human brain. In this sense, neural networks can be referred to as a type of network of neurons that resembles that network. The process helps to adapt according to the changing input and generates the best possible outcomes. Neurons, a mathematical function that gathers and categorises data following a distinctly unique design, are also included in neural networks. The three primary components of the neural network architecture are the input layer, the hidden layer, and the output layer (Figure 12.1).

The first layer that depicts an artificial neural network's process is the input layer. The systems' initial data is introduced into the input layer, which has artificial input neurons, where it will be

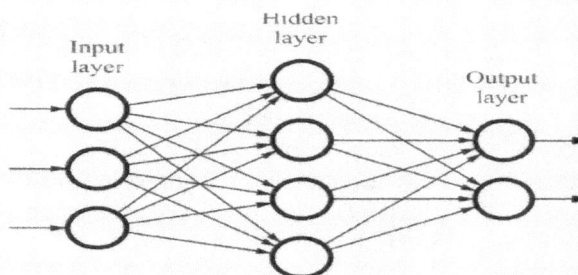

FIGURE 12.1 Components of neural network.

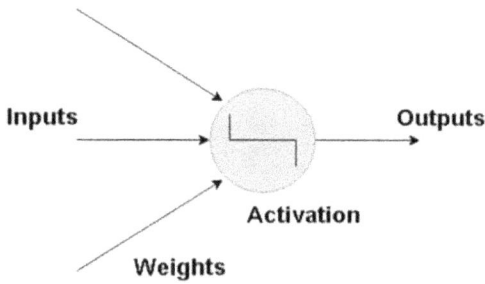

Inputs

Outputs

Activation

Weights

FIGURE 12.2   Working of activation function.

processed by further layers of artificial neural networks. The second layer of an artificial neural network design is a hidden layer that exists between the input and output. The hidden layer applies to the input region and controls output through activation processes. The input that is sent to the network is transformed nonlinearly by the hidden layer. The output layer, the third and last layer in the neural network, aids in producing the program's output. Understanding the fundamental principles of activation function is necessary since they are crucial in defining the operation of the hidden layer. Equations known as activation functions assist in predicting a neural network's output. According to whether each neuron's input is important to the model's prediction system, the functions associated with each neuron in the network assist determine whether it should be engaged or not (Figure 12.2).

By converting output values into a range of 0 to 1 or −1 to 1, the activation function aids in identifying the program's output. The linear activation function is the first of two different types of activation functions. Because these functions are aligned or presented in linear form, their output is not restricted to a certain range. The equation for the line would be affected equal to X and the range be from minus infinity. The issue with the linear activation function is they do not help us with the complexity of a problem or several common data parameters that are provided to neural networks (Figure 12.3).

To address the issue with the linear-activation function, the primary technologies must comprehend the functioning of a non-linear function. For the model to generalise or adapt to different types of details and to distinguish between the output, nonlinear functions are required. The model can generalise or adapt to a range of inputs and distinguish between the outputs with ease thanks to the non-linear function (Figure 12.4).

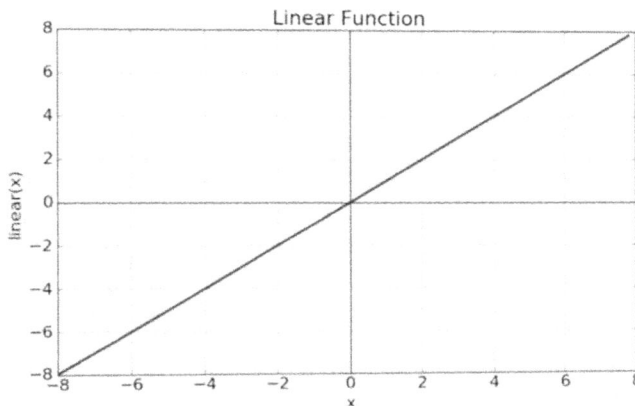

FIGURE 12.3   Linear activation function and the equation ranging from −infinity to + infinity.

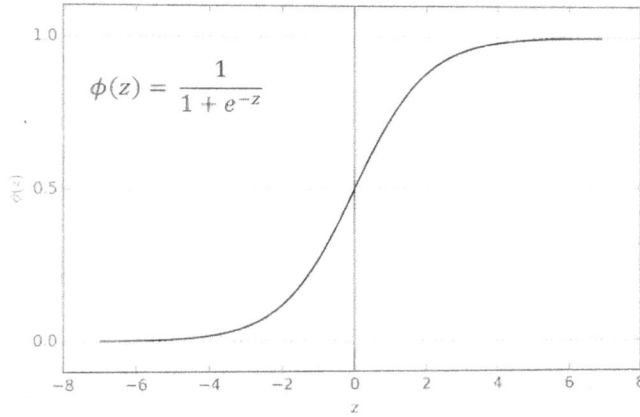

FIGURE 12.4 Non-linear activation function; the diagram shows how it becomes easy for the model to generalize or adapt to the variety of data and easily differentiate between the final output.

12.3.2 CHEST X-RAY OF DIFFERENT STAGES IN CASE OF PNEUMONIA

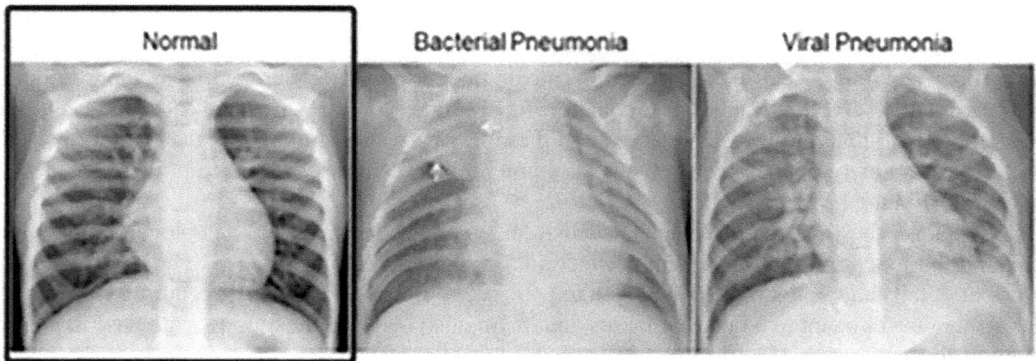

FIGURE 12.5 Chest x-ray without pneumonia.

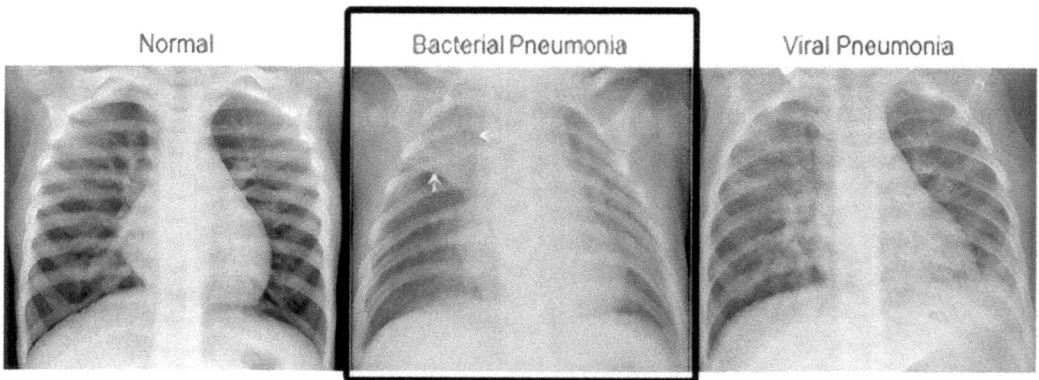

FIGURE 12.6 Chest x-ray infected with bacterial pneumonia [16,17].

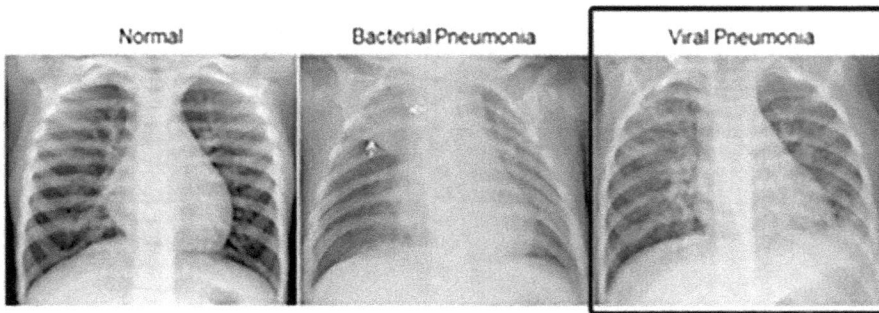

FIGURE 12.7 Chest x-ray infected with viral pneumonia.

12.4 PROPOSED METHODOLOGY

12.4.1 TECHNIQUES AND ARCHITECTURE OF DEEP LEARNING USED IN THE PROJECT AS A DIFFERENTIATING FACTOR

12.4.1.1 Neural Network

Neural networks employ a method akin to how the human brain works to find underlying linkages in a piece of data. It can be described as a computer system with interconnected nodes that operate similarly to brain neurons. Using algorithms, they can classify and group raw data, identify underlying patterns and connections, and learn and get better over time. The majority of pre-trained deep learning models are built using three crucial types of neural networks: artificial neural networks (ANNs), convolution neural networks (CNNs), and recurring neural networks (RNN) (Figures 12.5, 11.6 and 12.7) [18,19,20].

12.4.1.2 Artificial Neural Network (ANN)

Artificial neural networks are a branch of biologically inspired artificial intelligence that is brain-inspired. A biological neural network that forms the structure of the human brain serves as the basis for an artificial neural network, which is typically a computer network. Just like the human brain has interconnected neurons, an artificial neural network also has neurons that are linked together in different layers of the network. These neurons are called nodes. In the field of artificial intelligence, an artificial neural network attempts to replicate the neural network that constitutes the human brain so that computers are capable of comprehending the information and making judgments like humans do. Computers are programmed to operate like interconnected brain cells in artificial neural networks (Figure 12.8).

12.4.1.3 Recurring Neural Networks (RNNs)

An RNN is a specific type of neural network where the output of one phase is used as the input for the next. While the inputs and outputs of conventional neural networks are independent of one another, when predicting the next word in a sentence, for example, the previous words are necessary and are thus needed. Remember the previous words. So RNN was born to solve this problem by using a hidden layer. A hidden area that contains string information is the primary and most significant characteristic of RNNs. RNNs have a "memory" that houses all the data related to the computations. It employs the same settings for each input since it performs the same work on all inputs or hidden layers to get the conclusion. Unlike other neural networks, it lessens the complexity of the parameter set.

12.4.1.4 Convolution Neural Network (CNN)

Convolutions neural networks (CNNs) are a group of deep neural networks that focus on image processing and are therefore frequently employed in computer-vision applications like object

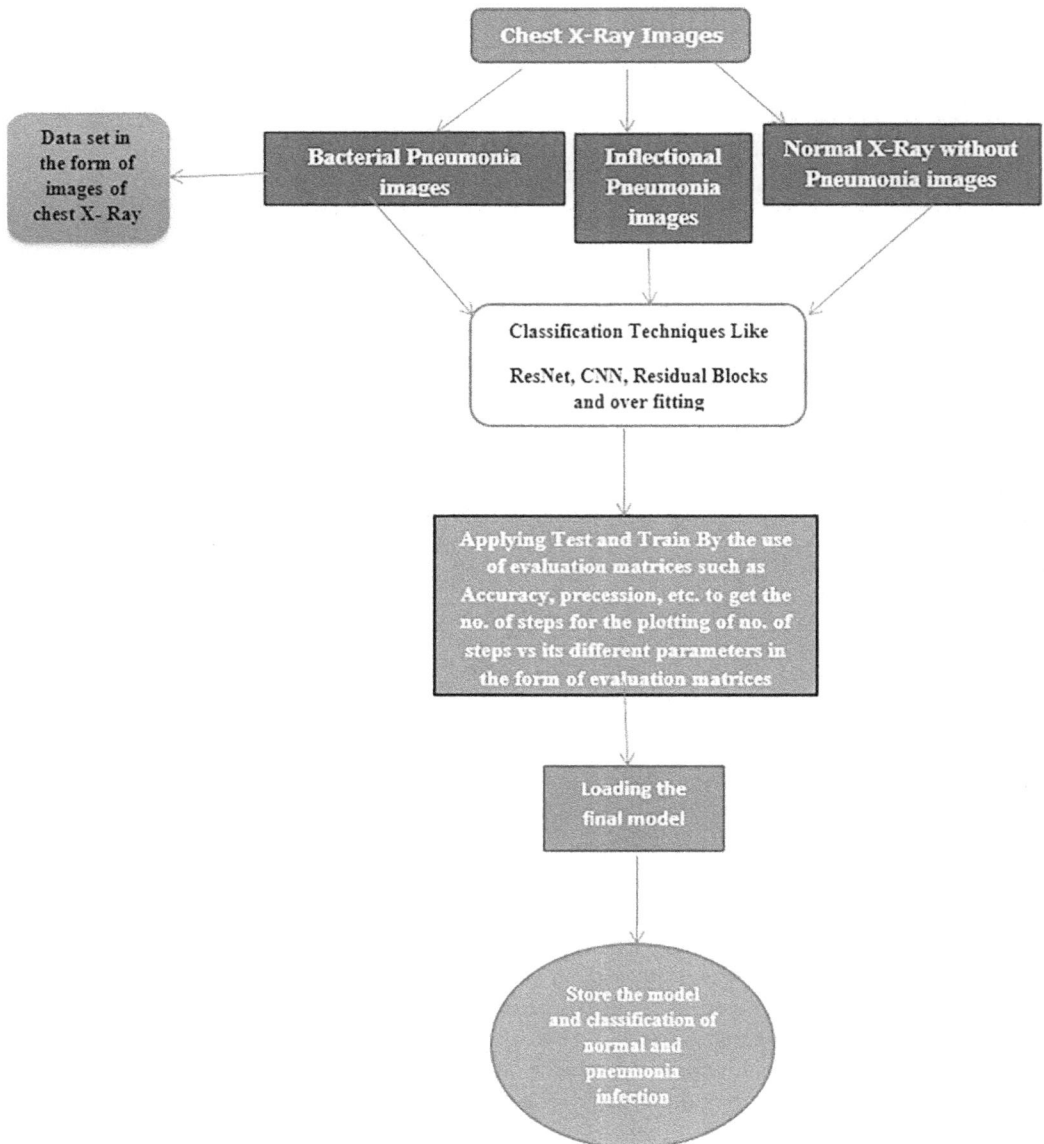

FIGURE 12.8   Proposed structure of pneumonia detection using x-ray images.

detection, neural transmission, and picture classification and clustering. CNN is arguably the oldest deep-learning architecture. CNN is used for handwritten postal code recognition and is of the relay network type. The capability of CNN to consider the feature's location is a significant advantage [20,21]. The intricate layers that give CNN its name is at the network's foundation. a combined layer that takes features out of the source picture. Each input map's size is reduced while still retaining important data thanks to a clustering layer. Multiple integrations and convolutional layers coupled in sequence make up the network architecture. A SoftMax layer is utilised for picture classification at the network level. The leaking gradient is the deeper CNNs' primary drawback. CNN's are well suited for image data classification because they automatically extract the invariant characteristics of the transformation and integration filtering from the input image. CNN's are

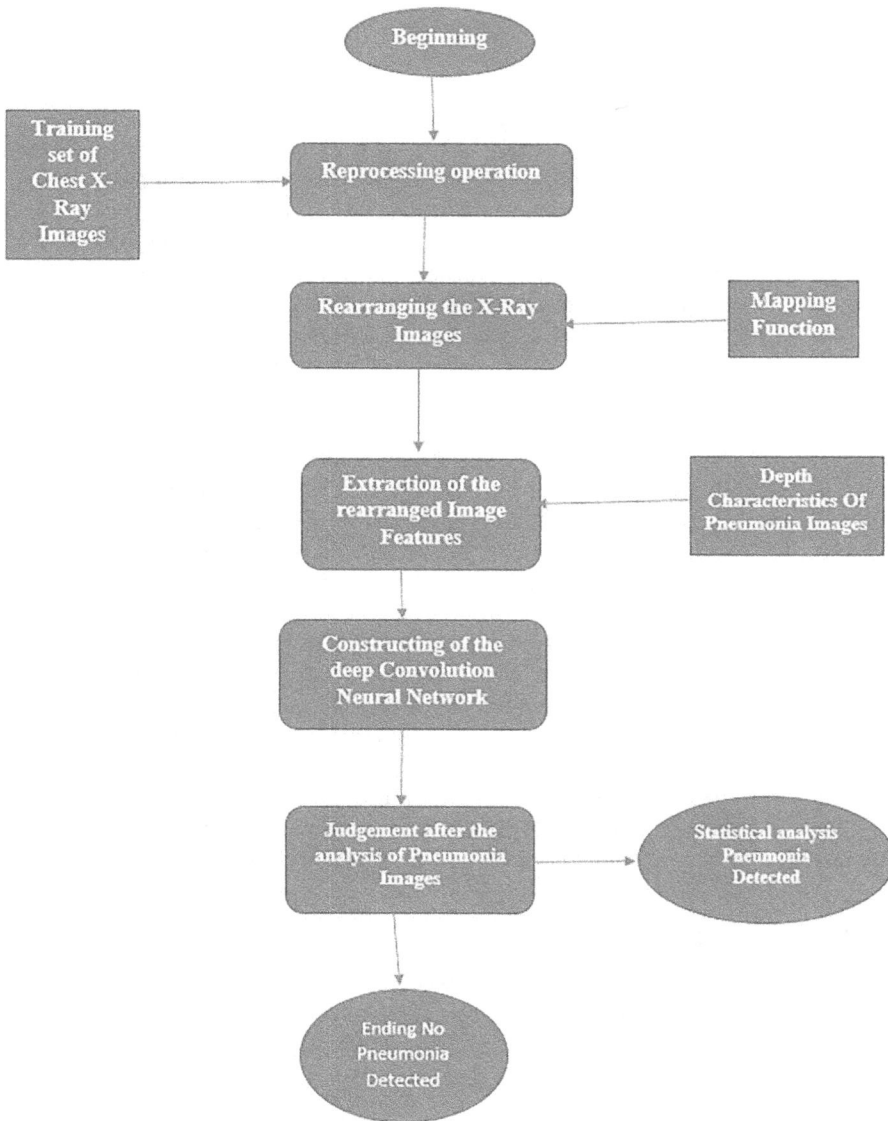

FIGURE 12.9 Structure of CNN used in pneumonia detection using x-ray images.

widely used by researchers because they are translation invariant and better than traditional image-processing methods for machine learning and image classification tasks (Figure 12.9).

12.4.1.5 ResNet

The suggested ResNet model is built on a residual-learning architecture, which boosts network deep-learning effectiveness. In contrast to the initial non-reference mapping in monotonically progressive convolutions, residual blocks in the ResNet model make it simpler to optimise the entire network, hence increasing the model's accuracy. These "ignored connections" or residuals carry out identity mapping with no additional parameters or increased computational complexity. Residual network (ResNet) is a cumulative neural network (CNN) architecture that overcomes the "leak gradient" problem, allowing to build of networks with thousands of convolutional layers, which perform better than other networks shallower.

12.4.1.6 The Ideology of Natural Language Processing (NLP)

Natural language processing (NLP) describes the spoken and written ways that individuals interact with one another. The procedure includes verbal and textual communication, which transmits a great deal of information. Daily themes chosen by people, their tonality, and word choice all add up to some kind of information that can be analyzed, and its value may be deduced from the supplied form of data. NLP is a branch of artificial intelligence that, in plain English, gives robots the ability to read, comprehend, and extract meaning from human language (AI). NLP allows people to converse with computers using a natural language, such as English. With improvements in data access and a rise in computing capacity, NLP is flourishing in the modern world. NLP is incredibly useful in industries like banking, journalism, and healthcare. Today, millions of data are produced through discussions, statements, or tweets; these data are unstructured and do not fit in a row-and-column format, making them challenging to alter and analyze. NLP enables the machines to analyze sentiment and even recognize speech figures like irony. Data can always be in the form of numbers since NLP can readily take raw language as an input and extract useful insights from it when dealing with textual data. NLP is in high demand right now on the market. The digital revolution is something none of the businesses wishes to ignore. Every company tries to take advantage of artificial intelligence. Businesses examine unstructured data to find trends and make data-driven choices, and a sizable percentage of that data is text data. Projects involving textual analytics are in high demand for NLP experts with professional skills. Diseases are identified and predictions are made. By identifying customer reviews and obtaining essential information from the reviews, the target customer can be identified based on what customers have to say about their products. Sentimental analysis can reveal a lot about the customer's preferences and motivating factors. Examples of sophisticated voice-driven interfaces that employ NLP to respond to vocal commands are Amazon's Alexa and Apple's Siri. By determining the skills of potential hires, NLP is also employed in the talent-recruiting process during both the search and selection phases. NLP technology is also used by autocorrect and autocomplete to display accurate items and results. The pneumonia-detection project plays a major role in image-processing techniques and achieves higher accuracy and better precision value. By using NLP, the process of automation and discovery of new emerging technologies can be easily done.

12.4.2 Methodologies Differentiating from Other Models

The figure mentioned above mentions the difference between plain networks vs Resnet, but there is not much difference in validation errors of plain 18 layers and Resnet 18. But the difference starts showing up when we use deeper models like Resnet 34 and Resnet 50. Also, the validation error for 34 layers Resnet is significantly lower compared to its plain counterpart. As shown in the figure mentioned above, issues using plain convolutional networks are the validation errors for two plain convolutional networks with 18 layers, and 34 layers. The error for a 34 layers network is higher compared to 18 layers and differences will keep increasing with the increase in the number of layers (Figure 12.10).

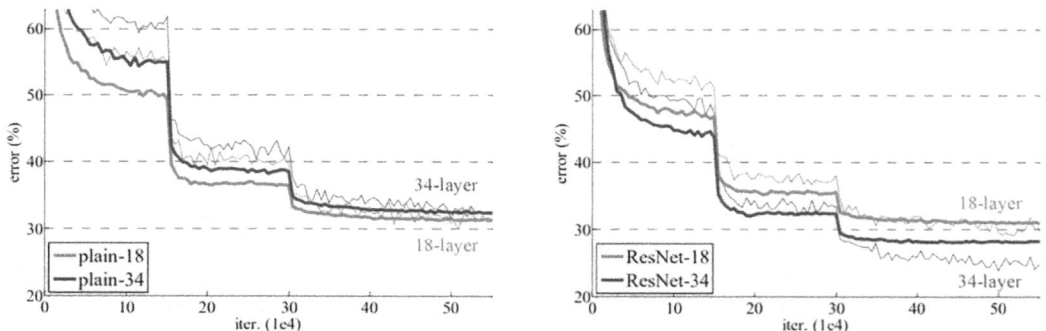

FIGURE 12.10 Comparison of plain networks vs Resnets.

12.4.3 Use of Another Modern Resnet

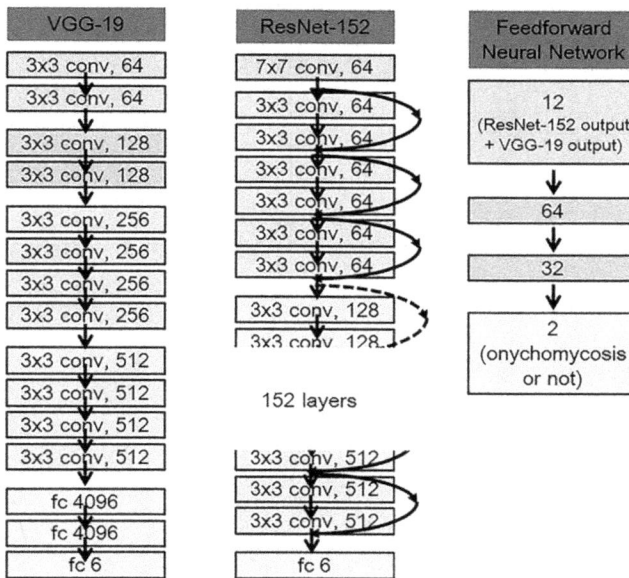

FIGURE 12.11 Deeper Resnet.

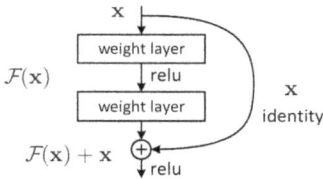

FIGURE 12.12 Diagram of residual block.

12.4.4 Residual Block-Responsible for Establishing Skip Connection

A residual block receives a layer's output and passes it on to additional layers. Additionally, it retains historical data, which is simply the identity function. The term "skip connection" is also used to describe this kind of connection (Figure 12.11 and Figure 12.12).

12.5 RESULTS AND DISCUSSION

When training of the model is done, the result of the training in a variable was obtained, which is known as history. History contains all the progress of the model and its metrics, such as training, accuracy, and loss, which are the default type of metrics. Also, parsing in precision and recall is done while training in the cell, and iteration is done. In the cell, iteration and recall are performed based on all metrics and plotting graphs for each metric in a subplot. The blue line is the progress of the metric on training data and the orange line is the progress on validation data. When precision and recall are required, the aim is to move validation progress to gradually moving higher and touch the training curve gradually. Here recall is the most important metric in medical problem statements. The formula for finding recall is – **True positive / (True positive + False negative).** The false negatives are the number of predictions that when predicted are normal, but in actual situations, it's pneumonia. The maximum recall is directly proportional to the minimum false

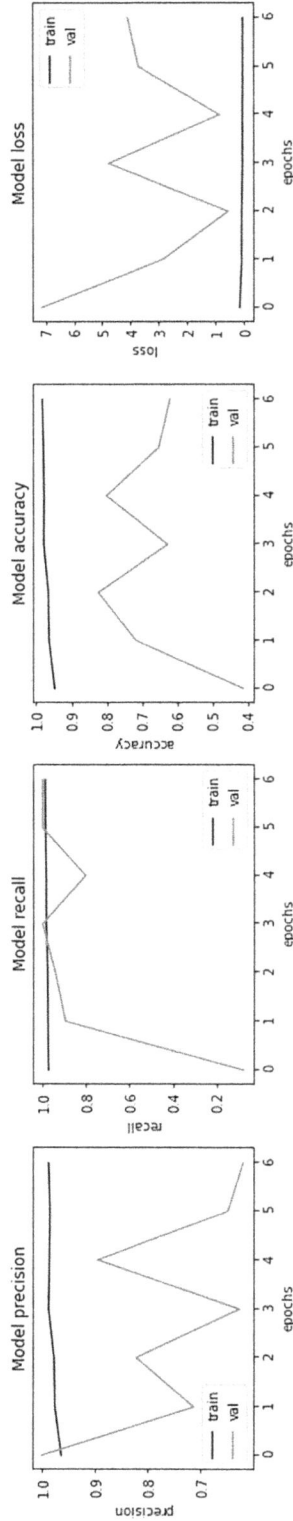

FIGURE 12.13   Plots based on different evaluation metrics.

TABLE 12.1

Number of Steps to Show the Evaluation Metrics Based on Different Parameters

Epochs (Steps)	Accuracy	Precision	Recall	Val Loss	Loss
1/8	0.9477	0.9637	0.9717	7.1131	0.1560
2/8	0.9638	0.9760	0.9752	2.8368	0.0928
3/8	0.9659	0.9777	0.99767	0.5668	0.0897
4/8	0.9787	0.9880	0.9832	4.7747	0.0589
5/8	0.9780	0.9866	0.9838	0.8688	0.0593
6/8	0.9795	0.9856	0.9869	3.7289	0.0510
7/8	0.9822	0.9881	0.9878	4.1027	0.0512

negatives. In this particular case, precision and recall, curves are following the trends nicely. The accuracy of the revalidation dataset also keeps increasing when training is done, and the loss keeps decreasing. This factor describes the learning ability of the model. For overfitting, there is a need to look at the lost graph. If the loss starts increasing and there is no indication of its coming down, then it is considered an overfitted model. Basically, by the following method's performance of the model is evaluated (Figure 12.13 and Table 12.1).

12.6 CONCLUSION

The project helps to talk about the working of google collab and its resources and how it can be implemented to solve high-level problems of deep learning and its various methodologies where the dataset is in the form of images, text, and videos. TensorFlow plays a major role in building convolutional neural networks. The identification and detection of pneumonia are done using the ResNet architecture and perform well. The model can be deployed to get real-time responses using APIs. The problem has around 7000 images, which were easy to process the data, but in the case of millions of data, there is a need to adopt advanced techniques to enhance the work of deep learning, which can be implemented by performing image recognition and classification techniques. The major key takeaway from the project is to utilize the data. It should be made balanced, and resampling techniques should be applied for the proper working of the deep-learning model. More things could be tried; medical problem statements are complex, and there's a high chance to miss some important points before solving the issue for proper implementation. Different companies make different x-ray scanners, and processing and working methods are different. To improve the existing dataset, x-rays from multiple hospitals and different machines can be collected. Using a deep-learning model, the project gives confidence to users to perform more classification tasks and image-processing tasks. For future purposes, augmentation can be used as its most tricky part in image processing. To use augmentations that do not affect pixel values like horizontal rotations, random image cropping can be done or minimally tested on blurry images. The main benefit of the project highlights how resnets work better than plain networks and helps in improving the model accuracy, as well show its implementation. Using deep learning, many lives can be saved from pneumonia infection and help people to live a healthy and prosperous life [9–21].

REFERENCES

[1] Nayak, S., Gourisaria, M. K., Pandey, M.; and Rautaray, S. S. 2019, May. Prediction of heart disease by mining frequent items and classification techniques. In 2019 International Conference on Intelligent Computing and Control Systems (ICCS) (pp. 607–611). IEEE.

[2] Rajpurkar, P.; Irvin, J.; Zhu, K.; Yang, B.; Mehta, H.; Duan, T.; Ding, D.; Bagul, A.; Langlotz, C.; Shpanskaya, K.; Lungren, M. P.; and Ng, A. Y. 2017. Chexnet: Radiologist-level pneumonia detection on chest x-rays with deep learning. arXiv preprint arXiv:1711.05225.

[3] Pankratz, D. G.; Choi, Y.; Imtiaz, U.; Fedorowicz, G. M.; Anderson, J. D.; Colby, T. V.; Myers, J. L.; Lynch, D. A.; Brown, K. K.; Flaherty, K. R.; Steele, M. P.; Groshong, S. D.; Raghu, G.; Barth, N. M.; Walsh, P. S.; Huang, J.; Kennedy, G. C.; and Matinez, F. J. 2017. Usual interstitial pneumonia can be detected in transbronchial biopsies using machine learning. *Annals of the American Thoracic Society (ATS)*, 14(11): 1646–1654.

[4] Caruana, R.; Lou, Y.; Gehrke, J.; Koch, P.; Sturm, M.; and Elhadad, N. 2015. Intelligible models for healthcare. In Proceedings of the 21st ACM SIGKDD International Conference on Knowledge Discovery and Data Mining (KDD '15) (pp. 1721–1730).

[5] Germany, D. S.; Goldbaum, M.; Cai, W.; Valentim, C. C. S.; Liang, H.; Baxter, S. L.; McKeown, A.; Yang, G.; Wu, X.; Yan, F.; Dong, J.; Prasad, M. K.; Pei, J.; Ting, M. Y. L.; Zhu, J.; Li, C.; Hewett, S.; Dong, J.; Shi, W.; Fu, X.; Duan, Y.; Huu, V. A. N.; Wen, C.; Zhang, E. D.; Zhang, C. L.; Li, O.; Wang, X.; Singer, M. A.; Sun, X.; Xu, J.; Tafreshi, A.; Lewis, M. A.; Xia, H.; and Zhang, K. 2018. Identifying medical diagnoses and treatable diseases by image-based deep learning. *Cell*, 172(5): 1122–1131.

[6] Xu, X.; Jiang, X.; Ma, C.; Du, P.; Li, X.; Lv, S.; Yu, L.; Chen, Y.; Su, J.; Lang, G.; Li, Y.; Zhao, H.; Xu, K.; Ruan, L.; and Wu, W. 2020. Deep learning system to screen coronavirus disease 2019 pneumonia. arXiv preprint arXiv:2002.09334.

[7] Rautaray S. S.; Pandey, M.; Gourisaria, M. K.; Sharma, R.; and Das, S. 2020. Paddy crop disease prediction-A transfer learning technique. *International Journal of Recent Technology and Engineering (IJRTE)*, 8(6): 1–6.

[8] Zech, J. R.; Badgeley, M. A.; Liu, M.; Costa, A. B.; Titano, J. J.; and Oermann, E. K. 2018. Variable generalization performance of a deep learning model to detect pneumonia in chest radiographs: A cross-sectional study. *PLOS Medicine*, 15(11): e1002683.

[9] He, K.; Zhang, X.; Ren, S.; and Sun, J. 2016. Deep residual learning for image recognition. In Proceedings of the IEEE Conference on Computer Vision and Pattern Recognition (CVPR) (pp. 770–778). Las Vegas, NV.

[10] Hastie, T.; and Tibshirani, R. 1995. Generalized additive models for medical research. *Statistical Methods in Medical Research*, 4(3): 187–196.

[11] Wang, X.; Peng, Y.; Lu, L.; Lu, Z.; Bagheri, M.; and Summers, R. M. 2017. Chest-xray8: Hospital-scale chest x-ray database and benchmarks on weakly-supervised classification and localization of common thorax diseases. *Journal of Engineering Science and Technology February 2021*, 16(1) Proceedings of the IEEE Conference on Computer Vision and Pattern Recognition. Honolulu, HI, 3462–3471.

[12] Nayak, S.; Gourisaria, M. K.; Pandey, M.; and Rautaray, S. S. 2019. Prediction of heart disease by mining frequent items and classification techniques. In International Conference on Intelligent Computing and Control Systems (ICCS) (pp. 607–611). Madurai, India.

[13] Kermany, D. S.; Goldbaum, M.; Cai, W.; Valentim, C. C. S.; Liang, H.; Baxter, S. L.; McKeown, A.; Yang, G.; Wu, X.; Yan, F.; Dong, J.; Prasadha, M. K.; Pei, J.; Ting, M. Y. L.; Zhu, J.; Li, C.; Hewett, S.; Dong, J.; Shi, W.; Fu, X.; Duan, Y.; Huu, V. A. N.; Wen, C.; Zhang, E. D.; Zhang, C. L.; Li, O.; Wang, X.; Singer, M. A.; Sun, X.; Xu, J.; Tafreshi, A.; Lewis, M. A.; Xia, H.; and Zhang, K. 2018. Identifying medical diagnoses and treatable diseases by image-based deep learning. *Cell*, 172(5): 1122–1131.

[14] Xu, X.; Jiang, X.; Ma, C.; Du, P.; Li, X.; Lv, S.; Yu, L.; Chen, Y.; Su, J.; Lang, G.; Li, Y.; Zhao, H.; Xu, K.; Ruan, L.; and Wu, W. 2020. *Deep Learning System To Screen Coronavirus Disease 2019 Pneumonia*. arXiv preprint arXiv:2002.09334.

[15] Simonyan, K.; and Zisserman, A. 2014. Very deep convolutional networks for large-scale image recognition. arXiv preprint arXiv:1409.1556.

[16] Wang, X.; Peng, Y.; Lu, L.; Lu, Z.; Bagheri, M.; and Summers, R. M. 2017. Chestx-ray8: Hospital-scale chest x-ray database and benchmarks on weakly-supervised classification and localization of common thorax diseases. *Pneumonia Detection Using CNN Through Chest X-Ray 875 Journal of Engineering Science and Technology February 2021*, 16(1) Proceedings of the IEEE Conference on Computer Vision and Pattern Recognition. Honolulu, HI, 3462–3471.

[17] Zhou, S., Zhang, X.; and Zhang R. 2019. Identifying cardiomegaly in ChestX-ray8 using transfer learning. MEDINFO 2019: Health And Wellbeing E-Networks For All. pp. 482–486.

[18] Huang, G.; Liu, Z.; Van Der Maaten, L.; and Weinberger, K. 2017. Densely connected convolutional networks. Proceedings of The IEEE Conference on Computer Vision and Pattern Recognition. (pp. 4700–4708).

[19] Selvaraju, R., Cogswell, M., Das, A., Vedantam, R., Parikh, D.; and Batra; D. 2017. Grad-cam: Visual explanations from deep networks via gradient-based localization. Proceedings of The IEEE International Conference on Computer Vision (pp. 618–626).

[20] Mahmud, T., Rahman, M.; and Fattah S. 2020. CovXNet: A multi-dilation convolutional neural network for automatic COVID-19 and other pneumonia detection from chest X-ray images with transferable multi-receptive feature optimization. *Computers in Biology and Medicine*, 122: 103869

[21] Antin, B., Kravitz, J.; and Martayan, E. 2017. Detecting pneumonia in chest X-Rays with supervised learning. *Semantic scholar. Org.*

13 AI Technique from Type CN2 Rule Induction for Industry 4.0 with Healthcare Problem

Samaher Al-Janabi, Ayad Alkaim, Noor Al-Janabi, and Ameer M

Department of Computer Science, Faculty of Science for Women (SCIW), University of Babylon, Babylon, Iraq

CONTENTS

13.1 INTRODUCTION

The World Health Organization (WHO) declared the pandemic of COVID-19 as an "international emergency," leading to the stopping of outside life all over the world, with thousands of lives lost rapidly. Then the world's scientists estimated the pandemic's scale to determine and illustrate that the virus is lethal and spreadable, way more than the normal flu. According to the reports situationally from the (WHO), those most susceptible to the risk of infection are old people and those who have cardiovascular hypertension, cancer, and respiratory disease; the reports referenced people who passed away in China, Italy, and Iran. Therefore, medical robots must assist in

DOI: 10.1201/9781003333081-13

controlling the spread of infection among people. There are many ways of checking, testing, fogging, and disinfecting, very different from, not even comparable to, ordinary cleaning procedures. Cleaning involves special techniques like cold fogging to kill viruses. Specific chemical solvents have been recommened, according to the National Environment Agency (NEA). This all adversely affects and poses danger to workers in cleaning companies, even though the procedures include precautionary measures; psychological damage to the working people is also a risk [1–3].

COVID-19 is a disease in which a new strain of coronavirus causes corona, the illness. The English name for the disease is derived as follows: CO is the first two letters of the word Corona, and VI, the first two letters of the word virus, and D, the first letter of the word disease, and this disease was previously called 19 novel. Coronavirus is a new virus associated with the same family of viruses as the virus that causes "severe acute respiratory syndrome (SARS)" and some types of common cold, and is rapidly spreading and infectious [4–8].

As the world turned to a strategy of social isolation, dedication to quarantine and contact through new media technologies to achieve the highest levels of safety from infection, the spread of the coronavirus pandemic contributed to changing the course of normal life and moving the world to new social phenomena that affected the nature and quality of social bonding and the usual human formations. Our society is therefore in desperate need of awareness of the rules of health awareness and knowledge of both the harms and benefits to proceed with sound health strategies. Health requires the integrity of the functional aspects of the person's bodily structures to prevent any deficiencies or defects that affect the individual's personality and actions, and thus, their ability to raise their level [9–11].

The main problem of this study can show as follows. Sickness and health are among the phenomena that have received the attention of all segments of society, especially in light of the pandemice, when coronavirus has swept the world and spread in every country. This spread has been accompanied by many measures taken by countries to besiege the virus and prevent its spread. These inclue the home quarantine that requires the commitment of families to stay in their homes. Because this is a precautionary and necessary measure to confront the virus, it has many consequences for families, which may affect their physical or mental health. It is very important at this stage to know the health measures necessary for families to take to promote health, confront the virus, and manage the coronavirus crisis. Accordingly, the problem of the study lies in the following main question:

- What is the level of health awareness in the Iraqi society about the era of the COVID-19 (corona) epidemic?
- To answer this question, the following sub-questions were asked:
- What is the level of health awareness in Iraqi society about the era of the COVID-19 (corona) epidemic?
- Are there statistically significant differences at the significance level ($\alpha \leq 0.05$) in the estimates of the respondent's responses to the level of health awareness in the Iraqi community about the era of the COVID-19 (corona) epidemic due to gender variables?

13.2 RELATED WORKS

Gregory Kahn et al., (2018) [12] developed an approach of the ordinary graph to reach a level that learns from their failure by interpolating both model-free and model-based methods. These learn from raw images and are efficient in sampling, such as from experiments on RC cars that can navigate through an indoor complex environment. This sounds similar to our work in finding effective and efficient high-quality representations for each node based on the given features, neighborhood, and structural information underlying the graph. The solutions should be designed to automatically extract and utilize any useful signals in the graph, whether by heuristic or systematic models.

Guang-Zhong Yang et al., (2020) [13]: Robots' main role in times such as the 2015 Ebola outbreak and the 2020 COVID-19 pandemic should be clear and effective. Efforts included the disinfection and delivery of food and medicines to help people monitor patients' condition and manage as well as prevent the disease. Solutions were developed and extended to many domains, such as mobile software connected to robots to retrace contacts of infected people and alert others, or decrease the cost and risk to the people who work to disinfect and clean the most touched surfaces. Our robot is one of those developed robots and smart devices/ software to pass through the pandemic.

Ki Ho Hong et al. (2020) [14], for the sake of knowing many of the general diagnostic methods and interpreting the results and selection of the specimens. All of those are keys to globalize the epidemiological studies' results, their level, and the (PUI: patient under investigations) to be change checked relating to the new information from the KCDC'S update. To make a robot and software deals with hygienic needs in the present time, we should be aware of all those aspects and headlines.

Nathaniel Després et al. (2020) [15], this method is working on micro-lattice architectures; those are generated by a compact genetic algorithm, connected to mechanical properties that are finite-elemental. They analyze the autoencoder trained to supervise the manner of graph representations on the micro lattices and the displace characteristics, and then the decoder generates micro lattices from desired properties. It then adds more graph convolutional layers to the graph. And the similarities with our work are where producing deeper networks and working on autoencoder-decoder methods on a genetic algorithm helps get to the representations and the result of the testing. Table 13.1 shows the comparison among the previous works based on five points, types of dataset, methodology used, evaluation measures, and advantages.

Fei Tian et al. (2017) [16], as soon as deep learning had been adopted in applications like speech recognition and image classification. This graph clustering works on a new method that uses k = means algorithm on the non-leaner embedding to the original graph and runs the algorithm to obtain results. It's working on autoencoder and spectral clustering, and it's more efficient than spectral clustering. It's similar to our work, using low computational complexity, and the form is linear to the number of nodes. It's tested and got results of various datasets of the graph, showing the proposed method, significantly the effectiveness of deep learning in graph clustering.

Trung Thien Pham et al., (2020) [17], caution and prevention against coronavirus by creating a chamber controlled by main system roles. Three subsystems include the automatic sanitization of the hands and checking the body temperature, getting to the final step to spray the whole body 360° with silver nano solvent. If the infrared sensor read that the body's temperature was more than 37, it would send it to the processor to be displayed on the screen. That is similar to the sanitizing part of our work, but we also have developed it as a transforming and medication teleport smart vehicle.

Zeashan Hameed Khan et al., (2020) [18], automatic devices and robots in the field of healthcare get wider and better. The International Federation of Robots (IFR) sees that it will increase from now on, and the robot must meet all of the dexterity, sterilization, operator safety, power requirement, and finally, the cost to be as efficient as the human need in such a time, while our robot is passing all of these conditions and difficulties.

As for what separates the current research from previous studies, it is reflected in the fact that it relies on health awareness that can be found in all age groups in Iraqi society, which, in most cases, can have negative implications.

This study is distinguished by its new theme, which relates to the degree of health knowledge of the COVID-19 (corona) epidemic in the Iraqi culture. The current analysis followed the descriptive and analytical approach, and the electronic questionnaire was used as an information-collection too. The study population and its sample consisted of all members of the Iraqi community from 2019 to 2020, and the researcher followed the available sample process.

13.2.1 CORONAVIRUS

It discusses the concept of the coronavirus (COVID-19), its patterns and symptoms, and the methods used to transmit this virus. It discusses how coronavirus infection can be avoided (COVID-19) (Figure 13.1).

TABLE 13.1

Compare Among the Previous Works

Author(s)	Dataset	Suggested Method	Evaluation Method	Advantages	Disadvantages
Gregory Kahn 2018 [12]	Real-world dataset	Having the robot maintain an internal map of the world	Localization and planning method (Learning-based method)	Approach outperforms single-step and N-step double Q-learning	Learning in large outdoor environments with dynamic obstacles present immense challenges
Guang-Zhong Yang 2020 [13]	Eye on all kinds of robotics in health and infectious diseases care	Checking and spotlighting on all the disinfection and human-assist methods	Compare the results of the method to the robots and devices using the same one	Makes sure that the robots developed to deal with cleanliness risks and unsuitable jobs for humans	Without the effort of researchers in such a field to specify the risk, we'll get back to ready robots for the next pandemic.
Ki Ho Hong 2020 [14]	Tests that are granted an (EUA) by the American food and drug admin.	CDC guidance and testing method	Using the respiratory specimens storing and shipping to compared to other places results	Doing the COVID-19 tests and distinguishing its symptoms from other respiratory system diseases.	The delay the systems take, also the uncertainty of the COVID-19 cause.
Nathaniel Despre's 2020 [15]	Learning dataset	Analysis and design of microlattices	Design of microlattice (compact genetic algorithm)	Reducing the time and resources required during the design process	Still in developing period and not specified for specific work
Fei Tian 2020 [16]	Several real-world datasets	Takes the sparse autoencoder as its building block	k-means algorithm	More efficient and flexible than spectral clustering, the computational complexity of autoencoder is much lower than spectral clustering	It is nonstraightforward to implement a sparse spectral method. And it does not work on non-linear method.
Trung Thien Pham 2020 [17]	Disinfectant system	Sanitizing testing and 360 spraying method	(BRQPS 10M-TDTA-C type NPN) sensor and JMNano silver solution	Hand washing, temperature testing, and disinfection with solution have an impact on H1N1, SARS viruses.	The system doesn't have an Android app or is not even remotely controlled.
Zeachan Hameed Khan 2020 [18]	Utilization of Robots in Healthcare	Robotics in medicine potentially and relation to COVID-19	Educating and sophisticated robots in healthcare fields	Reduce the number of infected people because of the management effectiveness of the COVID-19 virus.	Robots are not dependent, not even reliable and safe, compared to the human role

Severe acute respiratory syndrome coronavirus 2 (SARS-CoV-2)

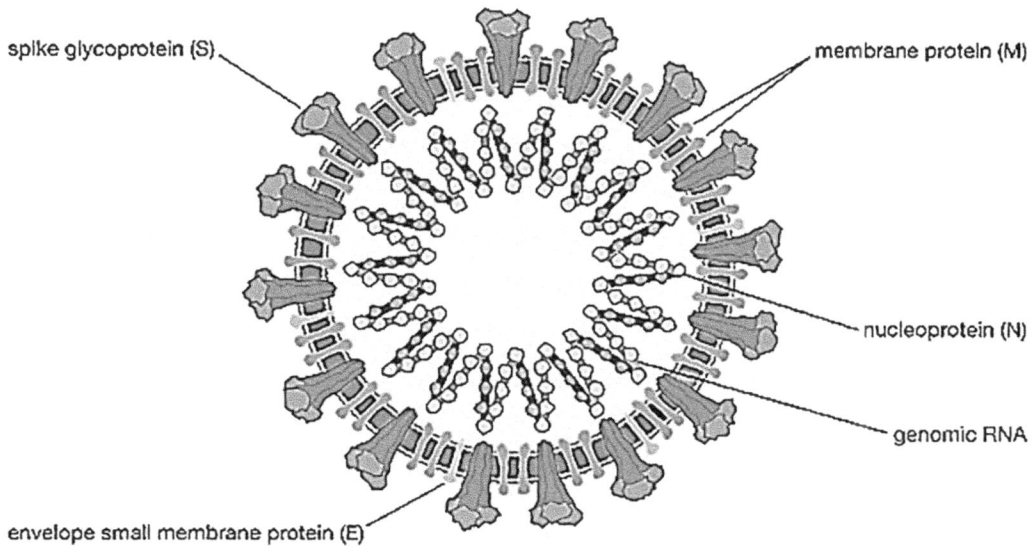

FIGURE 13.1   Coronavirus content.

13.2.2   CONCEPT OF CORONAVIRUS

The new virus was dubbed the MERS-CoV MERS Middle East Airborne Syndrome or Corona Novel, and the coronavirus is the sixth largest virus in the coronavirus family. It was named initially in some international papers as a variety of different names, including SARS or Saudi SARS. Recently, it was decided to be named «Coron» Corona Mers Middle East Respiratory Syndrome, a new virus, not identified in the past. But, it did not emerge from a vacuum, but from the respiratory syndrome, and from the acute coronavirus (SARS) in China in 2003 and spreading into 17 countries, triggering global panic, until it was quickly confronted In the Middle East Respiratory Syndrome [19,20] (Figure 13.2).

Coronavirus (COVID-19) 2019 is a new infectious disease described as 'pneumonia of unknown origin.' It was called acute respiratory syndrome (SARS-2) by the World Health Organization, despite the great efforts made by the Chinese government. It was first reported to have been described with rapid human transmission capabilities and a large varying number of deaths due to acute respiratory distress syndrome (ARDS) [21,22] (Figure 13.3).

13.3   CORONAVIRUS PATTERNS

There are three main epidemiological patterns of the virus:

- First: In cultures, sporadic cases occur, and we don't know the origin or infection of the virus.
- Second: It is a category of infections between members of the family; clusters and transmittal occur in most of these classes, but the infection tends to be determined by direct contact with the sick person in the family.
- Third: In France, Jordan, and Saudi Arabia, it is a group of infections in health facilities, and these trends have been identified. The infection in these groups is transmitted from person to person following the disease's introduction in a healthcare facility for treatment.

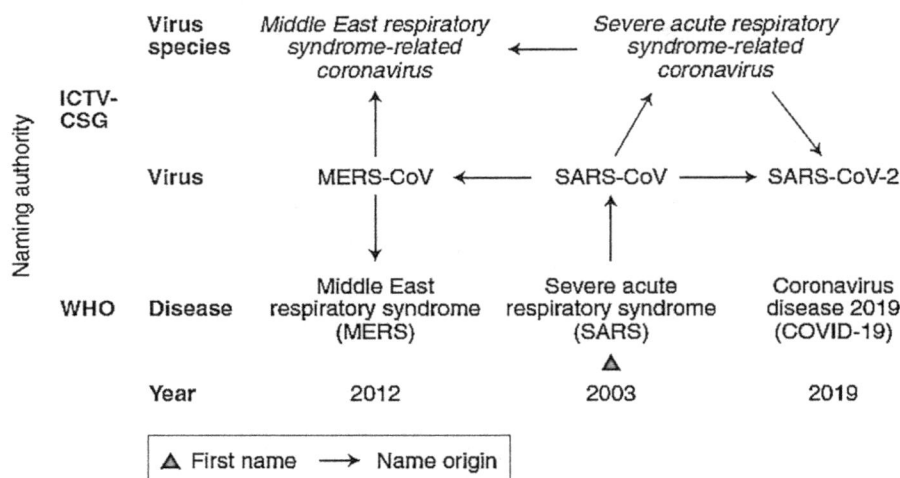

FIGURE 13.2   Coronavirus naming.

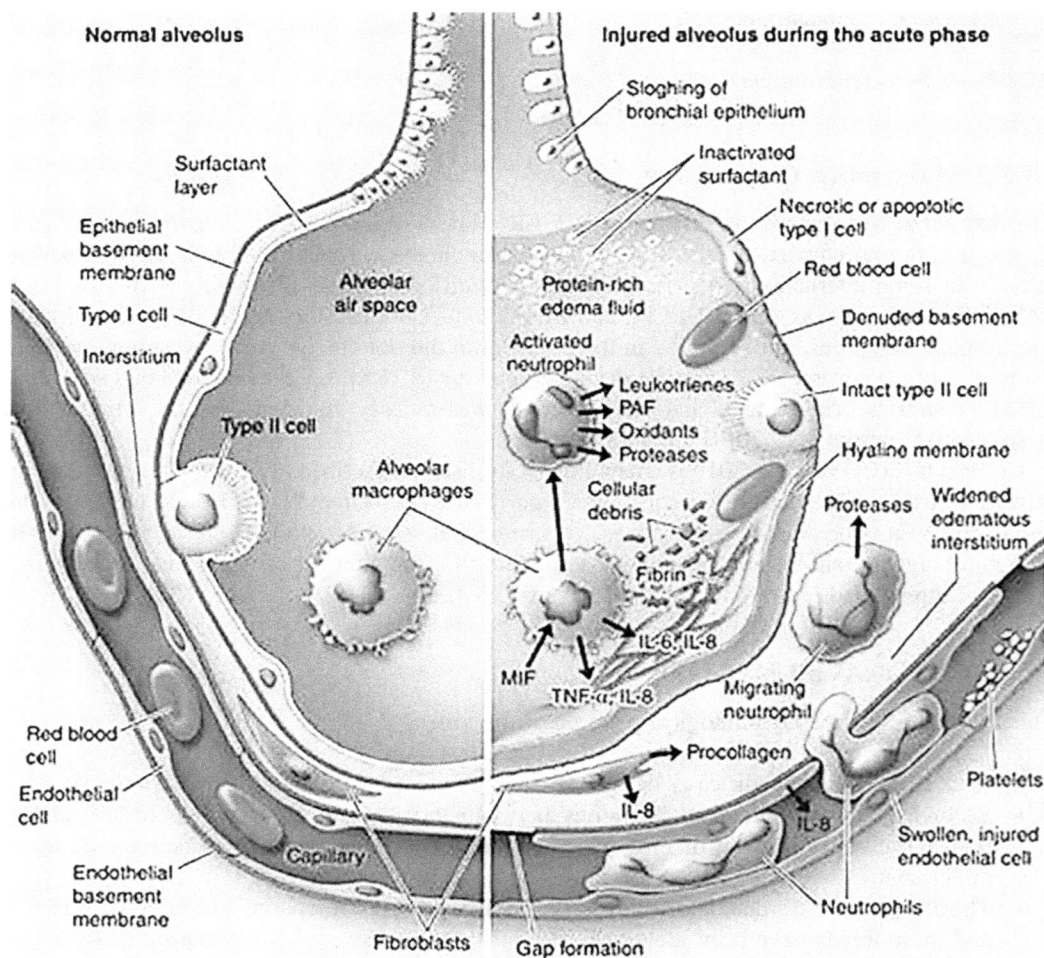

FIGURE 13.3   ARDS.

13.4 SYMPTOMS OF CORONAVIRUS

The most common symptoms of COVID 19 are fever, exhaustion, and dry cough, and pain, nasal congestion, runny nose, sore throat, and diarrhea can be encountered in some patients [23,24]. These symptoms typically begin gradually and become mild, and some people become infected without feeling ill. Some 16 to 21 percent of those infected with the virus, with a mortality rate of 2–3 percent, have become critically ill, according to the World Health Organization. The current estimate for virus replication is the average number of other individuals transmitted to a fully non-immune population by a person infected with the virus, around 3.77, which means that the rapid spread of the disease is imminent. It is important to classify infected individuals for quarantine procedures and care as soon as possible [25,26] (Figure 13.4).

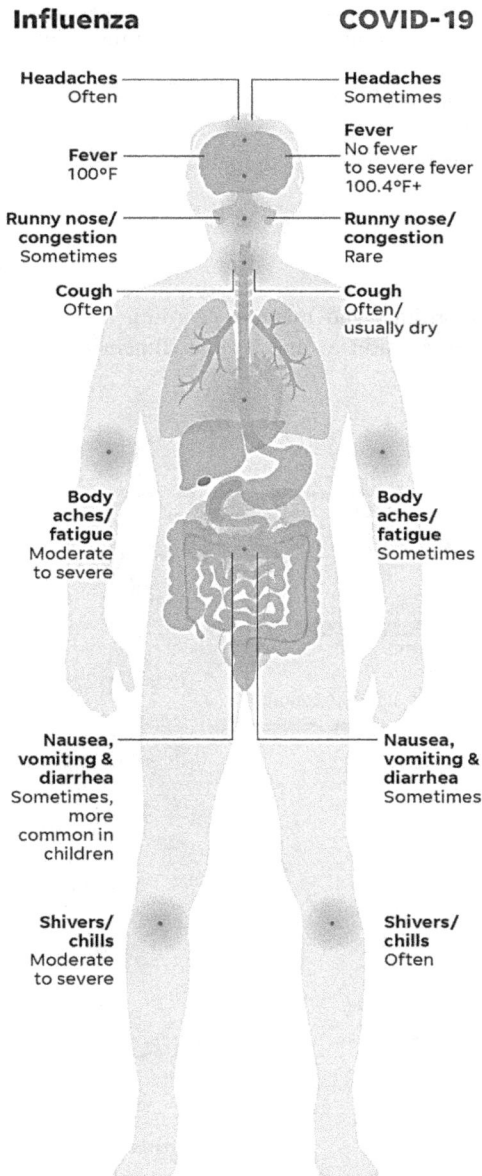

Influenza　　　　　**COVID-19**

Headaches — Often
Headaches — Sometimes

Fever — 100°F
Fever — No fever to severe fever 100.4°F+

Runny nose/congestion — Sometimes
Runny nose/congestion — Rare

Cough — Often
Cough — Often/usually dry

Body aches/fatigue — Moderate to severe
Body aches/fatigue — Sometimes

Nausea, vomiting & diarrhea — Sometimes, more common in children
Nausea, vomiting & diarrhea — Sometimes

Shivers/chills — Moderate to severe
Shivers/chills — Often

FIGURE 13.4 Coronavirus symptoms.

13.5   CORONAVIRUS TRANSMISSION METHODS

1. Transfer of aerosols through the respiratory system. Generally speaking, aerosols are very small water particles with a diameter greater than 5 microns. And the droplets that cause the disease from the contamination source reach the surface of the sensitive mucosa within a certain distance (one meter in general), then reach the respiratory system of the infected person. There are usually two key sources for the transmission of the droplets; they are [27–29]:
   - Coughing, sneezing, chatting.
   - Performing (immersion) surgery in the respiratory system, such as swallowing sputum or inserting a tube into the windpipe to hold it open, and so on to induce coughing and CPR.
2. Transmission of infection by direct contact. The transmission of infection through direct contact means that infections of infectious diseases, such as coughing and sneezing, are transmitted from one person to another via the mucous membrane of the body or the skin. There are two ways in which this can happen:
   - The transfer of blood or body fluids to the human body via the mucous membrane or the infected skin.
   - Transmission of infection by touching or shaking hands with pathogens such as coughing or sneezing (Figure 13.5).

13.6   RULE INDUCTION

Rule induction is one of the artificial-intelligence algorithms and machine-learning fields that learns from the data without getting to a programming solution to make more dimensions and

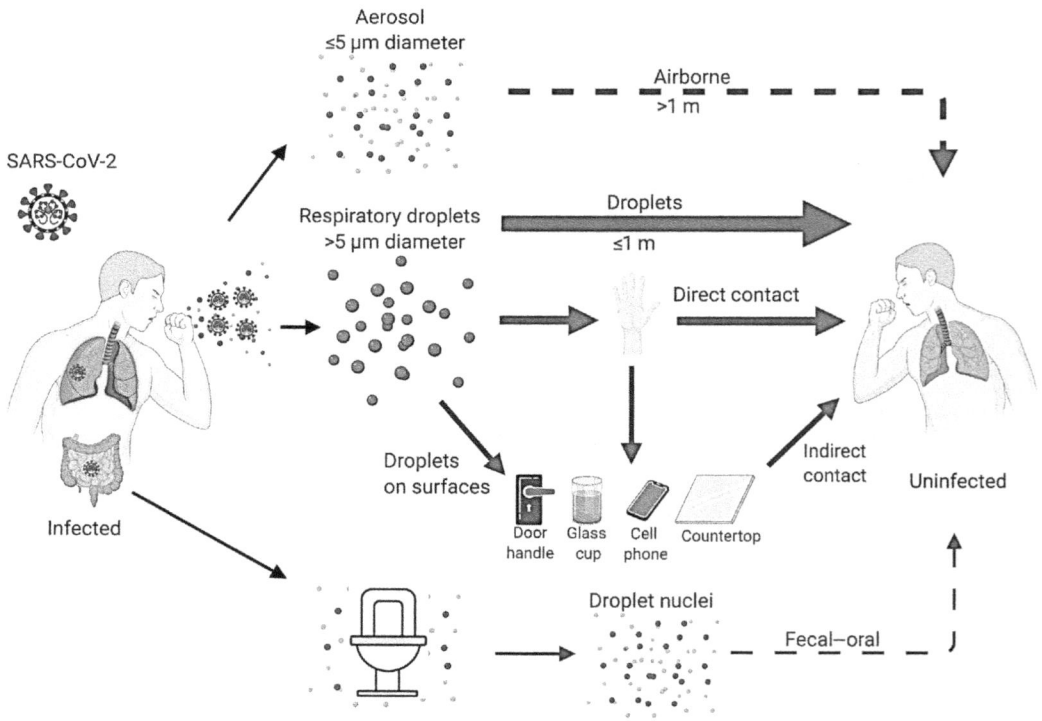

Trends in Immunology

FIGURE 13.5   Transmission method.

estimate all the classification and clustering. The benefit and the impact of the algorithm is big compared to the simplicity and easy-to-understand rules and depending on the if-then class conditions [30,31].

```
routine CN2(TrainingSet)
   let the ClassificationRuleList be empty
   repeat
      let the BestConditionExpression be
Find_BestConditionExpression(TrainingSet)
         if the BestConditionExpression is not nil
            then
               let the TrainingSubset be the examples covered by the
BestConditionExpression
               remove from the TrainingSet the examples in the
TrainingSubset
               let the MostCommonClass be the most common class of
examples in the TrainingSubset
               append to the ClassificationRuleList the rule
                  'if ' the BestConditionExpression ' then the class is '
the MostCommonClass
      until the TrainingSet is empty or the BestConditionExpression is nil
   return the ClassificationRuleList

routine Find_BestConditionExpression(TrainingSet)
   let the ConditionalExpressionSet be empty
   let the BestConditionExpression be nil
   repeat
      let the TrialConditionalExpressionSet be the set of conditional
expressions,
         {x and y where x belongs to the ConditionalExpressionSet and y
belongs to the SimpleConditionSet}.
      remove all formulae in the TrialConditionalExpressionSet that are
either in the ConditionalExpressionSet (i.e.,
            the unspecialized ones) or null (e.g., big = y and big = n)
         for every expression, F, in the TrialConditionalExpressionSet
            if
               F is statistically significant
                  and F is better than the BestConditionExpression
                  by user-defined criteria when tested on the TrainingSet
               then
                  replace the current value of the BestConditionExpression by F
      while the number of expressions in the
TrialConditionalExpressionSet > user-defined maximum
         remove the worst expression from the
TrialConditionalExpressionSet
      let the ConditionalExpressionSet be the
TrialConditionalExpressionSet
   until the ConditionalExpressionSet is empty
   return the BestConditionExpression
```

CN2 algorithm: To induce the rules in a (if, then) class, all simply and comprehensibly designing technique, the best choice is a cn2 classification algorithm.

13.7 PROPOSED SYSTEM

In this section, we will present the method used, the community and sample of the study, as well as the tools used for this study, as well as how to construct this tool and test its validity and reliability. The statistical methods used to process the data obtained are shown in the Figure 13.6.

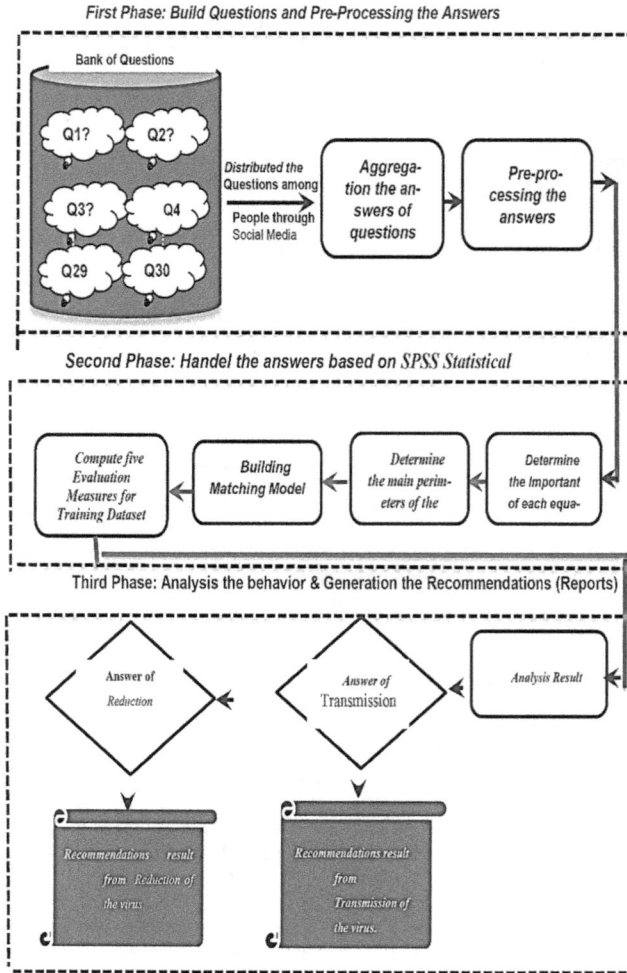

FIGURE 13.6   The phases conducted in our research.

13.8   STEPS OF ANALYSIS

The descriptive and empirical method is used to achieve the aims of the study by which it seeks to explain the phenomenon in question, "the degree of health consciousness in the community when some strange health phenomenon or crisis arises, such as the spread of a particular disease such as COVID-19 (corona)" in an accurate definition, and to convey it in terms and quantity by analyzing it.

- First, determine the gender (male or female).
- Second, a health understanding of symptoms is included the transmission and reduction of the virus:
    - Transmission of the virus, as shown in Table 13.2
    - Reduction of the virus, as shown in Table 13.3

TABLE 13.2
Questions Related to Transmission of the Virus

	Question	Yes	No
1	Can it spread the virus through the air?		
2	Is the virus passed on to the fetus from the pregnant mother?		
3	Is it possible to spread the virus to animals?		
4	Is eye rubbing a possibility of the virus transmitted?		
5	Do animals have the coronavirus transmitted at home?		
6	Is the doorstep the most vulnerable place for virus transmission?		
7	Is it spread by sexual intercourse?		
8	Is it through mosquito bites to spread the virus?		
9	Can an entity become contaminated with the disease by a person's stool?		
10	Is contact with the patient and flying droplets deemed the cause of their death or infectious diseases and loss of immunity for the elderly?		
11	Chance to spread the virus?		
12	Are sneezing and high temperatures a significant factor in disease risk?		
13	Is dry coughing and vomiting a sign of concern?		
14	A symptom of the disease is shortness of breath and weakness?		

TABLE 13.3
Questions Related to Reduction of the Virus

	Question	Yes	No
15	Does healthy eating help the reduction of virus infection for people with chronic diseases?		
16	Will the elderly regulate themselves after they have been injured?		
17	Is hand-washing with soap and antiseptic Dettol safer than chlorine for fear of killing the beneficial bacteria?		
18	Can hot liquids destroy the virus?		
19	Is SARS the same as COVID-19, and can it be avoided?		
20	Has malaria treatment shown some benefit in curing any cases in Iraq?		
21	Are children less likely to get sick due to their immune strength?		
22	Do the vaccines against pneumonia prevent the virus?		
23	Will consuming nutritious foods have a part to play in preventing the virus?		
24	Can saline help avoid daily rinsing of the nose?		
25	Are hand dryers available effective in removing the virus?		
26	Do UV sterilizers get rid of the virus?		
27	Are coronavirus-preserving antibiotics effective?		
28	Will spraying alcohol or chlorine on the body help to fully kill the virus?		
29	Can masks, after touching an infected human, be sterilized and re-used?		
30	Can you call a crisis cell if you suffer from the symptoms of the disease?		

13.8.1 COLLECTION OF DATA

The data group is established by posing different questions to all members of society, which are divided between issues related to the virus itself and methods of prevention and those related to the transmission of the virus, as we have already stated from all members of society.

TABLE 13.4

Distribution of the Sample Members According to the Study Variable

Variable	Category	Num	Percentage %
Sex	Male	493	27.8
	Female	1283	72.2
	Total	1776	100

With respect to the study sample, the available sample form, which is "one of the types of likelihood samples that guarantees an equal opportunity to appear for each of the individuals in the group in the sample," was used to select a total of (1776) individuals from the Iraqi group.

Table 13.4 displays the distribution of the study sample from the Iraqi population by study variable.

13.8.2 Tools Used for the Analysis

In this analysis, the questionnaire tool was used to gather information and data from sample individuals and, given the nature of the sample and its location, an electronic questionnaire (Google drive) was designed to facilitate its dissemination to the study sample participants. To perform the data analysis process, the causal networks used in the SPSS analytical software have been used to establish accurate logical recommendations that support the group [32,33]. Where the degree of the correlation between the responses was used to ensure their timing by measuring the Pearson coefficient for the correlation between the responses received, see (Table 13.5).

TABLE 13.5

Distribution of the Sample Members According to the Study Variable

Field	Q	Correlation Coefficient	Indication Level	Field	Q	Correlation Coefficient	Indication Level
Transmission of	1	0.392^{**}	0.005	**Reduction of**	15	0.288^{*}	0.042
the Virus	2	0.383^{**}	0.006	**the virus.**	16	0.417^{**}	0.003
	3	0.492^{**}	0.000		17	0.488^{**}	0.000
	4	0.571^{**}	0.000		18	0.364^{**}	0.009
	5	0.603^{**}	0.000		19	0.285^{*}	0.045
	6	0.306^{*}	0.031		20	0.355^{*}	0.011
	7	0.569^{**}	0.000		21	0.465^{**}	0.001
	8	0.295^{*}	0.037		22	0.499^{**}	0.000
	9	0.476^{**}	0.000		23	0.440^{**}	0.001
	10	0.490^{**}	0.000		24	0.378^{**}	0.007
	11	0.548^{**}	0.002		25	0.408^{**}	0.003
	12	0.389^{**}	0.005		26	0.287^{*}	0.043
	13	0.484^{**}	0.007		27	0.394^{**}	0.005
	14	0.490^{**}	0.000		28	0.433^{**}	0.000
					29	0.439^{**}	0.000
					30	0.480^{**}	0.000

Notes

* Correlation is statistically important at 5–007 = 0.05.

** Correlation is statistically relevant at the $\Delta = 0.01$ level of significance.

It is evident from (Table 13.5) above that all the scale paragraphs are statistically relevant at the level of 0.05 = 5–007 and 0.01 = 5–007.

13.9 ANALYSIS OF RESULTS

The goal of this study was to find out what the level of community health knowledge during an outbreak or a particular health problem was, so it was COVID-19 (corona), and specifically, the study in this chapter sought to address the questions of the study and its hypotheses. At the beginning, we will show the answer received from the person and how perform the coding of that response will handle it through SPSS [34,35].

13.10 RESULTS OF ANSWERING AND DEBATING THE STUDY'S FIRST QUESTION

This section will show the response to the first question, which stated:

13.10.1 In the Community, What is the Degree of Health Awareness?

For all their fields, the arithmetic averages and standard deviations were determined individually and collectively for the study sample estimates, where the results were as follows:

It is clear from the findings of (Table 13.6) that the level of health consciousness in the current output analysis as a whole originated at the average level, with an arithmetic mean (0.64) and a standard deviation (0.123). The "virus transmission symptoms" field came first in order of level, the dominant health field, with a mean (0.69) and a standard deviation (0.69). For the estimates of the study sample individuals, the arithmetic averages and standard deviations were determined on the paragraphs of each sector separately, where the results were as follows:

13.10.2 Field 1, Symptoms of Transmission of the Virus

To respond to the paragraphs of this area, the arithmetic means and standard deviations of the responses of the study sample individuals were used for each paragraph of the area, and the results were given as shown in the (Table 13.7).

The results of the table show that the question: "Is it spread by sexual intercourse?" It came first and then with a mean of 013, followed by the two questions: "Do the door handle the most vulnerable place for the transmittal of the virus?"

After getting the mean of 013 to the question A6: Is it spread by sexual intercourse?

We had to make our own experiments of the dependencies and behaviors of the A6 question, according to the other transmission questions. The community split into multi groups, then generated the rules using the form.

TABLE 13.6
AM and SD for Health Awareness Fields

S	Field	AM	SD	Seq
1	Transmission of the virus	0.69	0.152	1
2	Reduction of the virus	018	0.145	2
	Health awareness	0.64	0.123	–

TABLE 13.7

The Correlation Coefficient Between Ach of the Questionnaire Questions and the Total Degree of the Questionnaires

Question	Yes		no		AM	SD	Order
	seq	per	seq	per			
Can it spread the virus through the air?	776	43.7	1000	56.3	0.44	0.496	13
Is the virus passed on to the fetus from the pregnant mother?	1115	62.8	661	37.2	0.63	0.484	9
Is it possible to spread the virus to animals?	1005	56.6	771	43.4	017	0.496	12
Is eye rubbing a possible way to transmit the virus?	1550	87.3	226	12.7	0.87	0.333	4
Is the doorstep the most vulnerable place for virus transmission?	1602	90.2	174	9.8	010	0.297	2
Is it spread by sexual intercourse?	1652	93	127	7	013	0.255	1
Do pets have the coronavirus transmitted at home?	1047	59	729	41	019	0.492	11
Is it through mosquito bites to spread the virus?	1611	90.7	165	9.3	010	0.290	2
Can an entity become contaminated with the disease by a person's stool?	1439	81	337	19	0.81	0.392	5
Is contact with the infected person and flying droplets deemed?	1095	61.7	681	38.3	0.62	0.486	10
Are the cause of their death infectious diseases and loss of immunity for the elderly chance to spread the virus?	1239	69.8	537	30.2	0.70	0.495	6
Are sneezing and high temperatures an significant factor in disease risk?	525	29.6	1251	70.4	0.30	0.456	14
Is dry coughing and vomiting a sign of concern?	1233	69.4	543	30.6	0.69	0.461	7
A symptom of the disease is shortness of breath and weakness?	1230	69.3	546	30.7	0.69	0.461	7

13.10.3   IF Conditions Then Action

We see in (Figure 13.7) the result of 010, which refers to "Is the doorstep the most vulnerable place for virus transmission?" We also had to make our own experiments of the dependencies and behaviors of the A5 question according to the other transmission questions the community split into ten groups then generated the rules take the form

The results of the (Table 13.8) show the question "Do your disease suffer?" As I asked, "Do UV sterilizers kill the virus?" With a mean of 013 and a standard deviation of 0.252? "The most recent episode on my average is 0.17, a default is 0.377.

- IF (A_Q7 IS 1) THEN A_Q6 is 1
- IF (A_Q1 is 1) AND (A_Q2 is 1) AND (A_Q3 is 0) AND (A_Q4 is 1) AND (A_Q5 is 1) AND (A_Q7 is 1) AND (A_Q8 is 0) AND (A_Q9 is 1) AND (A_Q10 is 1) AND (A_Q11 is 1) AND (A_Q12 is 0) AND (A_Q13 is 0) AND (A_Q14 is 1) AND (Sex is Famel) THEN A_Q6 is 1
- IF (A_Q8 = 1) AND (A_Q9 = 0) AND (A_Q10 = 1) AND (A_Q11 = 1) AND (A_Q12 = 1) AND (A_Q13 = 0) AND (A_Q14 = 1) AND (Sex = Male) THEN A_Q6 is 1
- IF (A_Q7 is 0)) THEN A_Q6 is 0

- IF (A_Q1 IS 1) AND (A_Q2 IS 0) AND (A_Q7 IS 1) AND (A_Q11 IS 1) AND (A_Q14 IS 1) THEN A_Q6 is 1
- IF (A_Q1 is 2) AND (A_Q2 is 0) AND (A_Q3 is 1) AND (A_Q4 is 1) AND (A_Q5 is 1) AND (A_Q7 is 1) AND (A_Q8 is 1) AND (A_Q9 is 1) AND (A_Q10 is 1) AND (A_Q11 is 1) AND (A_Q12 is 1) AND (A_Q13 is 0) AND (A_Q14 is 1) AND (Sex is Male) THEN A_Q6 is 1
- IF (A_Q1 = 1) AND (A_Q3 = 1) AND (A_Q4 = 1) AND (A_Q5 = 0) AND (A_Q7 = 1) AND (A_Q8 = 1) AND (A_Q9 = 0) AND (A_Q10 = 1) AND (A_Q12 = 1) AND (A_Q13 = 0) AND (A_Q14 = 1) AND (Sex = Male) THEN A_Q6 is 1
- IF (A_Q1 is 1)) AND (A_Q7 is 0)) AND (A_Q14 is 1)) THEN A_Q6 is 1

- IF (A_Q11 IS 0) THEN A_Q6 is 1
- IF (A_Q1 is 1) AND (A_Q2 is 0) AND (A_Q3 is 1) AND (A_Q4 is 1) AND (A_Q5 is 1) AND (A_Q7 is 1) AND (A_Q8 is 1) AND (A_Q9 is 1) AND (A_Q10 is 1) AND (A_Q11 is 0) AND (A_Q12 is 1) AND (A_Q13 is 0) AND (A_Q14 is 1) AND (Sex is Male) THEN A_Q6 is 1

- IF (A_Q1 is 1) AND (A_Q2 is 0) AND (A_Q3 is 0) AND (A_Q4 is 0) AND (A_Q5 is 0) AND (A_Q7 is 1) AND (A_Q8 is 0) AND (A_Q9 is 1) AND (A_Q10 is 1) AND (A_Q11 is 0) AND (A_Q12 is 0) AND (A_Q13 is 0) AND (A_Q14 is 1) AND (Sex is Male) THEN A_Q6 is 1

- IF (A_Q2 IS 1) THEN A_Q6 is 1
- IF (A_Q8 is 1) AND (A_Q9 is 1) AND (A_Q10 is 1) AND (A_Q11 is 1) AND (A_Q12 is 1) AND (A_Q13 is 0) AND (A_Q14 is 1) AND (Sex is Male) THEN A_Q6 is 1
- IF (A_Q1 = 1) AND (A_Q3 = 1) AND (A_Q4 = 1) AND (A_Q5 = 0) AND (A_Q7 = 1) AND (A_Q8 = 1) AND (A_Q9 = 0) AND (A_Q10 = 1) AND (A_Q11 = 1) AND (A_Q12 = 1) AND (A_Q13 = 0) AND (A_Q14 = 1) AND (Sex = Male) THEN A_Q6 is 1

- IF (A_Q9 IS 1) AND (A_Q14 IS 0) THEN A_Q6 is 1
- IF (A_Q1 is 2) AND (A_Q2 is 0) AND (A_Q3 is 1) AND (A_Q4 is 0) AND (A_Q5 is 1) AND (A_Q7 is 1) AND (A_Q8 is 1) AND (A_Q9 is 1) AND (A_Q10 is 1) AND (A_Q11 is 1) AND (A_Q12 is 1) AND (A_Q13 is 0) AND (A_Q14 is 0) AND (Sex is Male) THEN A_Q6 is 1
- (A_Q8 = 1) AND (A_Q9 = 0) AND (A_Q10 = 1) AND (A_Q11 = 1) AND (A_Q12 = 1) AND (A_Q13 = 0) AND (Sex = Male) THEN A_Q6 is 1
- IF (A_Q9 is 1) THEN A_Q6 is 1

- IF (A_Q2 IS 1) AND (A_Q11 IS 0) THEN A_Q6 is 1
- IF (A_Q7 is 1) AND (A_Q8 is 0) AND (A_Q9 is 1) AND (A_Q10 is 1) AND (A_Q11 is 0) AND (A_Q12 is 1) AND (A_Q13 is 0) AND (A_Q14 is 0) AND (Sex is Male) THEN A_Q6 is 1
- IF (A_Q2 = 1) AND (A_Q5 = 0) AND (A_Q8 = 1) AND (A_Q9 = 0) AND (A_Q10 = 1) AND (A_Q11 = 1) AND (A_Q12 = 1) AND (A_Q13 = 0) AND (A_Q14 = 1) AND (Sex = Male) THEN A_Q6 is 1
- IF (A_Q2 is 1) AND (A_Q11 is 1) THEN A_Q6 is 1

FIGURE 13.7   Rules generation through split community into six groups based on A6 related to Transmission dataset.

TABLE 13.8

AM and SD for First Field Questions

Question	Yes		no		AM	SD	order
	seq	per	seq	per			
Does healthy eating help the reduction of virus infection for people with chronic diseases?	1632	911	144	8.1	012	0.273	3
Will the elderly regulate themselves after they have been injured?	856	48.2	920	51.8	0.48	0100	10
Is hand-washing with soap and antiseptic Dettol safer than chlorine for fear of killing the beneficial bacteria?	837	47.1	939	521	0.47	0.499	11
Can hot liquids destroy the virus, please?	693	39	1083	61	0.39	0.488	13
Is SARS the same as COVID-19, and can it be avoided?	793	44.7	983	55.3	0.45	0.492	12
Has malaria treatment shown some benefit in curing any cases in Iraq?	883	49.7	893	50.3	010	0100	8
Are children less likely to get sick due to their immune strength?	1172	66	604	34	0.66	0.474	6
Will consuming nutritious foods have a part to play in preventing the virus?	626	35.2	1150	64.8	0.35	0.478	14
Are hand dryers available effective in removing the virus?	1052	59.2	724	40.8	019	0.491	7
Do UV sterilizers get rid of the virus?	304	17.1	1472	821	0.17	0.377	16
Will spraying alcohol or chlorine on the body help to fully kill the virus?	454	25.6	1322	74.4	0.26	0.436	15
Do the vaccines against pneumonia prevent the virus?	1477	83.2	299	16.8	0.83	0.374	5
Can saline aid avoid daily rinsing of the nose?	869	481	907	51.1	0.49	0100	9
Are coronavirus-preserving antibiotics effective?	1618	91.1	158	81	011	0.285	4
Can masks, after touching an infected human, be sterilized and re-used?	1675	94.3	101	5.7	014	0.232	1
Can you call a crisis cell if you suffer from the symptoms of the disease?	1655	93.2	121	6.8	013	0.252	2

For the reduction part, we had to get the highly mean result of 017, which refers to "Do UV sterilizers kill the virus?"

We had to make our own experiments of the dependencies and behaviors of the A24 question according to the other transmission question to get the results, and checking them as Figure 13.8.

As we see in (Figure 13.8), the A24 pattern depends on the result of the compression and applying the rule on the other 15 questions' answers to get a tolerated new important A24 pattern; for the last rule, we had to make an (if_ then) condition. We had to make our own experiments of the dependencies and behaviors of the sex question.

- IF (A_Q15 is 0) AND (A_Q16 is 1) AND (A_Q17 is 0) AND (A_Q18 is 1) AND (A_Q19 is 0) AND (A_Q20 is 0) AND (A_Q21 is 1) AND (A_Q22 is 1) AND (A_Q23 is 0) AND (A_Q25 is 0) AND (A_Q26 is 0) AND (A_Q27 is 1) AND (A_Q28 is 0) AND (A_Q29 is 1) AND (A_Q30 is 1) THEN A_Q24 is 1

- IF (A_Q15 = 0) AND (A_Q16 = 0) AND (A_Q17 = 0) AND (A_Q18 = 1) AND (A_Q19 = 0) AND (A_Q20 = 0) AND (A_Q21 = 1) AND (A_Q22 = 0) AND (A_Q23 = 0) AND (A_Q25 = 1) AND (A_Q26 = 1) AND (A_Q27 = 0) AND_____ _____

- IF (A_Q20 IS 0) AND (A_Q29 IS 2) AND (A_Q30 IS 1) THEN A_Q24 is 0

- IF (A_Q15 is 1) AND (A_Q16 is 1) AND (A_Q17 is 0) AND (A_Q18 is 0) AND (A_Q19 is 0) AND (A_Q20 is 0) AND (A_Q21 is 0) AND (A_Q22 is 0) AND (A_Q23 is 0) AND (A_Q25 is 0) AND (A_Q26 is 0) AND (A_Q27 is 1) AND (A_Q28 is 0) AND (A_Q29 is 1) AND (A_Q30 is 1) THEN A_Q24 is 0

- IF (A_Q15 = 0) AND (A_Q16 = 0) AND (A_Q17 = 0) AND (A_Q18 = 1) AND (A_Q19 = 0) AND (A_Q20 = 0) AND (A_Q21 = 1) AND (A_Q22 = 0) AND (A_Q23 = 0) AND (A_Q25 = 1) AND (A_Q26 = 1) AND (A_Q27 = 0) AND (A_Q28 = 1) AND (A_Q29 = 1) THEN A_Q24 is 0

- IF (A_Q30 IS 1) THEN A_Q24 is 1

- IF (A_Q15 is 1) AND (A_Q16 is 1) AND (A_Q17 is 0) AND (A_Q18 is 0) AND (A_Q19 is 0) AND (A_Q20 is 0) AND (A_Q21 is 1) AND (A_Q22 is 1) AND (A_Q23 is 0) AND (A_Q25 is 0) AND (A_Q26 is 0) AND (A_Q27 is 1) AND (A_Q28 is 0) AND (A_Q29 is 1) AND (A_Q30 is 1) THEN A_Q24 is 1

- IF (A_Q15 = 0) AND (A_Q16 = 0) AND (A_Q17 = 0) AND (A_Q18 = 1) AND (A_Q19 = 0) AND (A_Q20 = 0) AND (A_Q21 = 1) AND (A_Q22 = 0) AND (A_Q23 = 0) AND (A_Q25 = 1) AND (A_Q26 = 1) AND (A_Q27 = 0) AND (A_Q28 = 1) AND (A_Q29 = 1) AND (A_Q30 = 1) THEN A_Q24 is 1

- IF (A_Q16 IS 1) AND (A_Q25 IS 0) AND (A_Q29 IS 1) AND (A_Q30 IS 1) THEN A_Q24 is 1

- IF (A_Q15 is 1) AND (A_Q16 is 1) AND (A_Q17 is 0) AND (A_Q18 is 0) AND (A_Q19 is 0) AND (A_Q20 is 1) AND (A_Q21 is 0) AND (A_Q22 is 0) AND (A_Q23 is 1) AND (A_Q25 is 0) AND (A_Q26 is 0) AND (A_Q27 is 1) AND (A_Q28 is 0) AND (A_Q29 is 1) AND (A_Q30 is 1) THEN A_Q24 is 1

- IF (A_Q15 = 0) AND (A_Q16 = 0) AND (A_Q17 = 0) AND (A_Q18 = 1) AND (A_Q19 = 0) AND (A_Q20 = 0) AND (A_Q21 = 1) AND (A_Q22 = 0) AND (A_Q23 = 0) AND (A_Q26 = 1) AND (A_Q27 = 0) AND (A_Q28 = 1) AND (A_Q29 = 1) AND (A_Q30 = 1) THEN A_Q24 is 1

- IF (A_Q16 is between (0 - 1)) AND (A_Q29 is between (0 - 1)) AND (A_Q30 is between (0 - 1)) THEN A_Q24 is 1

- IF (A_Q16 IS 1) AND (A_Q18 IS 1) AND (A_Q29 IS 1) AND (A_Q30 IS 1) THEN A_Q24 is 1

- IF (A_Q15 is 1) AND (A_Q16 is 1) AND (A_Q17 is 0) AND (A_Q18 is 1) AND (A_Q19 is 1) AND (A_Q20 is 0) AND (A_Q21 is 0) AND (A_Q22 is 1) AND (A_Q23 is 0) AND (A_Q25 is 0) AND (A_Q26 is 0) AND (A_Q27 is 1) AND (A_Q28 is 0) AND (A_Q29 is 1) AND (A_Q30 is 1) THEN A_Q24 is 1

- IF (A_Q15 = 0) AND (A_Q16 = 0) AND (A_Q17 = 0) AND (A_Q18 = 1) AND (A_Q19 = 0) AND (A_Q20 = 0) AND (A_Q21 = 1) AND (A_Q22 = 0) AND (A_Q23 = 0) AND (A_Q25 = 1) AND (A_Q26 = 1) AND (A_Q27 = 0) AND (A_Q28 = 1) AND (A_Q29 = 1) AND (A_Q30 = 1) THEN A_Q24 is 1

- IF (A_Q16 is between (0 - 1)) AND (A_Q18 is between (1 - 0)) AND (A_Q29 is between (0 - 1)) THEN A_Q24 is 1 _____

FIGURE 13.8 Rules generation through split community into eight groups based on A24 related to reduction dataset.

TABLE 13.9

The Results of the "T-test for the Two Independent Samples" - Gender

Fields		Gender		T-Test Value	Probable Value
		Male	Female		
Field1, Transmission of the virus	repeat	493	1283	−1.773	0.083
	means	0.68	0.69		
Field2, Reduction of the virus	repeat	493	1283	−1108	0.057
	means	017	019		

* "The T-value at the significance level of 0.05 and the degree of freedom of "1774" is 1.645".

13.10.3.1 Results of Addressing and Explaining the Second Question in the Analysis

To answer the second question, which said:

Are there statistically relevant variations at the level of ($\Delta \leq 0.05$) in the response estimates of the subjects?

Here we put forward the following hypothesis:

No statistically significant differences were found at the level of ($\Delta \leq 0.05$) in the population response estimates to the level of health knowledge due to the gender variable.

To check this hypothesis, the "T-test for the two independent samples" was used to assess whether there are statistically significant differences in the level of health knowledge among both males and females in the Iraqi population, and the results are shown in the Table 13.9.

From the results shown in (Table 13.9) above, it has been found that the likelihood value (Sig) corresponding to the "T-test for the two independent samples" is greater than the significance level (0.05 ≥ 5–007) for the two fields, and thus, it can be assumed that there are no statistically significant discrepancies in the population estimates assigned to the variable gender.

As a result, there is no disparity in the degree of people's response to the level of health awareness in Iraqi society because they are male and female, and this is due to the fact that people are aware of health awareness at the same level.

13.11 CONCLUSION AND RECOMMENDATIONS

This section will explain the main recommendations from this research: undertaking a research similar to the current research, which involves age, educational qualifications, and gender variables. Study on the health awareness variable of the coronavirus and its connection to quarantine. Building extension projects in various audio-visual and written media in newspapers and magazines, due to the efficacy of these means and the speed at which they disseminate information to match the speed of virus dissemination. Iraqi people are fairly sophisticated in the health-awareness field. There are no statistically significant differences at the significance level ($\alpha \leq 0.05$) in the estimates of the respondents' responses to the level of health awareness in the Iraqi community about the era of the COVID-19 (corona) epidemic due to the gender variable. Reduction ways are the main method to be in a safe from transmission of the coronavirus. There are great impact of coronavirus transmission methods, such as (sexual intercourse and contact with surfaces), less important to the other methods of virus transmission. There are many ways to reduce the virus, but there are priorities and some that are effective on the others, such as the (UV sterilizing).

ACKNOWLEDGEMENT

We, the authors want to thanks all the Anonymous Reviewers, Publishers and Editors of this project for their speedy response.

Consent for Publication

We, the author, the undersigned, give our consent for the publication of identifiable details, which can include photograph(s) and/or videos and/or case history and/or details within this chapter to be published by Bentham Science.

Conflict of Interest

We, the authors do not have any conflict of interest with respect to research, authorship and/or publication of this book chapter.

REFERENCES

[1]   H. Alahdal, F. Basingab, R. Alotaibi: An analytical study on the awareness, attitude and practice during the COVID-19 pandemic in Riyadh, Saudi Arabia, 2020, 10.1016/j.jiph.2020.06.015

[2]   S. Al-Janabi, A. Alkaim, E. Al-Janabi et al. Intelligent forecaster of concentrations (PM2.5, PM10, NO2, CO, O3, SO2) caused air pollution (IFCsAP). *Neural Comput & Applic*, 2021. 10.1007/s00521-021-06067-7

[3]   S. Al-Janabi, A. F. Alkaim: A nifty collaborative analysis to predicting a novel tool (DRFLLS) for missing values estimation, *Springer, Soft Comput*, Vol. 24, 2020, No. 1, pp. 555–569. 10.1007/s005 00-019-03972-x

[4]   S. Al-Janabi, A. Patel, H. Fatlawi, K. Kalajdzic, I. Al Shourbaji: Empirical rapid and accurate prediction model for data mining tasks in cloud computing environments, IEEE, 2014 International Congress on Technology, Communication and Knowledge (ICTCK), Mashhad, 2014, pp. 1–8. 10.1109/ICTCK.2014.7033495

[5]   S. Al-Janabi: Overcoming the Main Challenges of Knowledge Discovery through Tendency to the Intelligent Data Analysis, 2021 International Conference on Data Analytics for Business and Industry (ICDABI), 2021, pp. 286–294, 10.1109/ICDABI53623.2021.9655916

[6]   J. P. Nolan, L. Bossaert, R. Greif: European Resuscitation Council COVID-19 guidelines executive summary, 2020, 10.1016/j.resuscitation.2020.06.001

[7]   A. Kuckerts, L. Brandle, A. Gaudig: Startups in times of crisis- A rapid response to the COVID-19 pandemic, 2020, 10.1016/j.jbvi.2020.e00169

[8]   N. Magnavita, A. Sacco, F. Chirico: First aid during the COVID-19 pandemic, 2020, 10.1093/occmed/kqaa148

[9]   S. Al-Janabi, I. Al-Shourbaji, M. Shojafar, M. Abdelhag: Mobile Cloud Computing: Challenges and Future Research Directions, IEEE, 2017 10th International Conference on Developments in eSystems Engineering (DeSE), Paris, 2017, pp. 62–67. 10.1109/DeSE.2017.21

[10]   Y. Shu, M. Ghajar, E. Mitre: Spreading health awareness with resources and education libratians role in patient education, *A Case Study*, 2016, 10.1080/15323269

[11]   C.-C. Lai, T.-P. Shih, P.-R. Hsueh: Severe acute respiratory syndrome coronavirus 2 (SARS-COV-2) and coronavirus disease-2019; the epidemic and the challenge, 2020, 10.1016/j.ijantimicag.2020.1 05924

[12]   G. Kahn, A. Villaflor, B. Ding, P. Abbeel, S. Levine: Self-supervised Deep Reinforcement Learning with Generalized Computation Graphs for Robot Navigation, 10.1109/ICRA.2018.8460655

[13]   G.-Z. Yang, B. J. Nelson: Combating COVID-19 The role of robotics in managing public health and infectious diseases, *Science Robotics*, 10.1126/scirobotics.abb5589

[14]   K. H. Hong, S. W. Lee, H. J. Huh: Guidelines for Laboratory Diagnosis of Coronavirus Disease 2019 (COVID-19) in Korea, *Ann Lab Med*, 10.3343/alm.2020.40.5.351

[15] N. Després, E. Cyr, P. Setoodeh, M. Mohammadi: Deep Learning and Design for Additive Manufacturing: A Framework for Microlattice Architecture, 10.1007/s11837-020-04131-6

[16] F. Tian, B. Gao, Q. Cui, E. Chen, T.-Y. Liu: Learning Deep Representations for Graph Clustering, 10.1.1.720.6007

[17] T. T. Pham, M. H. Nguyen, N. S. Nguyen: The disinfectant solution system preventing SARS-COV=2 Epidemic, International journal of Scientific Engineering and Science: ISSN(online): 2456–7361

[18] Z. H. Khan, A. Siddique, C. W. Lee: Rpbotics Utilization for Healthcare Digitization in Global COVID-19 Management, *International Journal of Environmental Research and Public Health.*

[19] S. H. Ali: Miner for OACCR: Case of medical data analysis in knowledge discovery, IEEE, 2012 6th International Conference on Sciences of Electronics, Technologies of Information and Telecommunications (SETIT), Sousse, 2012, pp. 962–975. 10.1109/SETIT.2012.6482043

[20] S. Al-Janabi, M. A. Mahdi: Evaluation prediction techniques to achievement an optimal biomedical analysis, *Int. J. Grid and Utility Computing*, Vol. 10, 2019, No. 5, pp. 512–527.

[21] J. Sun, D. Taylor, E. M. Bolt: Causal network inference by optimal Causation Entropy, 2015, 10.1137/140956166

[22] S. Al-Janabi, A. Alkaim, A novel optimization algorithm (Lion-AYAD) to find optimal DNA protein synthesis, *Egyptian Informatics Journal*, Vol. 23, 2022, No. 2, pp. 271–290, 10.1016/j.eij.2022.01.004

[23] C. Kilpatrick, E. Tartari, J. Storr: Global hand hygiene improvement progress two surveys using the WHO hand hygiene self-assessment framework, 2018, 10.1016/j.jhin.2018.07.036

[24] O. Evrova, D. Kellenberger, C. Scalera: Impact of UV sterilization and short term storage on the in vitro release kinetics and bioactivity of biomolecules from electrospun scaffolds, 2019, 10.1038/s41598-019-51513-1

[25] S. Al-Janabi, A. F. Alkaim: A Comparative Analysis of DNA Protein Synthesis for Solving Optimization Problems: A Novel Nature-Inspired Algorithm, 2021. 10.1007/978-3-030-73603-3_1

[26] S. Al-Janabi, I. Al-Shourbaji: A Hybrid Image steganography method based on genetic algorithm, 2016 7th International Conference on Sciences of Electronics, Technologies of Information and Telecommunications (SETIT), Hammamet, 2016, pp. 398–404. 10.1109/SETIT.2016.7939903

[27] W. K. Leung, K.-F. To, N. Lee: Enteric involvement of Severe acute respiratory syndrome-associated coronavirus infection, 2020, 10.1016/j.gastro.2003.08.001

[28] M. J. Vincent, E. Bergeron, S. Benjannet: Chloroquine is a potent inhibitor of SARS coronavirus infection and spread, 2020, 10.1186/1743-422X-2-69

[29] Y. Arbel, C. F. Koff, A. Kerner: Can reduction in infection and mortality rates from coronavirus be explained by an obesity survival paradox? *An analysis at the US state-wide level*, 2020, 10.1038/s41366-020-00680-7

[30] J. Treur: Dynamic Modeling based on a temporal-causal network modelling approach, 2016, 10.1016/j.bica.2016.02.002

[31] W.-J. Guan, Zheng-yi: Clinical characteristics of 2019 novel coronavirus infection in China, 2020, 10.1101/2020.02.06.20020974

[32] B. Al-wassan, Y. Al-Amiri, M. Bouhaimed: Hand hygiene practices among nursing staff in public secondary care hospitals in Kuwait: self-report and direct observation, 2011, 10.1159/000324545

[33] M. A. Mahdi, S. Al_Janabi: A Novel Software to Improve Healthcare Base on Predictive Analytics and Mobile Services for Cloud Data Centers. In: Farhaoui Y. (eds) *Big Data and Networks Technologies. BDNT 2019. Lecture Notes in Networks and Systems*, vol 81, 2020. Springer, Cham, 10.1007/978-3-030-23672-4_23

[34] H. Al-Dmour, A. Salman, R. Al-Dmour: Influence of social media platforms on public health protection against the COVID-19 pandemic via the mediating effects of public health awareness and behavioural changes: intergrated model, 2020, 10.2196/19996

[35] A. S. Bhagavathula, J. Rahmani, A. Mahabadi: Novel Coronavirus(COVID-19) knowledge and perceptions: a survey of health care workers, 2019, 09.20033381

14 Artificial Intelligence Issues in Healthcare

Sapna M. Rathod and Nisarg C. Patel
APMC College of Pharmaceutical Education & Research, College Campus, Motipura, Himatnagar, Gujarat Technological University, Gujarat, India

Bhupendra G. Prajapati
Shree S.K. Patel College of Pharmaceutical Education & Research, Ganpat University, Gujarat, India

Jigna B. Prajapati
Acharya Motibhai Institute of Computer Application, Ganpat University, Ganpat, Gujarat, India

Sudarshan Singh
Department of Chemistry, Faculty of Science, Chulalongkorn University, Bangkok, Thailand

CONTENTS

DOI: 10.1201/9781003333081-14

14.1   INTRODUCTION

The superstar of industry and research, artificial intelligence (AI), is influencing every sphere of our civilization, including healthcare and medicine. Artificial intelligence (AI) was first used by McCarthy in 1955. It is defined as "the science and engineering of creating intelligent machines" [1]. The phrase suggests the least human involvement in the usage of a computer to simulate intelligent behaviour. According to the Cambridge Dictionary, AI encompasses a broader definition in this regard, namely as an interdisciplinary approach that uses concepts and tools from a range of disciplines, including computation, mathematics, logic, and biology, to address the challenges of comprehending, simulating, and duplicating intelligence and cognitive processes [2]. Science fiction is no longer the exclusive domain of artificial intelligence. It is regarded as having enormous societal and economic potential and being the most revolutionary technology of the 21st century and beyond. The large internet corporations have started a virtual competition for dominance in the field and are pouring billions of dollars into AI research. Healthcare has been highlighted as an early candidate to be changed by AI technology [3], along with other important industries like mobility and energy [4]. AI has been used in a variety of fields during the past 10 years, including search engines, machine-translation tools, and intelligent personal assistants. Along with the growing use of electronic health records (EHRs) and the quick development of life sciences, especially neuroscience, AI has also found many applications in the medical industry.

14.2   HEALTHCARE

When used in an attributional sense, healthcare frequently refers to actions taken, typically by qualified and certified professionals, to maintain or restore individual's physical, mental, or emotional well-being [5]. The healthcare system is complicated. One aspect is that they are made up of different components that operate well together. According to the World Health Organization, "organisations, people, and actions whose primary objective is to promote, restore, or sustain health" constitute a healthcare system (WHO). Furthermore, they are frequently described as being on a national basis, which greatly expands their reach and include all areas, all types of institutions, and various medicinal systems of providing healthcare [6].

14.3   AI IN HEALTHCARE

One of the most exciting fields for AI applications has long been medicine. Numerous clinical decision support systems have been proposed and created by researchers since the middle of the 20th century [7,8]. The 1970s saw a lot of success for rule-based approaches [9,10], which have been demonstrated to interpret ECGs, identify diseases [11], select the best treatments [12], offer understandings of clinical reasoning [13], and help doctors come up with diagnostic hypotheses in challenging patient cases [14]. However, rule-based systems can be fragile and expensive to construct since they require explicit representations of decision rules and human-authored revisions, much like any textbook.

Additionally, it is challenging to encode higher-order relationships between knowledge pieces written by various specialists, and the effectiveness of the systems is constrained by how complete past medical information is [15]. A system that combines deterministic and probabilistic reasoning to prioritise diagnostic hypotheses, hone in on important clinical context, and suggest treatment was also challenging to implement [16]. The challenges of AI in healthcare are depicted in Figure 14.1.

In recent years, several healthcare institutions have adopted AI-supported technologies to improve the level of patient care and the efficiency of available medical resources [17,18]. The knowledge-intensive healthcare industry has a lot of opportunity for innovation thanks to artificial intelligence (AI), which combines machine learning, natural language processing, and intelligent robotics [19,20]. In fact, a number of clinical and patient-facing applications [17] are now used in

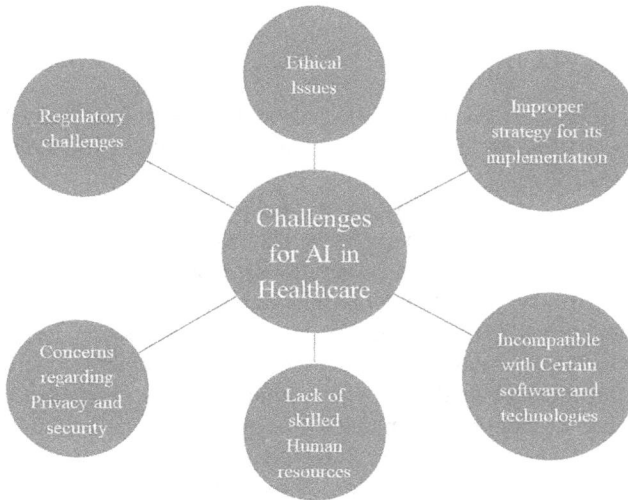

FIGURE 14.1 Challenges for artificial intelligence in healthcare.

healthcare. Included in this is GP at Hand, a Babylon health-powered application that analyses known symptoms and risk factors to offer accurate medical advice as well as tips about how to stay healthy [18]. Using Corti technology, the emergency dispatch procedure in Copenhagen is managed and optimised. To identify diabetic retinopathy in retinal fundus photographs [21] or image-related technologies, Google created a deep-learning algorithm. Supporting technologies for AI play a crucial role in enhancing clinicians' decision-making for diagnosis and treatment by learning and diagnosing from a massive volume of medical research and patients' treatment records [22–24]. The technology algorithms are utilised to assist radiologists in interpreting images while diagnosing breast cancer, according to Shiraishi et al. [25]. Additionally, it was claimed that the technology can identify skin cancer with greater accuracy compared to trained dermatologist [26]. Since the diagnosis is based on knowledge drawn from a sizable body of data and skill, it may be handled more rapidly and effectively [27]. Additionally, sophisticated virtual human models are also utilised to have the discussions necessary to identify and treat people with mental illnesses [28]. Figure 14.2, demonstrates various regulatory and ethical considerations for AI in healthcare.

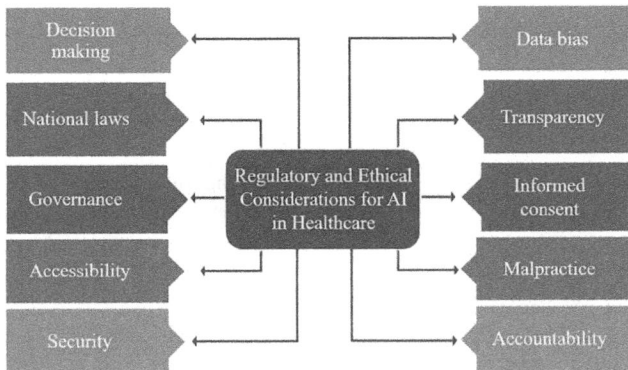

FIGURE 14.2 Regulatory and ethical considerations for AI in healthcare.

14.4 ELEMENTARY ISSUES

14.4.1 PRIVACY ISSUES

Many different types of data are currently collected on users by robots and AI systems. Although these data collecting entail a lot of work, the advantages of this collection technique may not immediately be apparent [29].

The medical industry is one of the significant fields where the problem of upfront privacy counts. This privacy is important, particularly in the US, one of the only countries that doesn't have universal healthcare and where pre-existing condition safeguards are still in jeopardy. The US has used HIPAA (The Health Insurance Portability and Accountability Act) as the basis for defining personally identifiable information (PII) and imposing limitations on its sharing since it was approved in 1996 [30]. While it has mostly focused on how businesses can exchange data with other businesses in the medical field and who within businesses can access the data, IT and development teams have frequently determined they are not covered by the judgment. According to the creators, complete data is required to create precise systems [31].

Compared to conventional health technology, AI has a number of distinctive qualities. Notably, they can occasionally be difficult or even impossible for human medical experts to supervise due to their propensity for specific sorts of errors and biases [32–35]. The latter is a result of the "black box" issue, in which learning algorithms' methods and "reasoning" may be partially or entirely opaque to human observers as they reach their decisions [36,37]. This opacity may also apply to how health and personal information is utilized and exploited if the appropriate controls are not regulated. Importantly, in response to this problem, numerous researchers have been studying on interpretable versions of AI that will make it easier to include into medical care [38]. Due to the unique properties of AI, the regulatory procedures utilised for approval and ongoing oversight will also need to be exceptional. Healthcare data privacy threats and benefits associated to artificial intelligence are shown in Table 14.1.

The concentration of technical innovation and knowledge in major tech corporations may cause public institutions to become more committed partner in the implementation of health technology. The Deep Mind case demonstrates that appropriate steps must be made to preserve patient agency and privacy in the context of these public-private partnerships, even though some of these patient privacy violations may have occurred in spite of current privacy acts, regulations and policies. AI present a unique difficulty because the algorithms usually require access to enormous amounts of patient data and may exploit that data in a number of ways over time [39], in addition to the possibility for general power abuses. The location and ownership of servers and computers that store and access patient health information are critical in these circumstances. Regulations should require that patient data be kept in the country from which it was attained, with very few exclusions. Strong

---

TABLE 14.1

Healthcare Data Privacy Threats and Benefits Associated to AI

AI's Threats for Data Privacy	AI's Scope for Data Privacy
Vulnerability to attacks on the integrity and privacy of data	Improving the use of data
AI-based re-identification of patients	Improved accountability for privacy violations
Data integrity and bias	Enhancing data exchange and productivity among doctors
Unintentional disclosure	
A lesser extent of ownership and management of data	
Less apparent understanding of individual's data privacy	
Using private health information outside of healthcare	
Privacy-related complications	

privacy protection is possible when organizations are fundamentally pushed to work together to assure data security by their own designs [40]. For the purposes of preserving privacy, commercial healthcare AI systems can be controlled; however, it introduces conflicting objectives. As we have observed, if businesses can make money off of the data or use it in other ways, and if the punishments for breaking the law are not severe enough to discourage such behaviour, they may not be highly motivated to enforce privacy protection. Due to these and other problems, request have emerged calls for more systemic oversight of big data medical studies and technologies [41].

Even in situations where "anonymization" is place, this reality might enhance the privacy dangers associated with giving private AI corporations power over patient health information. Additionally, it raises concerns about insurance, liability, and other practical matters that are distinct from situations in which governmental entities have direct ownership over patient information. Given the complex and variable level of the potential liability that corporate AI developers and support personnel may assume when working with large amounts of patient information, it will be necessary to create carefully drafted contracts that outline the roles and responsibilities of the parties involved as well as who will be responsible for any unintended consequences. Using generative data is one method AI system creators might be able to do away with lingering privacy worries. With no connection to actual people, generative models learn to produce realistic but synthetic patient data [42,43].

14.4.2 Security Issues

Most industries, from banking to entertainment, manufacturing to healthcare, have experienced data security breaches in recent years. According to a 2019 analysis, the average cost per stolen record was $150, and it took an average of 206 days to uncover a data breach and an additional 73 days to contain it. Healthcare is the solitary industry in the survey to indicate more internal (56%) than external (43%) reasons as the source of data breaches, with healthcare reporting the largest number of instances attributable to error, malware, and hacking (the remainder is caused by partners or multiple parties). The research itself underscores the particular difficulties faced by healthcare data: they are extremely sensitive and open to exploitation, while rapid access to accurate and current data is essential, particularly in emergency situations. The research proposes creating standards for the oversight of internal access to protected health information, minimising the possible effects of ransom ware on any particular network, and using full disc encryption as an efficient, affordable way to prevent data breaches in healthcare [44]. All forms of organisations are experiencing an increase in cyber-attacks globally, exposing private digital data to hacking and unauthorised access [45–47]. For instance, over 35,000 patients' medical details from all over India were exposed as a result of the hacking of a diagnostic laboratory database in Mumbai in 2016. Despite past invasions, the facility has not taken any precautions to protect the data [46]. The security and accuracy of AI solutions in the health industry must be guaranteed because the disclosure of particularly sensitive health information could have negative effects and endanger human lives. To process patient data securely, AI businesses must build safe infrastructure, India's privacy and security laws must be strengthened, and there must be rigorous security protocols and standards for breach notification [46]. The risks mentioned above are not specific to AI technologies, but it is widely acknowledged that the frequency and complexity of threats and data breaches in the healthcare and other sectors will increase with increased use of online tools and databases, including reliance on cloud solutions—some of which may fall under AI. Numerous initiatives to safeguard sensitive data are under way to combat these threats, utilising both conventional methods and, more recently, AI-based solutions.

14.4.3 Integrity Issues

The foundation of AI-driven healthcare is data. Data sets utilised to power AI solutions must be accurate and full for results to be reliable and objective [46]. To use machine-learning technology to optimise treatment, access to essential digital patient data is necessary [47]. Working with large data presents a number of difficulties, comprising unstructured data, absence of interoperability, and unorganised data [48]. Even if expensive infrastructure and AI tools can be implemented in resource-limited settings, their effectiveness may be limited by a non-existence of relevant historical health data and a general paucity of health data compared to industrialised markets [49]. It can be challenging and time-consuming to get high-quality datasets that can be utilised to train machine-learning algorithms to identify risk factors or provide clinical diagnosis for a number of illnesses pertinent to resource-poor settings. Digitizing health records may be more challenging because they are usually handwritten in various languages [50].

14.5   DATA COLLECTION

Given the diversity of the population and the increasing amount of unstructured data sets, data integrity calls for special attention. Data sets may contain particular cultural biases related to caste, age, gender, and sexual orientation. Therefore, it's crucial that the data and input sources used to train and inform the AI technology's algorithms come from a suitably wide and diversified population [46]. At a session on AI in India, AI and healthcare practitioners, start-ups, and thank tanks recognised this as a major issue in addition to data entry and tabulation problems [51].

14.6   DATA ANALYSIS

Large and complicated electronic health datasets that are difficult to manage with conventional software, hardware, and/or standard data management tools and processes are referred to as "big data" in the healthcare industry. Healthcare providers and other stakeholders in the healthcare delivery system can provide more thorough and insightful diagnoses and treatments when big data in healthcare is synthesised and analysed to uncover links, patterns, and trends [52]. Lack of an analytics system capable of collecting vast amounts of largely unstructured health data, performing sophisticated analysis fast, and launching actionable solutions is a barrier to the use of big data in healthcare. For instance, compiling and uploading all the data from the monitors in the intensive care unit, identifying important medical trends, and initiating a medical action [53]. Due to its sheer size, speed of management, range of data types, and volume, big data in healthcare is overwhelming [52].

14.7   REGULATION ISSUES

The Food and Drug Administration normally oversees the safety and efficacy of new and emerging medical technology and equipment (FDA). Whether the FDA genuinely has legal power over independently operating algorithms that are used to make (or assist in making) medical choices rests on the vague definition of what constitutes a "medical device." The FDA's long-standing claim that it does not control the practise of medicine may be in conflict with its regulation of black-box medical algorithms [54]. In other areas, the FDA has authority of over isolated algorithms and most likely in the context of linked technologies that could be more conveniently referred to as "medical devices," but there may be differences on this point [55]. However, certain algorithms will generate highly specific therapy predictions or suggestions, making the utilisation of clinical trials impossible. Even for algorithms that are susceptible to trials, the lengthy, cumbersome, and costly enterprise of clinical trials would greatly delay or even curtail the benefits of black-box medicine—quick, inexpensive shortcuts to otherwise inaccessible medical knowledge. Despite the fact that this may seem simple, technology used in the healthcare sector must adhere to a number of severe regulations. This is especially true for applications using cloud computing. As a result, a system should be created that considers how hospitals are set up, especially how healthcare providers want to use these models. The National Health Service, or NHS, in the United Kingdom (UK), for instance, adopted an AI chatbot-based triage system in 2019 [56]. The values of fair access that are synonymous with public health, however, have threatened to be displaced by the known and unknown consequences of making AI the standard for providing health services. While there are AI solutions for specialised or tertiary care institutions (particularly diagnostic assistance tools), few of these solutions successfully reach primary care settings. This is likely because of the high cost of development and operationalization, which prevents scale-friendly pricing [57]. Furthermore, the complexity of AI hinders its more widespread application by making key principles hard for people to understand and unreliable [58]. The decision paths of machine-learning algorithms are frequently too complex to be traced back and made understandable to their users without human intervention because they aggregate thousands of data points [59]. Due to its capability to learn pre-existing patterns in data, AI has come under fire for perpetuating biases against disadvantaged social groups that doctors would normally consciously rule out [60]. Concerns concerning potential bias associated with the use of AI in medical contexts (that is much harder to find and isolate) can have major repercussions in a medico-legal situation where culpability is difficult to determine and is instead shared [61].

The Health Insurance Portability and Accountability Act of 1996 ("HIPAA") [62] and other patient and individual privacy requirements around the world are major causes for concern. Access to patient data is only granted to those who need to handle patient data at a certain time for the patient's final care. A cloud-computing system that discloses data to the cloud is obviously unlawful as a result. This is not meant to imply that cloud-based software cannot be employed in the healthcare sector, but rather to highlight how beneficial it might be to upgrade a hospital's operating system. Cloud computing is projected to overtake on-premises technology in the near future because current EHR systems set the standard for the digital organisation, storage, and access of medical records. To adapt a specific system to the HIPPA and IT needs of a certain healthcare system, however, unique rules and regulations must be taken into account in the future [63,64]. Furthermore, as was already said, if the system used is too computationally intensive, the model itself may end up being unworkable because it can take hours to run on a laptop owned by a healthcare professional with inferior processing capacity. The speed and responsiveness of the regulatory system directly affect how quickly innovations are adopted. This regulatory framework needs to be adjusted regularly o promote the best advances while limiting healthcare costs [65]. Companies gain from regulatory certainty because certainty increases predictability and transparency. Furthermore, rules and standards can enhance product compatibility (interoperability for software products), which can lead to cost reductions [66]. The most effective strategy for dealing with this challenge will probably be less rigid and more flexible, involving a little less premarket oversight (focused on procedural safeguards like the calibre of the data used, the development methods, and the validation procedures) along with strict post-market oversight as these algorithms are implemented in clinical care. Recently, the FDA has shown interest in this strategy. Naturally, this is easier said than done; for example, post-market drug surveillance is tremendously difficult to implement. One appealing alternative would be for the FDA to collaborate with other highly developed healthcare organisations to enable ways to deliver them essential and useful information. Hospitals, insurance companies, and physician specialty societies all have an interest in ensuring the implementation of black-box algorithms to benefit patients (and, potentially, their bottom lines). Competing programmers might also be interested, particularly in identifying issues with current algorithms. These complex entities may also be able to conduct evaluations and produce performance data, particularly if they are used in clinical care. Many algorithm developers are hesitant to disclose that kind of information with any other parties, even if it is necessary to carry out this type of joint governance obligation. To enable those other organisations to participate in the regulation of black-box medications, the FDA may play the function of a central hub for information sharing. However, it remains largely unclear how exactly this concept might come to pass.

14.8 SOCIETAL ISSUES

14.8.1 Human Surveillance Issues

Starting off, human substitution is a frequent issue when examining the effects of AI. Many functions or jobs may be carried out by intricate lines of code that can be educated using the vast amounts of data amassed. To the cost of a thorough grasp of AI's more commonplace capabilities, the myth of a "workless future" appears to have taken hold in mainstream descriptions of the technology. Recognizing the legal implications of the digital transformation in terms of surveillance and the delicate balance that must be struck between real organisational needs and worker protection has not been helped much, admittedly, by the overstatement surrounding the advent of breakthrough technologies [67,68]. Therefore, the subtle potential of AI and algorithms, which could lead to a model of control and appraisal without an intuitive relationship between what is done while "logged-in" and how it is appraised, should potentially alarm the public more than the number of jobs lost through advanced automation. Zuboff has been discussing the possibility of technology "informating" work for a while now. This process of datafication has been ongoing for some time, and it has become more useful than ever because highly standardised organisational patterns are once again becoming prevalent [69].

More troubling still is the fact that while implementing these applications, artificial intelligence is adding a new chapter to the long history of pervasive worker surveillance, which is now based on call logs, screenshots, eye tracking, facial recognition software, smartphone sensors, and even smart glasses and smart glasses sensors. However, AI's "marriage of convenience" of already established authoritative practises is its key quality that sets it apart from other kinds of monitoring systems [70]. Simple indicators for purportedly "data-driven" or "evidence-based" personnel management decisions, such as the quantity of emails sent, the list of websites visited, cookies, or the number of documents and apps opened, may be found, which can result in new kinds of anticipatory conformity, both before and after hiring [71,72].

Recruiting, compensation, and even firing decisions made by managers may become increasingly computerised, experts warn, which may give way to discriminatory prejudices more frequently, maintain social segregation, and undermine humanity and fairness. Simply said, advances in AI technology expand the potential for digital monitoring and hierarchical management in a way that has never been possible before and isn't even desirable [73]. However, the negative effects do not end there. For entry-level prospects, what may start as an online screening "ends with the alteration of practically every facet of hiring, performance assessment, and management." All of this may be accomplished using systems that, once created and calibrated, operate automatically and collect large volumes of detailed information about employee behaviour from various sources, frequently far more than is required. Additionally, workforce analytics powered by AI may acquire predictive abilities by deriving "non-intuitive and unverifiable" assumptions from data [74]. AI thereby affects autonomy, moral reasoning, independence, and privacy, which is particularly important in a culture where the historically strong division between personal and professional life is eroding. The potential for algorithms to become uncontrollably efficient exists when they are trained to become more effective. Additionally, a lack of openness may contribute to the deviance and misconduct of employees. AI apps frequently gain from a purportedly participative character that promotes information sharing without friction in exchange for minimal benefits like reputation or promotions. In connection to gamified internal initiatives, the underlying working culture likewise promotes personal measurement and self-tracking [75]. Concurrently, while the dangers of the "devil's bargain" [76], which consumers must enter into in exchange for unrestricted access to services that appear to be free and are supported by a glittering promise of connectivity, convenience, personalization, and innovation, have largely been exposed and countered [77], it has received less attention how feedback mechanisms, surveillance, and data—now viewed as crucial organisational components—are changing the power dynamics in the workplace.

14.8.2 SOCIETAL ISSUES

Risks associated with using AI for social benefit are generally relatively similar to those associated with more commercial uses. One of the main hazards is that authorities and others who have access to AI's tools and tactics could misuse them maliciously, harming people, organisations, and society as a whole. AI can be used maliciously to endanger people's digital safety, financial security, equity, and fair treatment, in addition to their physical and emotional safety. Although there may be fewer commercial risks than those that could potentially harm for-profit corporations, improper use for organisations frequently involves risks to their brand and legal compliance. Malicious uses of AI could endanger infrastructure, political stability, economic stability, national security, and labour markets. One major distinction between the dangers connected to commercial and non-commercial goals is how labour displacement affects workforce and workers. In the world of for-profit AI, the possibility of worker displacement dominates most of the public discussion. Examining our use case collection reveals that many of the applications of AI for social good may provide less of a risk. In fact, as mentioned in the earlier discussion of bottlenecks, a lack of individuals with the necessary skills and technical know-how tends to hinder AI's implementation for socially beneficial purposes. For instance, if AI were to improve access to healthcare or education, this might have a positive impact on the employment of physicians, nurses, and educators. When using AI solutions for social good, as we discuss below, four key kinds of risk were identified through a review of our use case library. They are impartiality and bias, privacy, secure use, and "explainability"—the capacity to pinpoint the specific feature or combination of data that influences a certain judgement or prediction. Risk kinds and their severity vary greatly from situation to case. Every domain carries some level of risk, but generally speaking, our analysis reveals that the risk is greatest in the domains where data are sensitive and forecasts identify specific individuals, such as economic empowerment, education, equality, health, and security. In other fields, including crisis response, inaccurate AI offers significant concerns. For instance, incorrect location predictions for missing people could have disastrous consequences. Based on insights from our discussions with domain experts and AI experts, the exhibit's scoring was determined. We ranked individual use cases from low too high for each of the five categories—risk of bias, risk of privacy violation, risk of unsafe use of the AI solution, level of explainability required to reduce or mitigate risks, and considerations of the risk of negative effects on the workforce and workers—to develop the risk profiles [78]. There are several immediate ways in which the social impact of artificial intelligence can be felt in healthcare:

a. ***Practitioner well-being and support*** – The harsh reality of modern medicine is that it is hectic, taxing, stressful, and frequently overwhelming. For practitioners, the need to deliver excellent care while handling exceptionally heavy workloads never goes away. They are exhausted and overworked. AI algorithms have been developed to minimise errors brought on by fatigue. AI is constantly awake. It never stops exploring the data and examining the images. By having a pair of eyes that never shut, the medical sector can gain from an additional safety net that supports their workloads and daily lives more successfully.

b. ***Rapid diagnosis and urgent detection*** – In several applications, AI has advanced significantly, but particularly in the field of stroke detection. When it comes to patient outcomes, algorithms' capacity to expedite the start of treatment or to alert doctors to potential risk regions can make all the difference. The social impact of artificial intelligence in healthcare is outstanding in this case since a patient may receive prompt, life-saving therapy before suffering the full effects of a stroke or at a pace that lessens those effects, leading to a dramatically improved quality of life.

c. ***Improved radiology capabilities*** – Radiologists need critical support, and products like Aidoc have been on the market long enough to demonstrate their worth in this regard. These AI solutions are gaining traction on a global scale as a result of their demonstrated value addition. They are created to expedite processes, reliably monitor staggering image volumes, and alert practitioners of potential patient concerns.

14.9 UNEMPLOYMENT EFFECTS

People's fear of losing their jobs as a result of the rise of AI in healthcare has slowed down the adoption of AI among healthcare professionals. According to the majority of federal governments and policymakers, as AI grows more prevalent, occupations will become unproductive and the economic goal of job growth will suffer. On the other hand, it is anticipated that as AI becomes more widely used, career opportunities will expand and there will be a significant demand for fresh talent. Many professions, like nursing and rehabilitation, call for the uttermost compassion and human emotions, which AI cannot yet replicate. Rather than replacing care delivery, AI is used to enhance it in healthcare organisations. Moreover, if AI in healthcare develops further, more employment for new skill sets would be developed.

A larger volume of care could be supplied thanks to AI because of higher productivity and cheaper treatment costs. Higher earnings and more employment prospects would follow from this. It is erroneous to believe that AI would displace healthcare professionals; instead, it may enhance the need for a skilled workforce and boost productivity in areas like diagnostics, patient engagement, and precision medicine. AI is now filling in holes in healthcare services that have been found. The world is undergoing a healthcare professional shortage that is only getting worse due to its expanding population. By 2035, the World Health Organization (WHO) projects that there will be a shortage of roughly 13 million healthcare professionals worldwide [79]. Furthermore, it has been difficult to teach doctors and other health professionals because there is still a significant shortage of skilled trainers worldwide. In addition to potentially replacing certain administrative occupations, such as those related to patient interaction and the upkeep of medical records, AI may also lead to a rise in the demand for specialised specialists.

According to high-level projections, automation and AI might change or destroy one-fourth of American jobs. Entire job segments could become extinct as AI develops and more duties fall into the category of things that can be easily automated. Manufacturing, agribusiness, catering services, commerce, transportation & logistics, and hospitality are the industry's most likely to be impacted by automation. If a recession is on the horizon, it might hasten this trend toward automation as financially strapped companies look for ways to cut expenses. A lot of these professions might not follow the traditional model of full-time employment, which is another possibility. Instead, it's estimated that additional firms will nurture their remote workforces and rely heavily on contractors to fill the majority of their staffing gaps [79].

14.10 IMPLEMENTATION ISSUES

14.10.1 DATA COLLECTION

Our discussion of data collecting is based on a survey [80] by one of the authors but has been updated and revised using information from a tutorial [81]. There are three basic methods for gathering data. First, the issue of finding, enhancing, or producing new datasets is known as data acquisition. The second issue is data labelling, which is the process of annotating data in a way that is instructive so that a machine learning model can learn from it. Since labelling is expensive, there are a number of approaches to apply, including crowdsourcing, poor supervision, and semi-supervised learning. Finally, rather than collecting or labelling data from start, one can improve existing data and models if they already exist.

The unavailability of comprehensive open collections of medical data is a major barrier to the adoption and deployment of AI in healthcare in India. Legal issues and other factors can make it challenging to access healthcare datasets. Start-ups in particular face difficulties with this because bigger players frequently already have access to these data [82]. As a result, start-ups frequently rely on publicly accessible datasets from the US, Europe, and other regions [81,82]. As a result, the usefulness of deploying AI in healthcare is compromised because it does not take Indian consumers into account [83–85]. Using free data from other sources frequently leads to algorithms that reveals their unfairness and the creation of solutions tailored to a certain population [82,86]. It would be necessary to take into consideration these biases in the use of AI approaches and to retrain solutions on Indian data, particularly when it comes to drug discovery and genomics [84,85,86].

14.10.2 RELEVANCE

The development of robust and beautiful computational models has become easier with the development of more open-source and advanced statistical software. However, if models are simply created with technology answers in mind, they can easily be created to address a problem that doesn't exist or is unimportant. Alternatively, the solution offered by a specific model won't interest the technology's intended consumers, such as a practising physician in a clinic. A prime example of this issue is the enhanced capacity to identify mental disease based on more accurate and reachable maps of the brain connect [87]. Given a dataset with patient data on schizophrenia, a machine-learning specialist might create a model to diagnose schizophrenia as their initial step. Nevertheless, current medical practises are already quite adept at such identification; therefore, they would prefer to understand other issues offers additional profitable pathways for ML applications, like predicting modulatory therapy responses for schizophrenia [88]. As a result, thinking about such problems from a strictly computer science or statistical perspective inevitably restricts the potential of a given project.

Instead, the final consumers of the technology should be incorporated right from the start of the model's creation. The goals of research and development ought to be based on what the medical community has already recommended as important directions for future work on therapeutic breakthroughs. ML tools, for instance, can simplify the patient information provided in a particular pathological state and then present statistical anomalies that can be used by doctors to make more educated decisions for clinical treatment [89,90]. Rather than attempting to forecast an illness that can already be readily detected in clinical therapy, this is preferable.

14.10.3 SAMPLE SIZE

Most analytical approaches share the issue of sample size concerns. Inflated findings could be discovered by comparing a model's output to a control sample after it has been built and trained with a small sample size. As a result, when used in a novel, clinical setting, the model's accuracy could drop and it could malfunction. This is due to the possibility that a model, given the small sample size, will produce results that are just the consequence of chance. This must be considered to obtain reliable results. For ML systems to be taught in an era where data is more readily available, datasets must be huge and diverse. Even though it will likely require the harmonisation of data from several centres, this component is crucial if we are to trust that our models are robust enough to consistently offer meaningful results at various time points and in various contexts. A recent systematic review examined 62 complete research reporting novel machine-learning (ML) models for the diagnosis or prognosis of COVID-19 utilising chest x-ray and/or computed tomography data. It was discovered that the majority of the studies had issues with the small sample sizes used to train the models. Around 2,000 data points were used in more than half of the diagnostic-focused studies (19/32) among the 62 models examined. Compared to rare brain malignancies that may require years of poor data collection, COVID-19 has seen more than 2 million cases to date [91]. Therefore, it is not surprising that, when utilised in the intended context, a model built to represent a complex biological process based on just 2,000 data points may yield false results. ML models can be updated and improved over time to produce performances that are more dependable and accurate, unlike genuine medical devices. Models can be retrained with bigger sample sizes when new data becomes available for the best field performance. As a result, it may be necessary to take a model out of clinical practise, retrain it, test it using the more recent data that is now available, and then reintroduce it into the appropriate context. However, given the growing need for data, it's critical to contemplate the probability that an ML modeller might get and exploit patient-unconsented data. It is challenging to determine which data was used once the new data has been assimilated into the model and the model has been used in the field. Patient consent issues with expanding data may be resolved by implementing a certificate expressing patient approval in each image, like using non-fungible tokens (NFTs) [92,93].

14.10.4   DISCRIMINATORY BIASES

The propensity of AI technology to increase our pre-existing social prejudices in clinical practise is perhaps the worry. There may be issues with discriminatory bias when a model performs well on a particular sample of patient data but badly on different subgroups of people. For instance, ML-based apps are increasingly focusing on creating algorithms that can assist doctors in identifying and treating skin issues [93]. Recent research indicates that one of the primary causes of the racial inequities in access to healthcare, which are increasingly being reported, is the underrepresentation of race and skin tone in medical textbooks [94]. In spite of these issues, deep-learning (DL) image-based classifier algorithms commonly remain to train on low-quality datasets that frequently contain one-dimensional data (for example, primarily lighter skin photos). To reflect this, medical schools have revised the textbook illustrations [95]. These algorithms will also transfer whatever biases that were present in the initial datasets by outperforming the image type they were trained on. In the end, this cycle poses the danger of catastrophic failures with particular people groups. Examining three commercially available facial recognition algorithms (Microsoft, Face++, and IBM) based on intersectional studies of gender and race indicated that gender categorization error rates varied as high as 34.7 percent in darker-skinned females and 0.8 percent in lighter-skinned men [96]. All patients with a variety of skin types should be included for the potential future benefits of these algorithms, even when some diseases, such melanoma in non-Hispanic white individuals, are more common in specific races or genders [97]. Due to the fact that DL algorithms are currently being developed and there has been an increased focus on classification performance across gender and race, we are motivated to ensure that they can be used to successfully remove healthcare inequities based on demographics [98].

14.10.5   EMERGENCE OF NEW TRENDS

Given the current state of the world's affairs and the recent SARS-CoV-2 epidemic, this subject in focus. ML techniques have been widely used in the past to forecast changes in seasonal illnesses like influenza, to assist hospitals in better planning for medical supply needs like bed capacity, and to effectively inform the public and governments about the most prevalent strains that are currently circulating. This is due to the fact that several viruses frequently change and create a diversity of strains every annum, yet vaccinations can only protect against certain of the more common variants. In such a scenario, ML technologies can be used to accurately predict which strains will be most prevalent in following seasons, allowing for the inclusion of such strains in upcoming seasonal vaccines [95]. A new pandemic, for example, can cause unforeseen environmental changes that radically affect the environment's landscape and, as a result, modify how two variables may be represented using the new environmental parameters. These models can potentially cause harm if a continuous monitoring system is not in place since the results are no longer valid.

Similar modifications and upgrades are frequently made to medical equipment, such as functional magnetic resonance imaging (fMRI) scanners, to enhance its diagnostic and visualisation capabilities. However, magnetic field inhomogeneity, which has poor interscanner dependability, could cause variations in the relative blood oxygen level-dependent (BOLD) signal strength between various scanners, such as a 3 Tesla vs. a newer 7 Tesla [96].

14.10.6 DIAGNOSIS

Since Stanford created MYCIN to identify blood-borne bacterial infections in the 1970s, the diagnosis and treatment of sickness has been a prominent focus of AI. They did not significantly outperform human diagnosticians, and they did not integrate well into clinical procedures or medical record systems. The media has recently focused heavily on IBM's Watson because of its focus on correctness of medicine, particularly cancer detection and treatment. Natural language processing and machine learning are both employed by Watson. However, clients' initial eagerness for this utilisation of the technology started to diminish as they realised how difficult it was to educate Watson how to treat certain types of cancer [97] and to incorporate Watson into care processes and systems. Watson uses application programming interfaces (APIs) to provide "cognitive services," including as speech and language, vision, and machine-learning-based data analysis programmes. There is no one product called Watson. Instead, it is an assortment of these services [98]. Although the majority of observers believe the Watson APIs are technically capable, treating cancer was an desperately ambitious goal. Competition from free "open source" programmes offered by some companies, like Google's Tensor Flow, has hurt Watson and other proprietary programmes as well. The implementation of AI is difficult for many healthcare organisations. Rule-based systems integrated into EHR systems lack the accuracy of more algorithmic systems based on machine learning, despite being widely used, especially at the NHS [99]. These rule-based clinical decision support systems frequently can't handle the explosion of data and knowledge based on genetic, proteomic, metabolic, and other "omic-based" approaches to care, and it is challenging to keep up with them as medical knowledge develops. Even though it occurs more frequently in IT companies and research labs than in healthcare settings, the situation is starting to shift [100]. It is uncommon for a research facility to assert that it has created a method for leveraging AI or big data to diagnose and treat a condition as accurately as medical professionals. Even if some of them also use other types of pictures, including retinal scanning or precision medicine based on genetics, many of these studies are focused on radiological image analysis [101]. Tech firms and startups alike are assiduously tackling the same issues. In order to develop big data prediction algorithms that can alert clinicians to high-risk illnesses like sepsis and heart failure, Google, for instance, is working with health delivery networks Numerous startups are striving to create algorithms for AI-derived image interpretation, including Google, Enlitic, and many others. Jvion offers a "clinical success machine" that identifies people who are most susceptible to negative side effects, as well as those who are most likely to gain from recommended therapies. Each of these could give clinicians decision help as they look for the right patient diagnosis and care. Companies that specialise in this strategy include Foundation Medicine and Flatiron Health, both of which are currently acquired by Roche. Machine learning models for "population health" are also being used by healthcare payers and providers to identify groups that are more likely to develop certain diseases or accidents, or to have hospital readmission [101]. These models are nonetheless capable of producing precise forecasts even while they occasionally lack all the necessary data that could increase their predictive ability, such as the socioeconomic status of the patient. Some EHR businesses have begun to incorporate limited AI functions (beyond rule-based clinical decision support) into their solutions; however, these are still in the early stages. Providers will either have to wait until EHR suppliers add additional AI capabilities, or they will have to undertake large integration efforts on their own [102].

14.10.7 ETHICAL ISSUES

Examining the ethical concerns related to this impending paradigm change is necessary given the growing use of AI-powered technology in healthcare. The "Principles of Biological Ethics" by Beauchamp and Childress introduce four important principles: autonomy, beneficence, no maleficence, and justice [103], and are a frequently used and well-fitting ethical framework when evaluating biomedical ethical dilemmas. Although there are several bioethical frameworks available, principlism is a highly helpful basic practical framework that is well-accepted in both research and medical settings [103]. Explainability has significance for both patients and doctors with regard to autonomy. Informed consent, which is an independent, typically written authorisation with which the patient offers a doctor permission to conduct a specific medical act, is one of the main safeguards of patients' autonomy [104]. The foundation of proper informed consent is complete and intelligible disclosure of the nature and potential hazards of a medical procedure, as well as no undue interference with the patient's free choice to undergo the procedure. Currently, there is no ethically accepted position on whether informed consent should entail disclosure of the employment of a mysterious medical AI algorithm. The autonomy of patients may be compromised, the doctor-patient relationship may suffer, patients' trust may be jeopardised, and clinical recommendations may not be followed if the employment of an opaque AI system is not disclosed. If a patient discovers after the fact that a doctor's recommendation came from an opaque AI system, they may reject the advice, and they may also legitimately want an explanation—which, in the case of an opaque system, the clinician would not be able to supply. Therefore, opaque medical AI may offer a barrier to the delivery of accurate information, potentially jeopardising informed consent. Therefore, it's crucial to uphold appropriate ethical and explainability criteria to protect the informed consent's autonomy-preserving function. It is important to address the possibility for opaque AI to promote paternalism by limiting patients' ability to express their expectations and preferences for medical operations [105]. Shared decision-making calls for complete patient autonomy, but complete autonomy can only be realised if the patient is offered a wide range of worthwhile options to select from. In this approach, patients' opportunities to express their autonomy over medical procedures are reduced as opaque AI becomes more important to medical decision-making. The difficulty with opaque CDSS, in particular, is that it is still unknown whether and how the model considers patient values and preferences. The use of "value-flexible" AI that gives the patient options could help to address this situation. The value of patients, for whom a "reduction of suffering" is more significant, may not be aligned, for instance, with AI systems that are designed with "survival" as the desired objective. Last, but not least, when a decision is reached, patients must have confidence and autonomy in the AI system to determine whether or not to follow its recommendations [105]. If the AI model is opaque, then this is not feasible. As a result, systems that enable critical medical decision making from both the patient's and the clinician's perspectives must be understandable. The ideas of beneficence and non-maleficence are related, but they also provide insight into a number of other issues, such as explainability. Physicians are urged by beneficence to maximise patient benefits. Therefore, it is expected of doctors to use AI-based technology in a way that encourages the best outcome for the specific patient. However, in order to give patients, the best possible options to support their health and wellness, doctors must be able to fully utilise the system. This shows that physicians are knowledgeable about the system beyond its application to robotic tasks in a specific clinical use case, enabling them to evaluate the system's output. Explainability in the form of graphics or explanations in natural language enables physicians to make confident therapeutic decisions without having to rely exclusively on an automated output.

They can evaluate the results produced by the system critically and decide for themselves whether they appear reliable. This enables them to, if needed, modify predictions and advice to account for specific situations. As a result, doctors can use their clinical judgement to indicate potentially unsuitable interventions in addition to lowering the danger of inspiring false optimism or producing false despair. This becomes much more crucial when we consider a difficult-to-resolve scenario in which a doctor and an AI system disagree. Fundamentally, this is a matter of epistemic authority, and it is unclear at this point how medical practitioners can determine whether they can fully rely on a black box model's epistemic authority to accept its result. According to Grote et al. [106], there is little epistemic evidence for deference in the situation of opaque AI. Furthermore, they contend that when faced with a "black-box" system, clinical decision assistance may actually work against rather than in favour of doctors' abilities. Doctors might be forced to practise "defensive medicine," in this case, to avoid being questioned or held accountable. The autonomy of doctors would be seriously threatened in such a circumstance. Additionally, doctors will infrequently have the opportunity to thoroughly examine the reasons why their clinical judgement conflicts with the AI system. Therefore, in the clinical context, focusing solely on a performance outcome is insufficient. The best outcomes for patients can only be anticipated from healthcare practitioners who are capable of making knowledgeable choices regarding when to employ an AI-powered CDSS and how to interpret its findings [106]. Thus, it is difficult to see how any "black box" application might achieve goodness in the connection of medical AI.

14.11 CONCLUSION

The medical sector has been promised a wide range of fresh and possible uses for AI that will improve the calibre and provision of healthcare services. Despite the impressive progress made in recent years, many applications have not yet reached their full potential in clinical settings due to their inability to produce repeatable and dependable outcomes in addition to the widespread scepticism of these technologies in the medical field. Informed consent, high standards of safety and effectiveness, cyber resilience and cybersecurity, algorithmic fairness, an adequate level of transparency and regulatory oversight, high levels of safety and resilience, and an ideal liability regime for AIs are all significant factors that must be considered to successfully develop an AI-driven healthcare system with the motto "Health AIs for All of Us."

REFERENCES

[1] Sniecinski, I & Seghatchian, J (2018). Artificial intelligence: a joint narrative on potential use in pediatric stem and immune cell therapies and regenerative medicine. *Transfusion and Apheresis Science*, 57(3), 422–424.
[2] Tran, BX, Vu, GT, Ha, GH, et al. (2019). Global evolution of research in artificial intelligence in health and medicine: a bibliometric study. *J Clin Med*, 8(3), 360. 10.3390/jcm8030360
[3] Davenport, T & Kalakota, R (2019). The potential for artificial intelligence in healthcare. *Future healthcare journal*, 6(2), 94–98. 10.7861/futurehosp.6-2-94
[4] IPPR. (June 15, 2018). Better Health and Care for All: A 10-Point Plan for the 2020s. https://www.ippr.org/research/publications/better-health-and-care-for-all
[5] Gilson, L (2003). Trust and the development of health care as a social institution. *Social Science & Medicine*, 56, 1453–1468. https://www.merriam-webster.com/dictionary/health%20care
[6] Miller, RA (1994). Medical diagnostic decision support systems–past, present, and future: a threaded bibliography and brief commentary. *J. Am. Med. Inform. Assoc.*, 1, 8–27.
[7] Musen, MA, Middleton, B, & Greenes, RA in *Biomedical Informatics* (eds. Shortliffe, EH & Cimino, JJ) 643–674 (Springer, London, 2014).
[8] Shortliffe, E *Computer-Based Medical Consultations: MYCIN* Vol. 2 (Elsevier, New York, 2012).
[9] Szolovits, P, Patil, RS, & Schwartz, WB (1988). Artificial intelligence in medical diagnosis. *Ann. Intern. Med.*, 108, 80–87.
[10] de Dombal, FT, Leaper, DJ, Staniland, JR, McCann, AP, & Horrocks, JC (1972). Computer-aided diagnosis of acute abdominal pain. *Br. Med. J.*, 2, 9–13.
[11] Shortliffe, EH et al. (1975). Computer-based consultations in clinical therapeutics: explanation and rule acquisition capabilities of the MYCIN system. *Comput. Biomed. Res.*, 8, 303–320.
[12] Barnett, GO, Cimino, JJ, Hupp, JA, & Hoffer, EP (1987). DXplain. An evolving diagnostic decision-support system. *JAMA*, 258, 67–74.

[13] Miller, RA, McNeil, MA, Challinor, SM, Masarie, FE Jr, & Myers, JD (1986). The Internist-1/Quick Medical Reference Project — status report. *Western J. Med.*, 145, 816–822.

[14] Berner, ES et al. (1994). Performance of four computer-based diagnostic systems. *N. Engl. J. Med.*, 330, 1792–1796.

[15] Szolovits, P & Pauker, SG (1978). Categorical and probabilistic reasoning in medical diagnosis. *Artif. Intell.*, 11, 115–144.

[16] Lee, S & Lee, D (2020). Healthcare wearable devices: An analysis of key factors for continuous use intention. *Serv. Bus.*, 14, 503–531.

[17] Lee, D (2018). Strategies for Technology-driven Service Encounters for Patient Experience Satisfaction in Hospitals. *Technol. Forecast. Soc. Chang.*, 137, 118–127.

[18] Ramesh, A, Kambhampati, C, Monson, J, & Drew, P (2004). Artificial Intelligence in Medicine. *Ann. R. Coll. Surg. Engl.*, 86, 334–338.

[19] Safavi, K & Kalis, B (2019). How AI can Change the Future of Health Care. *Harv. Bus. Rev.* Available online: https://hbr.org/webinar/2019/02/how-ai-can-change-the-future-of-health-care (accessed on 15 June 2020).

[20] Aruba. (2017). IoT Heading for Mass Adoption by 2019 Driven by Better-than-Expected Business Results. Available online: https://news.arubanetworks.com/press-release/arubanetworks/iot-heading-mass-adoption-2019-driven-better-expectedbusiness-results (accessed on 10 April 2020).

[21] Amato, F, López, A, Peña-Méndez, E, Vaňhara, P, Hampl, A, & Havel, J (2013). Artificial Neural Networks in Medical Diagnosis. *J. Appl. Biomed*, 11, 47–58.

[22] Bennett, C & Hauser, K (2013). Artificial Intelligence Framework for Simulating Clinical Decision-Making: AMarkov Decision Process Approach. *Artif. Intell. Med.*, 57, 9–19.

[23] Dilsizian, S & Siegel, E (2014). Artificial Intelligence in Medicine and Cardiac Imaging: Harnessing Big Data and Advanced Computing to Provide Personalized Medical Diagnosis and Treatment. *Curr. Cardiol. Rep.*, 16, 441.

[24] Shiraishi, J, Li, Q, Appelbaum, D, & Doi, K (2011). Computer-aided Diagnosis and Artificial Intelligence in Clinical Imaging. *Semin. Nucl. Med.*, 41, 449–462.

[25] Esteva, A, Kuprel, B, Novoa, R, Ko, J, Swetter, S, Blau, H, & Thrun, S (2017). Dermatologist-level Classification of Skin cancer with Deep Neural Networks. *Nature*, 542, 115–118.

[26] Rigby, M (2019). Ethical Dimensions of Using Artificial Intelligence in Healthcare. *AMA J. Ethics*, 21, E121–E124.

[27] Luxton, D (2014). Artificial Intelligence in Psychological Practice: Current and Future Applications and Implications. *Prof. Psychol. Res. Pract.*, 45, 332–339.

[28] Bartneck, C, Lütge, C, Wagner, A, & Welsh, S (2021). *Privacy Issues of AI. In: An Introduction to Ethics in Robotics and AI. SpringerBriefs in Ethics.* Springer, Cham. 10.1007/978-3-030-51110-4_8

[29] Teich, DA "Artificial Intelligence and Data Privacy – Turning A Risk Into A Benefit." Forbes. Accessed November 3, 2022. https://www.forbes.com/sites/davidteich/2020/08/10/artificial-intelligence-and-data-privacy--turning-a-risk-into-a-benefit/

[30] Murdoch, B (2021). Privacy and artifcial intelligence: challenges for protecting health information in a new era. *BMC Med Ethics*, 22, 122. 10.1186/s12910-021-00687-3

[31] Dietterich, T (1995). Overftting and undercomputing in machine learning. *ACM Comput Surv.*, 27(3), 326–327.

[32] Mukherjee, S A.I. versus M.D. The New Yorker. Annals of Medicine, April 3, 2017 Issue. 2017. https://www.newyorker.com/magazine/2017/04/03/ai-versus-md. [accessed Jul 27 2022].

[33] Cuttler, M (2019). Transforming health care: how artifcial intelligence is reshaping the medical landscape. *CBC News.* https://www.cbc.ca/news/health/artificial-intelligence-health-care-1.5110892. [accessed Jul 27 2022].

[34] Char, DS, Shah, NH, & Magnus, D (2018). Implementing machine learning in health care—addressing ethical challenges. *N Engl J Med.*, 378(11), 981.

[35] Hashimoto, DA, Rosman, G, Rus, D, & Meireles, OR (2018). Artifcial intelligence in surgery: promises and perils. *Ann Surg.*, 268(1), 70–76.

[36] Bocchi, C & Olivi, G (2021). Regulating artifcial intelligence in the EU: top 10 issues for businesses to consider. https://www.jdsupra.com/legalnews/regulating-artificial-intelligence-in-3639576/. [accessed Jul 27 2022].

[37] Ahmad, MA, Eckert, C, & Teredesai A (2018). Interpretable machine learning in healthcare. In: Proceedings of the 2018 ACM international conference on bioinformatics, computational biology, and health informatics. pp. 559–560.

[38] He, J, Baxter, SL, Xu, J, Xu, J, Zhou, X, & Zhang, K (2019). The practical implementation of artifcial intelligence technologies in medicine. *Nat Med.*, 25(1), 30–36.

[39] Canadian Association of Radiologists (CAR) Artifcial Intelligence Working Group. (2019). Canadian Association of Radiologists white paper on ethical and legal issues related to artifcial intelligence in radiology. *Can Assoc Radiol J.*, 70(2), 107–118.

[40] Vayena, E & Blasimme, A (2018). Health research with big data: time for systemic oversight. *J Law Med Ethics.*, 46(1), 119–129.

[41] Yoon, J, Drumright, LN, & Van Der Schaar, M (2020). Anonymization through data synthesis using generative adversarial networks (ads-gan). *IEEE J Biomed Health Inform.*, 24(8), 2378–2388.

[42] Baowaly, MK, Lin, CC, Liu, CL, & Chen, KT (2019). Synthesizing electronic health records using improved generative adversarial networks. *J Am Med Inform Assoc.*, 26(3), 228–241.

[43] Torra, V & Navarro-Arribas, G (2016). Big data privacy and anonymization. In: Lehmann A, Whitehouse D, Fischer-Hübner S, Fritsch L, Raab C, editors. *Privacy and identity management. Facing up to next steps. Privacy and identity 2016. IFIP advances in Information and Communication Technology*, vol. 498. Cham: Springer.

[44] Ajmera, P & Jain, V (2019). Modelling the barriers of Health 4.0–the fourth healthcare industrial revolution in India by TISM. *Operations Management Research*, 12, 129–145. 10.1007/s12063-019-00143-x

[45] Kamble, SS, Gunasekaran, A, & Sharma, R (2018). Analysis of the driving and dependence power of barriers to adopt industry 4.0 in Indian manufacturing industry. *Computers in Industry*, 101, 107 – 119. 10.1016/j.compind.2018.06.004

[46] Walach, E (2022). Council Post: Overcoming AI Barriers In Health Care. *Forbes*. Accessed November 3. https://www.forbes.com/sites/forbestechcouncil/2018/07/11/overcoming-ai-barriers-in-health-care/

[47] Gujral, G, Shivarama, J, & Mariappan, M (2019). Artificial Intelligence (AI) and Data Science for Developing Intelligent Health Informatics Systems. In Proceedings of the Ntional Conference on AI in HI & VR, SHSS-TISS Mumbai.

[48] USAID (2019). *Artificial Intelligence in Global Health: Defining a Collective Path Forward.* Washington, DC: USAID. https://www.usaid.gov/sites/default/files/documents/1864/AI-in-Global-Health_webFinal_508.pdf [accessed Jul 27 2022].

[49] Wahl, B, Cossy-Gantner, A, Germann, S, & Schwalbe, NR (2018). Artificial intelligence (AI) and global health: how can AI contribute to health in resource-poor settings? *BMJ global health*, 3(4), e000798. https://gh.bmj.com/content/3/4/e000798

[50] Mohandas, S (2017). AI and healthcare in India: Looking forward. Roundtable Report. The Centre for Internet and Society, India. https://cis-india.org/internet-governance/files/ai-and-healthcare-report, [accessed Jul 27 2022].

[51] Raghupathi, W & Raghupathi, V (2014). Big data analytics in healthcare: promise and potential. *Health Information Science and Systems*, 2(3). https://www.researchgate.net/publication/272830136_Big_data_analytics_in_healthcare_Promise_and_potential, [accessed Jul 27 2022].

[52] Jagdev, G & Singh, S (2015). Implementation and Applications of Big Data in Health Care Industry. *International Journal of Scientific and Technical Advancements (IJSTA)*, 1(3), 29–34.

[53] Zettler, P (June 1, 2015). Toward Coherent Federal Oversight of Medicine. *San Diego Law Review* 52(2), 427. https://digital.sandiego.edu/sdlr/vol52/iss2/6.

[54] Price, W (December 1, 2017). Regulating Black-Box Medicine. *Michigan Law Review* 116(3), 421–474.

[55] Health, Center for Devices and Radiological. (October 3, 2022). Medical Device Accessories - Describing Accessories and Classification Pathways. U.S. Food and Drug Administration, https://www.fda.gov/regulatory-information/search-fda-guidance-documents/medical-device-accessories-describing-accessories-and-classification-pathways

[56] Melisande Rouge. (December 2019). The Cost of AI in Radiology: Is it Relly Worth it?. European Society of Radiology, AI Blog. [accessed Jul 27 2022].

[57] Ronald, Y & Alì, GS (April 24, 2019). *What's Inside the Black Box? AI Challenges for Lawyers and Researchers*. Cambridge University Press. 10.1017/S1472669619000021

[58] Rai, A (2020). Explainable AI: from Black Box to Glass Box. *Journal of the Academy of Marketing Science*, 48, 137–141, December 17, 2019. 10.1007/s11747-019-00710-5.

[59] Howard, A & Borenstein, J (2018). The Ugly Truth About Ourselves and Our Robot Creations: The Problem of Bias and Social Inequity. *Science and Engineering Ethics*, 24, 1521–1536, September 21, 2017. 10.1007/s11948-017-9975-2.

[60] Price, WN (November 2017). Artificial Intelligence in Health Care: Applications and Legal Implications. *The SciTech Lawyer*, 14(1).

[61] Tariq, RA & Hackert, PB (2021). *Patient Confidentiality*. StatPearls. Treasure Island (FL), StatPearls Publishing Copyright © 2021, StatPearls Publishing LLC.

[62] Chard, K, Russell, M, Lussier, YA, Mendonça, EA, & Silverstein, JC (2011). A cloud-based approach to medical NLP. *AMIA Annu Symp Proc.*, 2011, 207–216.

[63] Schweitzer, EJ (2012). Reconciliation of the cloud computing model with US federal electronic health record regulations. *J Am Med Inform Assoc.*, 19, 161–165.

[64] Steg, H & Thumm, N (July 2001). Single-Market Regulation and Innovation in Europe's medical devices industry. *International Journal of Technology Assessment in Health Care*, 17(3), 10.1017/S0266462301106136.

[65] Katz, ML & Shapiro, C (1985). Network Externalities, Competition, and Compatibility. *The American Economic Review*, 75(3), 424–440. Accessed April 27, 2020. www.jstor.org/stable/1814809.

[66] Farrell, J & Saloner, G (1986). Installed Base and Compatibility: Innovation, Product Preannouncements, and Predation. *The American Economic Review*, 76(5), 940–955. Accessed May 14, 2020. www.jstor.org/stable/1816461

[67] For an overview, see Brishen Rogers, *Beyond Automation: The Law & Political Economy of Workplace Technological Change* 24 (Roosevelt Institute Working Paper, 2019), *available at* https://ssrn.com/abstract=3327608

[68] Danaher, J (2016). *The Threat of Algocracy: Reality, Resistance and Accommodation*, 29 PHIL. & TECH. 245.

[69] Ajunwa, I, Crawford, K, & Schultz, J (2017). *Limitless worker surveillance*, 105 CAL. L. REV. 102. Ifeoma Ajunwa, *Algorithms at Work: Productivity Monitoring Platforms and Wearable Technology as the New Data-Centric Research Agenda for Employment and Labor Law*, ST. LOUIS U. L. J. 63 (2018).

[70] Solon, O (Nov. 6, 2017). *Big Brother isn't just watching: workplace surveillance can track your every move*, GUARDIAN, https://www.theguardian.com/world/2017/nov/06/workplace-surveillance-big-brother-technology

[71] Ball, K (2010). *Workplace surveillance: an overview*, 51 LAB. HIST. 87.

[72] Schubert, C & Hütt, M-T (2019). *Economy-on-demand and the fairness of algorithms*, 10 EUR. LAB. L.J. 3.

[73] Peck, D (Dec. DATE 2013). *They're Watching You at Work*, THE ATLANTIC, https://www.theatlantic.com/magazine/archive/2013/12/theyre-watching-you-at-work/354681/

[74] Swan, M (2013). *The quantified self: Fundamental disruption in big data science and biological discovery*, 1 BIG DATA 85.

[75] Davis, NJ (2007). *Presumed assent: The judicial acceptance of clickwrap*, 22 BERKELEY TECH. L.J. 577.

[76] Adler-Bell, S & Miller, M (Dec. 19, 2018). *The Datafication of Employment. How Surveillance and Capitalism Are Shaping Workers' Futures without Their Knowledge*, THE CENTURY FOUNDATION, https://tcf.org/content/report/datafication-employment-surveillance-capitalism-shaping-workers-futures-without-knowledge/?agreed=1

[77] Brundage, M et al. (February 2018). *The malicious use of artificial intelligence: Forecasting, prevention, and mitigation*. Future of Humanity Institute.

[78] https://www.mindfieldsglobal.com/blog/impact-of-ai-on-jobs

[79] Roh, Y, Heo, G, & Whang, SE (2019). *A survey on data collection for machine learning: a big data - AI integration perspective*. IEEE TKDE.

[80] 90 Whang, SE & Lee, J-G (2020). Data collection and quality challenges for deep learning. *Proc. VLDB Endow.*, 13(12), 3429–3432.

[81] Paul, Y, Hickok, E, Sinha, A, et al. (2018). Artificial intelligence in the healthcare industry in India. *Bengaluru: The Centre for Internet and Society (India)*. Available online: https://cis-india.org/internet-governance/files/ai-andhealtcare-report

[82] Haider, H (2020). *Barriers to the adoption of artificial intelligence in healthcare in India*. Brighton: Institute of Development Studies (UK). Available online: https://opendocs.ids.ac.uk/opendocs/handle/20.500.12413/15272

[83] India's bid to harness AI for healthcare. Factor Daily 2019 April 4. Available online: https://factordaily.com/ai-forhealthcare-in-india/. Accessed Nov 7 2020.

[84] 94 Panch, T, Pearson-Stuttard, J, Greaves, F, et al. (2019). Artificial intelligence: opportunities and risks for public health. *Lancet Digit Health*, 1, e13–e14.

[85] Dhanabalan, T & Sathish, A (2018). Transforming Indian industries through artificial intelligence and robotics in industry 4.0. *J Mech Eng*, 9, 835–845.

[86] Dadario, NB, Brahimaj, B, Yeung, J, & Sughrue, ME (2021). Reducing the cognitive footprint of brain tumor surgery. *Front Neurol.*, 12, 711646. 10.3389/fneur.2021.711646

[87] Ren, H, Zhu, J, Su, X, Chen, S, Zeng, S, Lan, X, et al. (2020). Application of structural and functional connectome mismatch for classification and individualized therapy in Alzheimer disease. *Front Public Health*, 8, 584430. 10.3389/fpubh.2020.584430

[88] Poologaindran, A, Profyris, C, Young, IM, Dadario, NB, Ahsan, SA, Chendeb, K, et al. (2022). Interventional neurorehabilitation for promoting functional recovery post-craniotomy: A proof-of-concept. *Sci Rep.*, 12, 3039. 10.1038/s41598-022-06766-8

[89] Stephens, TM, Young, IM, O'Neal, CM, Dadario, NB, Briggs, RG, Teo, C, et al. (2021). Akinetic mutism reversed by inferior parietal lobule repetitive theta burst stimulation: can we restore default mode network function for therapeutic benefit? *Brain Behav.*, 11, e02180. 10.1002/brb3.2180

[90] Roberts, MD, Aix-Covnet, Driggs, M, Thorpe, J, Gilbey, M, Yeung, S, et al. (2021). Common pitfalls and recommendations for using machine learning to detect and prognosticate for COVID-19 using chest radiographs and CT scans. *Nat Mach Intell*, 3, 199–217. 10.1038/s42256-021-00307-0

[91] Han, SS, Kim, MS, Lim, W, Park, GH, Park, I, Chang, SE, et al. (2018). Classification of the clinical images for benign and malignant cutaneous tumors using a deep learning algorithm. *J Invest Dermatol.*, 138, 1529–1538. 10.1016/j.jid.2018.01.028

[92] Louie, P & Wilkes, R (2018). Representations of race and skin tone in medical textbook imagery. *Soc SciMed.*, 202, 38–42. 10.1016/j.socscimed.2018.02.02335. Adamson AS, Smith A. Machine learning and health care disparities in dermatology. JAMA Dermatology. (2018) 154:1247–48. doi: 10.1001/jamadermatol.2018.2348

[93] Krishnan, A, Almadan, A, & Rattani, A (2020). Understanding fairness of gender classification algorithms across gender-race groups. 2020 19th IEEE International Conference on Machine Learning and Applications (ICMLA).

[94] Hayati, M, Biller, P, & Colijn, C (2019). Predicting the short-term success of human influenza a variants with machine learning. bioRxiv. 10.1101/609248

[95] Zhao, N, Yuan, LX, Jia, XZ, Zhou, XF, Deng, XP, He, HJ, et al. (2018). Intra- inter-scanner reliability of voxel-wise whole-brain analytic metrics for resting state fMRI. *Front Neuroinform*, 12, 54. 10.3389/fninf.2018.00054

[96] Buchanan, BG & Shortliffe, EH (1984). *Rule-based expert systems: The MYCIN e xperiments of the Stanford heuristic programming project*. Reading: Addison Wesley.

[97] Frank, X (2019). Is Watson for Oncology per se Unreasonably Dangerous?: Making A Case for How to Prove Products Liability Based on a Flawed Artificial Intelligence Design. *American Journal of Law & Medicine*, 45(2–3), 273–294. 10.1177/0098858819871109

[98] Davenport, TH (2018). *The AI Advantage*. Cambridge: MIT Press.

[99] Right Care Shared Decision Making Programme, Capita. (2012). *Measuring shared decision making: A review of research evidence*. NHS. www.england.nhs.uk/wp-content/uploads/2013/08/7sdm-report.pdf

[100] Chmidt-Erfurth, U, Bogunovic, H, Sadeghipour, A *et al.* (2018). Machine learning to analyze the prognostic value of current imaging biomarkers in neovascular age-related macular degeneration. *Opthamology Retina*, 2, 24–30.

[101] Aicha, AN, Englebienne, G, van Schooten, KS, Pijnappels, M, & Kröse, B (2018). Deep learning to predict falls in older adults based on daily-Life trunk accelerometry. *Sensors*, 18, 1654.

[102] Low, LL, Lee, KH, Ong, MEH *et al.* (2015). Predicting 30-Day readmissions: performance of the LACE index compared with a regression model among general medicine patients in Singapore. *Biomed Research International*, 2015, 169870.

[103] Beauchamp, TL (2008). *Principles of biomedical ethics. Paperback May-2008*. New York: Oxford University Press.

[104] Faden, RR & Beauchamp, TL (1986). *A history and theory of informed consent*. Oxford: Oxford University Press.

[105] McDougall, RJ (2019). Computer knows best? The need for value-flexibility in medical AI. *J Med Ethics.*, 45, 156–160.

[106] Grote, T & Berens, P (2019). On the ethics of algorithmic decision-making in healthcare. *J Med Ethics*. 10.1136/medet hics-2019-105586

15 Wearable Technologies in AI and Smart HealthCare

Animesh Singh Yadav, Garima Srivastava, and Shikha Singh
Department of Computer Science & Engineering, Amity School of
Engineering & Technology, Lucknow Amity University, Uttar Pradesh,
India

CONTENTS

15.1 INTRODUCTION

A growing variety of innovative services and rising customer needs are driving today's rapid growth of the information and communications technology (ICT) sector. In general, thanks to consumers and widespread adoption of the Internet of Things (IoT), there have been enormous increases in the number of connected handheld devices every year. The Internet of Things (IoT) devices are small, reasonably priced, and very diverse in terms of their design, function, and application. They have had a significant impact on the advancement of the telecommunications industry, not only by introducing new long-range wireless technologies and defining new standards for availability and reliability, but also by forcing network operators and vendors to redesign the entire ecosystem by switching from traditional human-generated traffic to more diverse IoT traffic.

The terms wearables, wearable devices, or wearable technology refer to small electronic and mobile devices, computers with wireless communications capability that are integrated into gadgets, accessories, or clothing that can be worn on the human body, or even invasive versions such as micro-chips or smart tattoos. The main advantage over current smartphones and tablets is that wearables can offer a variety of monitoring and scanning features, including biofeedback or other sensory physiological functions like those connected to biometry. Since they are convenient, seamless, portable, and can provide hands-free access to electronics, wearables can continually measure such values, subject to their battery limitations [1,2].

Wearable technology has advanced significantly during the past few years. All objects that can be worn by people are considered wearable, including watches, eyeglasses, chest straps, rings, and prosthetic sockets. Along with implanted, ambient, and stationary medical equipment used in hospitals, wearable devices are part of the Internet of Medical Things (IoMT). As seen in Figure 15.1, these devices often connect to a network and communicate remotely with mobile devices. To continually monitor numerous human signals, wearable technology may contain several types of sensors, such as temperature sensors, accelerometers, optical sensors, and biometric sensors. Depending on the application, some of these sensors' values are occasionally regarded as appropriate [3,4], even if they are not currently as precise as those from stationary equipment in hospitals. AI is being applied to

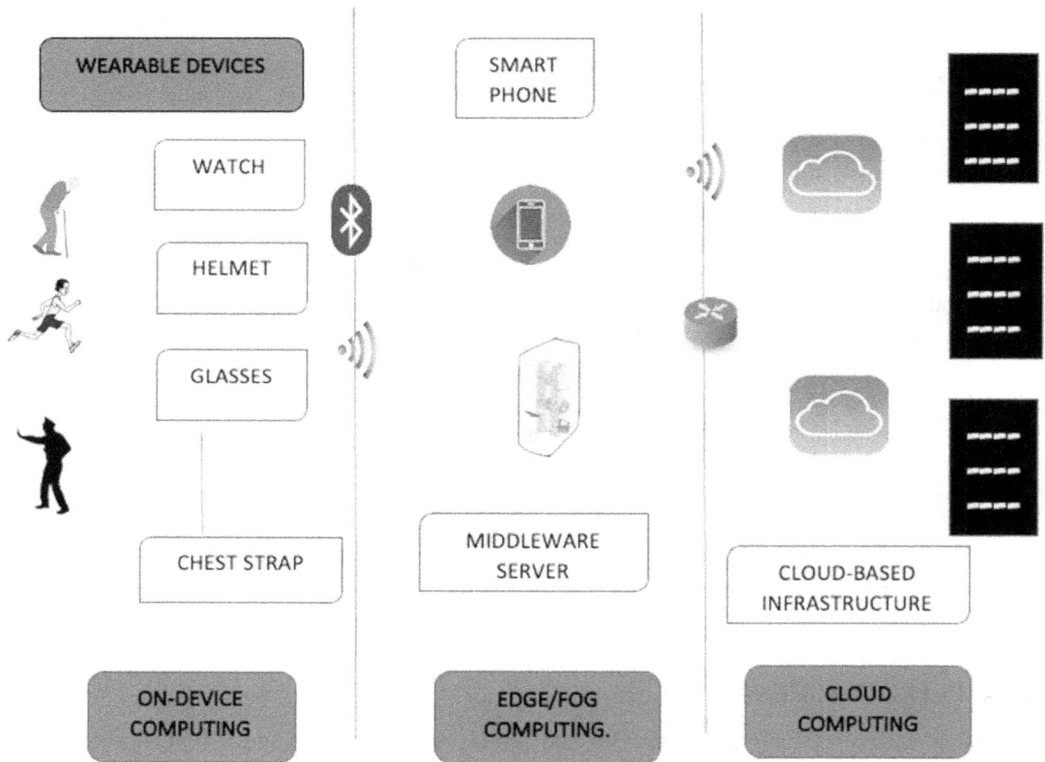

FIGURE 15.1   Wearable device application model [5–17].

wearables in the healthcare sector in several ways to enhance quality of life. Take, for instance, the Google Brain initiative's study on the AI-powered diagnosis of diabetic eye illness. In this system, neural networks are used as a learning tool by mathematical algorithms built on Deep Learning to master a specific activity through practise and self-correction [5–8]. Over 100 human-graded fundus images that depict different degrees of retinal bleeding brought on by elevated blood sugar levels were used to train this mathematical system. Each image is assigned a severity grade by the algorithm, and then a comparison is made with a previously established grade from the training set. Then, parameters are slightly changed to reduce the inaccuracy on that image. The algorithm learns how to correctly calculate the diabetic retinopathy severity from the pixel intensities of the image for each image in the training set by repeatedly performing this process for each image in the training set [9–12].

Few machine-learning applications for wearable devices have entered the market despite this extensive research effort and the extraordinary development in the use of wearable devices, notably smart watches [13,14,15]. Examples include the Apple Watch's irregular rhythm notification feature [16,17,18], which received FDA approval in 2018 with a long list of cautions and warnings (https://www.accessdata.fda.gov/cdrhdocs/reviews/DEN180044.pdf), and Eko's heart murmur detection algorithm, which was just recently published [19], which is actually for an electronic stethoscope rather than a personal wearable device. Additionally, several of the wearable monitoring devices that were assessed in [20] and used for monitoring are no longer on the market. The use of machine-learning techniques in the field of wearable technology still faces several difficulties.

The organization of the chapter is as follows. The background information about the topic is discussed in next section. The requirement for IoMT, wearable devices and the various human body signals utilized in wearable device research are described in the section 15.3. Furthermore, references to some of the most current research articles published in each field are used to assess and categorize applications for machine learning in IoMT and are discussed in detail as two case studies in section 15.5 and section 15.6, respectively. Various challenges that machine-learning research for wearable devices faces are covered in Section 15.7, along with pertinent privacy and security issues for IoMT applications and potential solutions from the literature. Finally, Section 15.8 presents the conclusion and future scope of the investigation.

15.2   LITERATURE SURVEY

Real-time monitoring of various physiological signs has sparked the research and development of a variety of wearable and implantable systems in response to the expanding global population and the rising demand for access to healthcare. The term "connected health" (CH) refers to a new paradigm for managing one's health and way of life that is facilitated by technology. It is implicitly a multi-disciplinary technological area designed to offer preventative care and remote medical assistance. CH supports engineering, systems, and applications connected to health by utilizing a digital information structure based on the internet, sensors, communications, and intelligent procedures.

The technologies most likely to change future health care and lifestyles are being viewed as wearables, hearables (in-ear devices), and nearables (neighbouring devices that interact with wearables) incorporated into the broader notion of Internet of Things (IoT). The smartphone, which is now a pervasive intrusive technology, was the catalyst for this shift. Most modern wearables and nearables come with a variety of high-tech sensors. To improve the features of fully portable medical laboratories, many sensor types driven by advanced analytics are now being investigated. The user experience in typical assisted living settings is improved by the seamless integration of these metrics in smartphone apps that enable timely delivery of tailored information.

The growing presence of wearables in consumer electronics exhibits that emphasize self-care and health management is a sign of the devices' growing significance. The International Data Corporation estimates that 172.2 million wearable units were sold in 2018, and this number is projected to rise, considerably fuelling the IoT market's revolution. The road to seamless physiological monitoring is being paved by developments in wearable technology and user acceptance of already available consumer wearable devices.

In the past 10 years, numerous research have been published that elaborate on the usage of wearables and sensors in assisted living settings, CH, and wellness and fitness apps. These studies offer crucial information for developing future CH systems, pointing out advantages as well as drawbacks, obstacles, and user feedback. However, few studies provide a broad overview of the type and scope of published research in that area. For the purpose of improving simplicity of use, comfort, and noninvasiveness of monitoring physiological vital signs and occasionally psychological or emotional state, which may be identified by analysing data from multiple sensors, the wearable device domain is currently being investigated. Following the enormous technical advancements in system on chip (SoC) design, wearable gadget development and adoption have surprisingly attained significant growth rates in recent years. According to Grand View Research's industry report on the wearable technology market (https://www.grandviewresearch.com/industry-analysis/wearable-technology-market), the size of the wearable device market was estimated at USD 32.63 billion in 2019 and is anticipated to grow rapidly in the coming years. According to Statista (https://www.statista.com/statistics/487291/global-connected-wearable-devices/), there will soon be 1 billion globally linked wearable devices. Smart watches, armbands, chest straps, shoes, helmets, glasses, lenses, rings, patches, fabrics, and hearing aids are a few examples of wearable technology [21]. Any object that is installed on the body qualifies as a wearable device because it may employ a variety of sensors to collect noninvasive data from the body. In literature, many well-known signals and indicators tare read from the human body to determine the vital signs and other details about the subject's health or mental condition. Examples of these sensors include the skin temperature sensor used in [22,23] and the electrodermal activity (EDA) sensor, also referred to as the galvanic skin response (GSR) sensor, which is used on the skin to record the skin conductance that changes depending on the subject's sympathetic state [4]. Another illustration is the employment of an electrocardiogram (ECG) sensor in [24–27] to record electrical changes in the skin that correlate to heartbeats.

15.3 POPULAR WEARABLE DEVICES

1. **Smart watches:** Watches with connectivity, such as the Apple Watch or Samsung Galaxy Watch, that allow users to answer calls, monitor their fitness, sleep, and other activities.
2. **Smart rings:** Smart rings are pieces of tech jewellery that combine the features of a smart watch with jewellery. There are several good possibilities for rings, but they haven't quite found their niche. The two very popular examples of smart rings are:-
   a. The NFC Opn is the best smart ring currently available, and it looks like something out of a science fiction film. Although it's not yet as functional as a smart watch, it's also less expensive, with options starting at $20. This ring manages apps, locks and unlocks your door, transfers data, and never, ever requires a charge. It is available with shipping from the U.K.
   b. The Oura Ring: The Oura Ring is really a magic ring, so you might start referring to it as "my precious" because of how lovely it appears. Sorry, Gollum, it won't turn you invisible, but it does offer helpful health information on things like sleep and daily activity. In addition, the Oura monitors a number of biometrics that many other wearable technology gadgets do not, warning you when something is out of the ordinary.
3. **Smart clothing:** Smart clothing is constructed of tech-infused fabrics that can shuffle your music or track your biological data.
4. **Advanced medical tech:** Wearable electrocardiograms (ECGs) that transmit your heart rhythm to a cardiologist and other life-saving on-body equipment are examples of advanced medical technology.

a. **Sensor for Core Body Temperature:**
Heat training can increase your level of fitness or prepare you for enduro races, marathons, and Iron Man events. Your success in heat training can be aided by a core body temperature sensor. Extreme sportsmen had to use invasive techniques like electronic pills or probes to measure the parameter until as recently as 2020.

b. **Training Breathing with Airofit ProBreathing:** exercises are a crucial practise for people with asthma, athletes who are serious about increasing their lung capacity, and people who are recovering from COVID-19. Your lung function can be improved with the help of the Airofit Pro Breathing Trainer and companion app, which will enable you to breathe more quickly and effectively.

c. **Pacemaker:** A pacemaker is a tiny device that is implanted in the chest to assist in heartbeat regulation. It serves as a safeguard against the heart beating too slowly. The placement of a pacemaker in the chest necessitates surgery. The term "pacemaker" can also refer to a cardiac pacing device.

5. **Head Mounted Displays:** VR headsets and other displays that provide a more immersive gaming or web browsing experience are known as head-mounted displays (HMDs).

15.4 WEARABLE DEVICES AND ML

Machine learning refers to getting wearable technology to respond or make decisions for a certain scenario without explicit programming. According to the kind of training data that is available, machine learning is typically categorized as either supervised, unsupervised, semi-supervised, or reinforced. Data examples with either labels or no labels are used to encode past experience learning. For data with labels, the target variable may be either categorical or numerical. Machine learning is used for a variety of tasks, including clustering for unlabelled data, regression for numerical labels, and classification for categorical target output variables.

Over the past 10 years, there has been an increase in the amount of applied research looking at how machine learning techniques might be used to monitor health, care for the elderly, and track fitness utilizing the bodily signals outlined in the previous subsection. Fall detection, seizure detection, vital sign monitoring and prediction, and activity recognition for tracking fitness or recognizing daily activities of people are some of the topics that caught the attention of researchers. Additionally, wearable technology has been studied for applications such as stress monitoring, heart rate arrhythmia detection, and rehabilitation.

In epilepsy, ML methods have a wide range of potential applications, from seizure prediction and surgical planning to diagnosis and medication selection. For instance, automated seizure diagnosis using ML algorithms from diagnostic scalp EEG has proven useful. The usage of 14 ML can also help clinicians choose the best course of treatment. Deep learning has recently been applied to the automatic selection of electrical stimulation parameters following training on a sizable database of patient EEG features and associated treatment outcomes. ML has also been applied with retrospective data to precisely predict medication resistance, antiepileptic drug effectiveness, surgical results, and the efficacy of treatment. On the basis of retrospective data, the aforementioned research has yielded encouraging findings, although there are still few instances of ML being successfully used in clinical epileptology. Figure 15.2, shows Healthcare tasks performed with the help of artificial intelligence and machine learning.

15.5 FACIAL EXPRESSION RECOGNITION DEEP TRANSFER LEARNING USING A HIGHLY IMBALANCED DATASET: A CASE STUDY

15.5.1 BACKGROUND AND OBJECTIVE

The requirement for agents to identify and adapt to users' emotional states has been widely recognized, despite the rapid advancements in human-computer interaction (HCI) and unrelenting

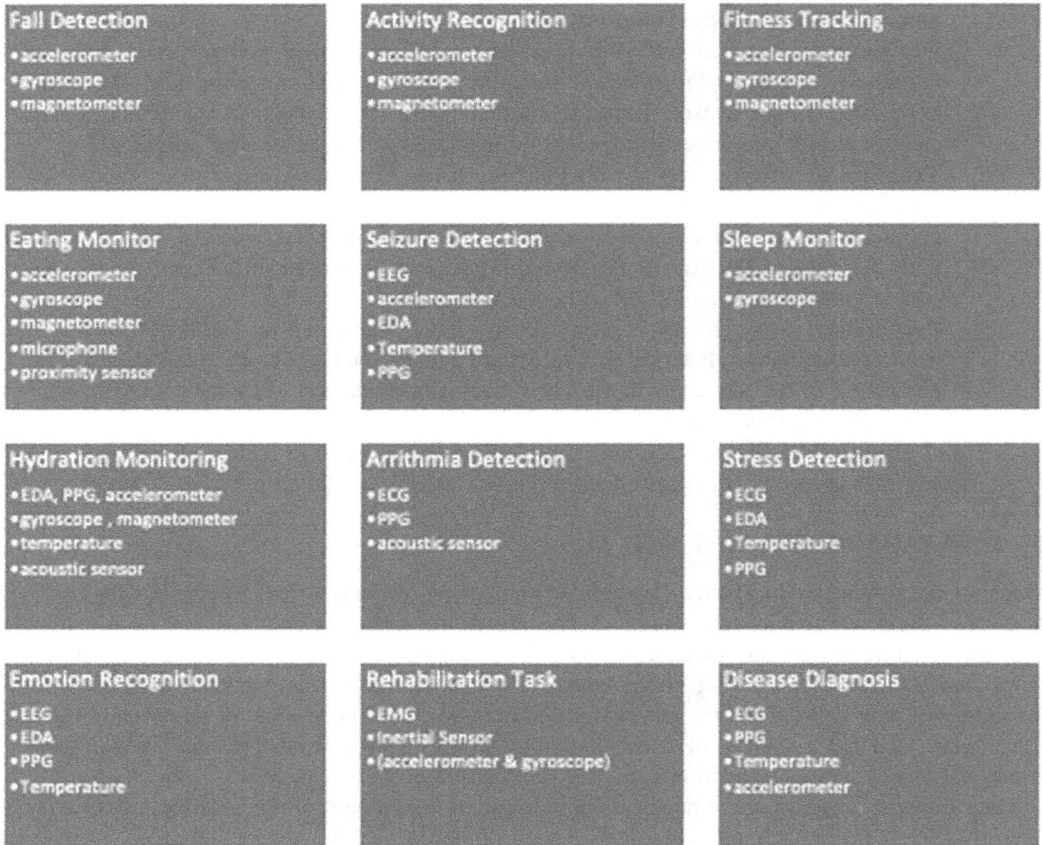

FIGURE 15.2 Healthcare tasks performed with the help of artificial intelligence/machine learning [5].

efforts to enhance user experience with computer systems. Since a link between the two was suggested in Eysenck's personality model, which argues that Neurotics are more sensitive to external stimuli while Extraverts are accompanied by low cortical arousal, research on the relationship between personality and affect has been ongoing.

Much affective research have sought to support Eysenck's paradigm, but few have looked at affective correlates of qualities outside extraversion and neuroticism. Furthermore, studies in social psychology have generally focused on non-verbal social behavioral indicators when examining personality, and there have been very few attempts to model personality traits using emotional behavior.

15.5.2 CNN ARCHITECTURE AND TRAINING

For general-purpose picture categorization and localization, CNNs like the well-known Alex Net were developed. Figure 15.3 depicts the fundamental operation of CNN. Both Task 1 (Classification) and Task 2 of the ImageNet LSVRC-2012 were decisively won by it (Localization and Classification). Five convolutional layers make up the neural network, followed by three globally linked layers (max-pooling layers in the first, second, and fifth convolutional layers). Rectifier Linear Units (ReLU) are used by Alex Net to introduce non-linearity rather than the hyperbolic tangent function (tanh) as activation. HUD (hidden-unit dropout) is also used to reduce overfitting in the globally linked layers. Initially, AlexNet was created to carry out a categorization

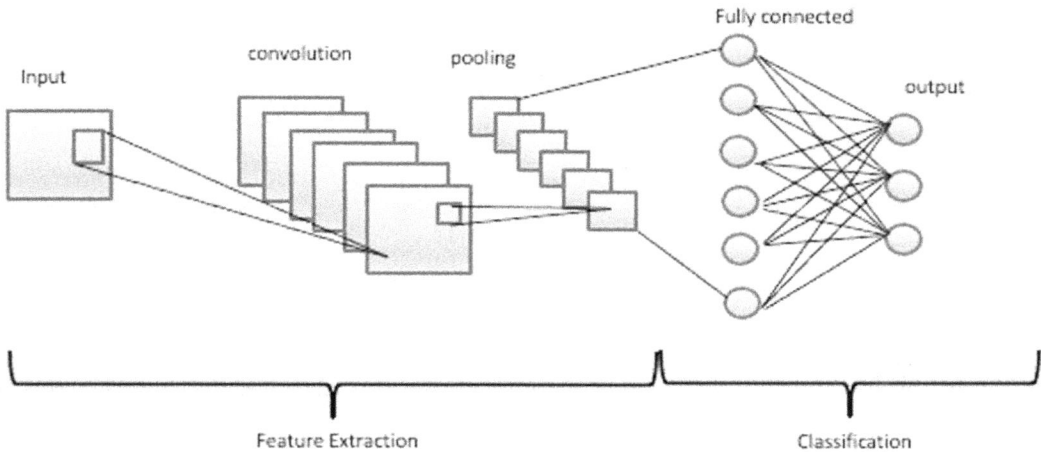

FIGURE 15.3 Working of CNN model [28].

between 1000 classes (a 1000-way softmax layer produces the output). Here, we added a single unit with a linear activation function to create two twin CNNs (to perform regression). The valence and arousal of CNNs were trained to be assessed independently. Training (60%) and validation (40%) sets of AffectNet pictures were created. Using Mini-Batch Gradient Descent (MBGD) with a batch size of 16, learning rate of 0.001, and Nesterov momentum of 0.9, we chose mean square error (MSE) as the loss function and trained the net. Over the whole training set, the training cycled 50 times. In terms of valence and arousal, the net obtained RMSE values of 0.279 and 0.242 over the validation set, respectively.

15.5.3 FINE TUNING

Following the training of the CNNs on a large dataset, we could benefit from two aspects: a) the ability of the nets to extract features (i.e., the pre-trained convolutional layers); and b) the current configuration of the task-related (dense) layers, which could be used as a starting guess for the fine-tuning phase to facilitate convergence. We used the following procedures on each CNN to achieve this goal. First, we divided the network into its dense and convolutional components (including the flatten layer). With the exception of the previously computed weights that served as initialization for the fine-tuning training, we now only operated on the dense layers, considering them as a new net. This made it possible to "freeze" the convolutional part's learning process and conduct additional tests in which the weights and bias were changed only in the dense region. In order to get the characteristics of each sample, the frozen convolutional part is employed.

15.5.4 POOL-BASED SAMPLING TECHNIQUES

15.5.4.1 Greedy Sampling

Exploring the feature space of the unlabeled pool is the foundation of the GS basic algorithm, GSx. In this study, we only examined one passive sampling strategy. The identical processes are followed by its counterpart, GSy, although that program's goal is to investigate the pool's output space. Since our goal was to update the regression model only after choosing all the samples that needed to be questioned and since the pre-trained regression model is already accessible in the fine-tuning scenario, we used a reduced version of the latter. These approaches' fundamental concept is the exploration of the feature and output spaces, respectively, using Euclidean distance calculations between samples. The element closest to the centroid of the set of elements to be labelled is chosen as

TABLE 15.1
Some Classifications About AffectNet

	Valence	Arousal
RMSE	0.37	0.41
CORR	0.66	0.54
SAGR	0.74	0.65
CCC	0.60	0.34

the initialization phase's beginning element and added to the output set (labelled set). After that, each candidate sample's minimum distance from the labelled set is calculated, and the element chosen at each stage of the iterative phase is the one with the greatest computed value.

15.5.5 AFFECT NET DATABASE

The most comprehensive collection of categorical and dimensional affect models is found in Affect Net (Affect from the Internet). Three search engines are queried to gather emotion-related terms, which are then annotated by skilled human labelers. This section discusses how to search the internet, how to analyze face photos and extract facial landmarks, and how to annotate facial expression, valence, and arousal of affect.

Affect Net uses 1250 emotion-related keywords in six different languages to search three major search engines and get more than 1,000,000 facial photos from the internet. Arousal and valence levels as well as the existence of seven distinct facial expressions were manually tagged in around half of the photos that were found. The outcomes of our experiments on the validation set using our standard operating procedures trained on the training set are shown in the Table 15.1 [29].

15.5.6 RESULTS

The results are summarized in below graphs (Figure 15.4).

According to the findings, valence and arousal differ significantly from one another. The first test for valence yielded subpar results (average RMSE = 0.37), demonstrating how challenging it is to learn valence only from subjective input. The pre-trained net (Transfer 0% Labeling) produced superior results (average RMSE = 0.14), indicating that the network trained on the AffectNet database (the transferred knowledge) enabled us to develop a very effective model able to generalise positive and negative valence across all individuals. In contrast, the pre-trained net performed horribly when it came to arousal (average RMSE = 0.22) while the net fed with subject-specific data performed much better. This shows that it is more difficult to generalize the correct recognition of arousal levels because it is more dependent on the specific subject. Indeed. The inherent properties of valence and arousal as well as the various types of training data employed can both be used to explain these discrepancies. In general, valence seems to be harder to learn from subject-specific data than arousal (see "No Transfer" scenario). Arousal is particularly confused by the transition from an in the wild context to a controlled one, even if it has no detrimental effects on the learning process for valence.

15.6 THE USAGE OF STATISTICAL LEARNING METHODS ON WEARABLE DEVICES AND A CASE STUDY: ACTIVITY RECOGNITION ON SMARTWATCHES

This study's objectives are to investigate the application of statistical learning techniques to wearable technology and to carry out an experimental investigation for the identification of human

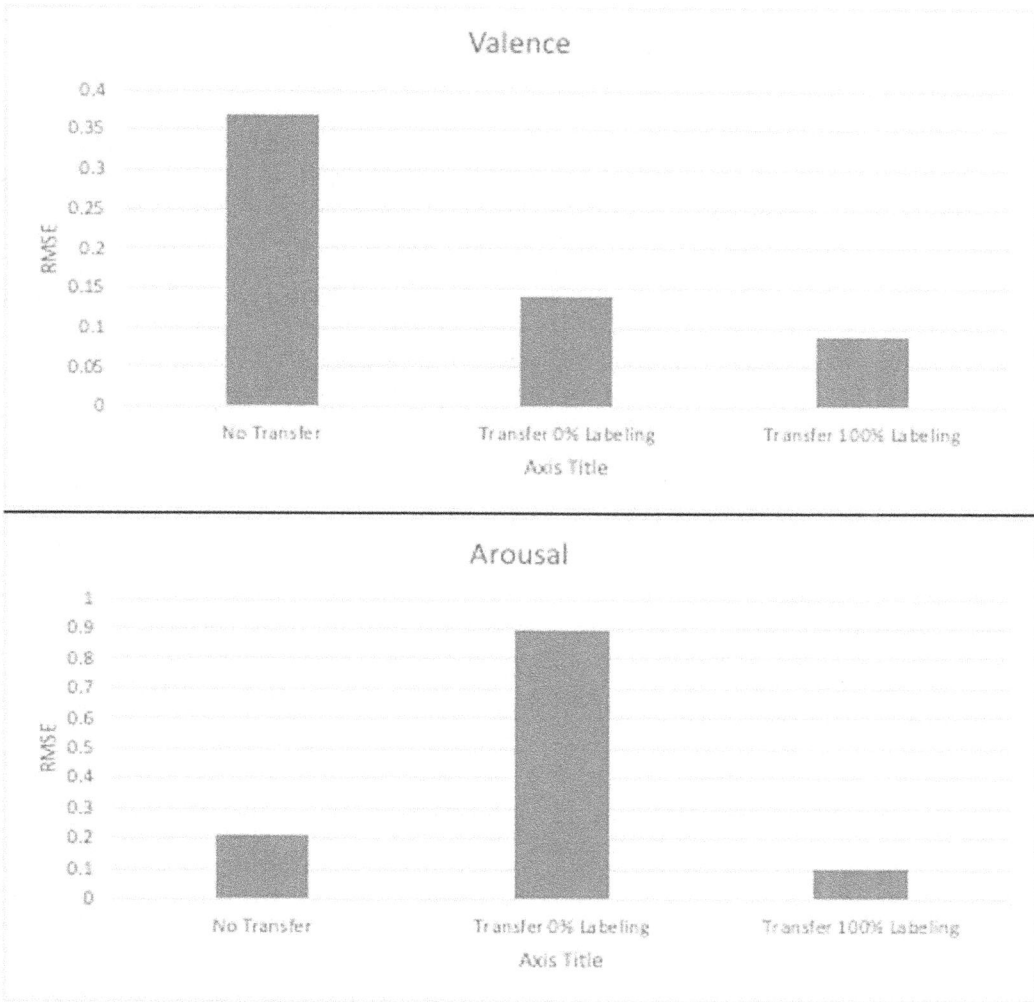

FIGURE 15.4 Average transfer learning results (RMSE) between subjects for valence and arousal, in three different transfer-learning settings.

activities using information from wristwatch sensors. To accomplish this goal, mobile applications that run on smartwatches and smartphones have been created to collect training data and quickly identify human activity. Some 500 patterns of data were collected at intervals of four seconds for each activity—walking, typing, stationary work, running, standing, writing on a board, brushing teeth, cleaning, and writing—using these applications. The performance of the created dataset was examined using various statistical learning methods, including Naive Bayes, k closest neighbor (KNN), logistic regression, Bayesian network, and multilayer perceptron.

15.6.1 OVERVIEW OF STATISTICAL LEARNING

There are numerous supervised and unsupervised tools for drawing conclusions from data in statistical learning. In several fields, including public policy, health, astrophysics, and business, supervised statistical learning is generally used as a statistical model to estimate or forecast an output using pertinent inputs. Unsupervised statistical learning allows for the learning of correlations and data structure without having to see the output. In this study, supervised learning methods (Naive Bayes, logistic regression, Bayesian network, k nearest neighbor (kNN) and multiplayer Perceptron) are used for activity recognition. The Naive Bayes approach is used in supervised learning tasks, where classes are known in the training phase and predictions of classes are realized in the test phase, to learn and represent probabilistic information from data with clarity and ease. The output of the input layer and all intermediate layers are exclusively submitted to the higher layer, making the multilayer perceptron a feedforward structure of artificial neural networks. A layer of perceptrons is meant by "layer" in this context. There is no restriction on the total number of perceptrons or hidden layers. Logistic regression is used to describe and test suppositions about associations between class variable and other related predictor variables by estimating probabilities using a logistic function. Logistic regression can be binomial, ordinal or multinomial.

Bayesian networks are one of the graphical models that use probability. In Bayesian networks, graphical structures are used to represent the knowledge about a hazy subject. Particularly, in the graph, variables are represented as nodes and probabilistic dependencies between the variables are shown as edges. Using well-known computational and statistical techniques, the values of the graph's edges can be determined. The model structure of the Bayesian Network used for the research in the case study is shown in Figure 15.5. Variables are standard deviations and averages of x-, y- and z-axis of accelerometer sensor.

15.6.2 Activity Recognition on Smartwatches Using Statistical Learning Method

This work uses accelerometer sensor data to conduct activity recognition. In addition to the force of gravity, an accelerometer measures the acceleration force in m/s^2 that is imparted to a device along each of the three physical axes shown in Figure 15.6.

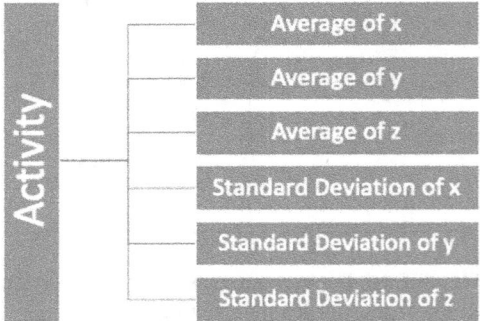

FIGURE 15.5 The model structure of the Bayesian network [30].

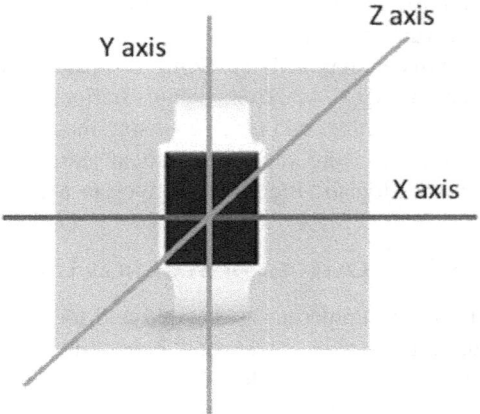

FIGURE 15.6 Smartwatches accelerometer axes [30].

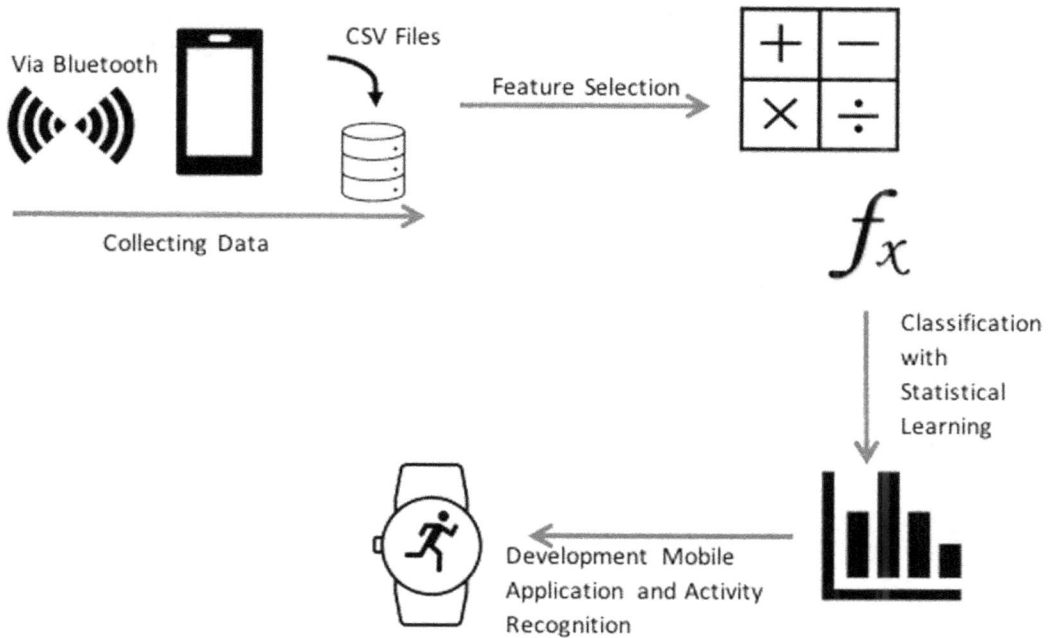

FIGURE 15.7   Flowchart of activity recognition [30].

For nine different daily activities, the amplitude of the accelerometer's x-axis changes according depending upon the type of activity (typing, writing, writing on board, walking, running, cleaning, standing, brushing teeth and stationary). Smartwatch accelerometer signals are used to detect activity using statistical learning techniques. The flowchart for activity recognition, shown in Figure 15.7, shows the procedures involved in data collection, feature selection, classification, and development of wristwatch applications. The following subsections provide details on these actions.

15.6.3   CLASSIFICATION WITH STATISTICAL LEARNING METHODS

The WEKA Toolkit, which includes these approaches, is used to assess the extracted features using a variety of statistical learning methods (Naive Bayes, kNN, logistic regression, Bayesian network, and multilayer perceptron). The other half of the data is used for testing after the training portion. Data are divided at random for testing and training purposes. The comparison of evaluation criteria for statistical learning methods, including accuracy rates, F-measure, ROC area, and root mean squared error (RMSE), is shown in Table 15.2. The accuracy of a test is measured by the F-measure. The

TABLE 15.2

The Accuracy Rates, F-Measure, ROC Area, Root Mean Squared Error Values of Statistical Methods [30]

Methods	Accuracy Rates	F-Measure	ROC Area	RMSE
Naive Bayes	81.33	0.819	0.974	0.1644
Bayesian Network	91.55	0.916	0.993	0.1242
kNN (k = 3)	89.68	0.896	0.971	0.135
Logistic regression	85.55	0.854	0.977	0.1507
Multilayer perceptron	74.57	0.734	0.957	0.1937

formula for the F-measure is provided in Eq (15.1). The letters FN, FP, TP, and TN stand for the numbers of false negatives, false positives, true positives, and true negatives, respectively.

$$\text{F-measure} = \frac{2x\frac{tn}{tp+fp}x\frac{tp}{tp+fp}}{\frac{tp}{tp+fn} + \frac{tn}{tp+fp}}. \tag{15.1}$$

The RMSE of a model prediction with respect to the estimated variable X-model is defined as the square root of the mean squared error are given in equation 15.2.

$$RMSE = \sqrt{\frac{1}{n}x\sum_{i=1}^{n}(X_{obs,i} - X_{model,i})^2}. \tag{15.2}$$

ROC (receiver operating characteristic) area is also known as area under curve (AUC) is calculated as in Eq. (15.3)

$$AUC = \frac{1}{mn}\sum_{i=1}^{m}\sum_{j=1}^{n}1_{pp}. \tag{15.3}$$

Here, the statistical methods for human activity recognition on smartwatches are investigated. It is determined by looking at the accuracy rates in Table 15.2 that the Bayesian network method is the most effective strategy for the study's dataset. Through this research, it is possible to comprehend how to categorize human activities utilizing sensor data and statistical learning techniques. For nine different activities, a single set of accelerometer sensor data is used. The studies for human activity recognition can be improved in the future by using various sensors, such as the heart rate monitor, ambient light, GPS, and gyroscope, to detect more activities by increasing the number of classes (handshake, smoking, drinking, etc.), or to separate more complex parts of activities (such as walking hands in pockets, walking hand in hand, etc.).

15.7   CHALLENGES FOR ML APPLICATION ON WEARABLE DEVICES

In the modern world, smartwatches that can connect to smartphones are frequently used as wearable technology. Wearables will likely take on a variety of shapes in the future, each one created for a particular need. Wearable technology that can assist humans in doing their responsibilities will rule the planet of the future. Sharing the information gathered allows them to market in the shortest amount of time possible and contributes to profit maximization. Other facets of life, such as those in the medical, geographic, or private domains, can be generalized by using it. To assist in the precise identification of diseases, wearables can disseminate the data they acquire in the form of text, video, audio, or other specified forms.

In general, the Cross-Industry Standard Process for Data Mining Cycle (CRISP-DM 1999) is used to develop machine-learning systems. Since virtually no ML model is guaranteed to be 100% accurate, the development-to-deployment process involves many challenges in gathering the data, choosing the best features, choosing the libraries and framework, evaluating the trained model(s), selecting the best model, and relying on the ML model decision. Healthcare ML learning models must be created to generalize well, deal with untried examples, take into account individual differences, analyze the results carefully, and communicate them.

There are many challenges that developers of a machine learning application for a wearable device should take care of in addition to the usual challenges facing any machine learning application regarding the used data and model. All of these challenges are shown in Figure 15.8 and are presented in the following subsections, along with how they affect the options available to developers.

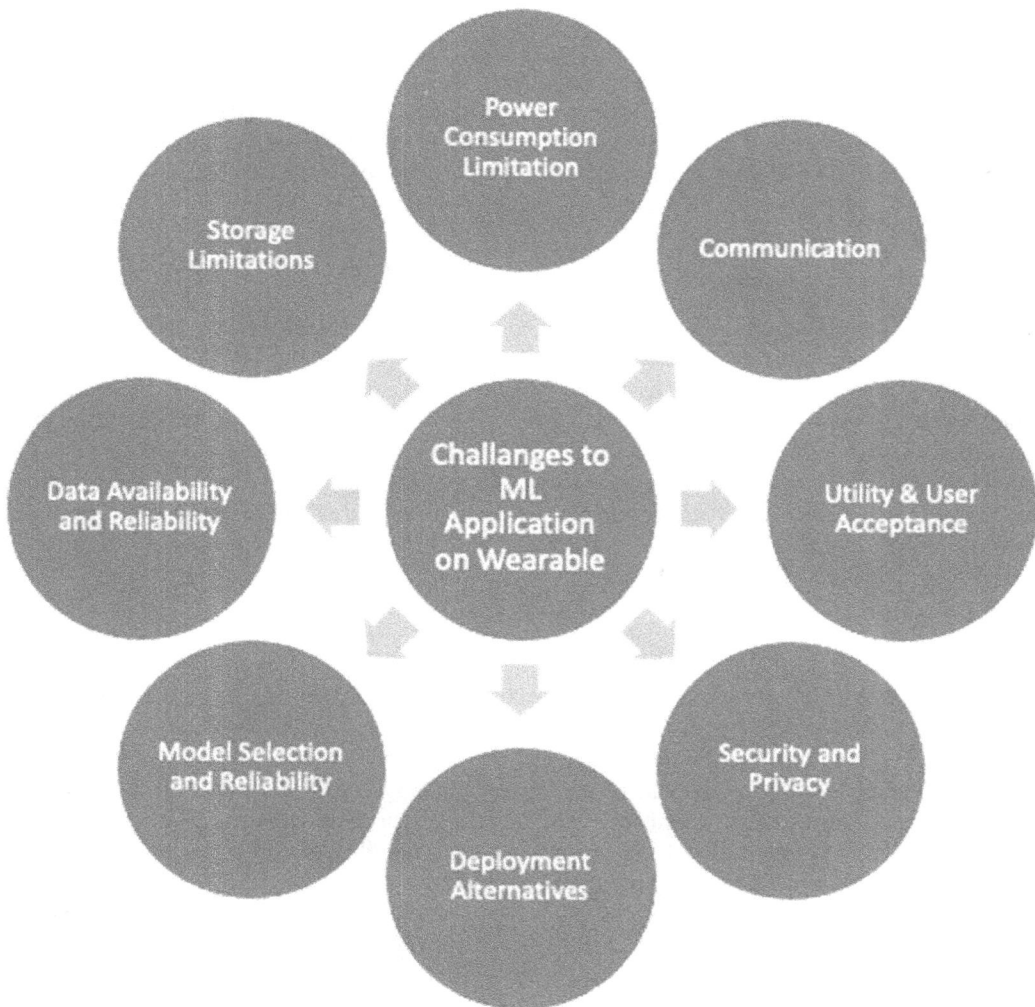

FIGURE 15.8 Challenges for ML on wearable devices [30].

15.7.1 Data Availability and Reliability

Since human health is the goal, wearable technology data must also be trustworthy, with clear assurance and alerts to seek medical assistance if any concerns arise. The authors of [31] looked into the potential sources of error in a variety of wearable optical heart rate sensors. They investigated heart rate and PPG data from wearables of both consumer and research-grade while engaging in various activities for people with various skin tones. Their research revealed that accuracy did not differ statistically among skin tones, but there were notable disparities between devices and activity kinds, with an average absolute inaccuracy of 30% more than at rest. The reliability of data in healthcare is so important for the patient and physician to rely on the device readings to take the most appropriate medical decision, which may in some cases threaten the life of a human.

15.7.2 Model Selection & Reliability

By testing the model with data that has not been used in training, cross-validation techniques are thought to be one method for accurately evaluating the accuracy of machine-learning models. The authors of [32] analyzed research studies that utilized either record-wise or subject-wise cross-validation. In their research, they used simulation data and a publicly accessible dataset for activity detection to discover that record-wise cross-validation overestimates the predictive power of machine-learning algorithms. This outcome is consistent with the research results in [33]. Differently, some of the authors in [34] critiqued the work in [32] with the claim that record-wise cross-validation can be applied because no within-subject dependence between observations can be found.

15.7.3 STORAGE LIMITATION

The viability of deploying a machine-learning application on a wearable device or an edge device depends on a number of variables, including the device's size, the data size (the number of features and duration of physiological data used for prediction), the model's complexity (the number of parameters and layers), and whether batch or real-time processing is used. For the same amount of parameters and layers, a high accuracy model frequently requires more memory than a model with a lower accuracy. Depending on the machine learning application, certain machine learning models (especially those that include image inputs) might reach up to an order of 100 megabytes or even a gigabyte, which cannot fit on the best wearable device coupled with the memory required to execute the computations.

15.7.4 DEPLOYMENT ALTERNATIVES

By analyzing sensitive private data on a local gateway, filtering it, and compressing it instead of doing it on a cloud out of the user's control, edge computing can reduce data transfer to the cloud, which in turn reduces power consumption and improves privacy. The scale of the machine learning model, the number of data streams to be utilized for training and testing, the demand for online training and real-time prediction, and the computational resources required for training and testing all play a role in this. The flexibility of storage and the scalability of computational resources on demand are the key benefits of adopting cloud computing.

Other factors that affect the choice of which deployment option to choose when developing wearable machine learning applications include data drift (how data distribution may change over time) and continuous integration and delivery. With some operations unique to machine-learning applications, such as data collection, cleaning, and pre-processing, continuous (re)training of the ML model, and continuous (re)deployment of the updated model to the device, the edge nodes, or the cloud service, the development process for wearable machine-learning-based software requires the same steps as for any software [35].

15.7.5 USER ACCEPTANCE

The device's use in daily life is a key determinant of user adoption. [36] identifies design standards for wearable technology. For instance, developing a wearable should take into account the diverse gender requirements, adhere to the anatomical structure of the human body, and utilise materials that are both comfortable for the body and do not irritate the skin. Additionally, it should be used in a fluid environment and must be as simple to use as feasible without requiring extensive setup or configuration.

15.7.6 POWER CONSUMPTION

Due to their generally short battery lives, wearable technology's primary drawback is power consumption. The necessity to transmit physiological data captured by the device's sensors to the cloud in order to carry out computations on the cloud has a significant impact on the power consumption for machine-learning applications on wearable devices. The best commercial smart watch battery life, which detects walking and running activities and provides an approximation of the heart rate and oxygen saturation, lasts only a few weeks at the time this article was written. In reality, this might be much lower and as little as a few hours for wearables that continuously monitor numerous vital indicators to warn users of anomalous circumstances (e.g., alerting for abnormal heart rhythm or detecting fall).

The elements that affect the power consumption in wearable devices include the board, its components of different biosensors and their sampling rate, the operating system and other software running on the board, the wearable display, the rate of logging data on the device, and the amount of data transmitted over the communication channel (e.g., Bluetooth or Wi-Fi) to be sent to the edge/cloud.

15.7.7 COMMUNICATION

When using an edge computing approach, the wearable device and the edge device can communicate internally using one of the following standards: Bluetooth, Zigbee, RFID, NFC, and UWB. Because it uses so little power, lightweight Bluetooth is frequently used [37,38]. However, the Bluetooth protocol only permits up to seven devices to connect to a device at once, and in practise, when there are many connections to a smartphone, performance suffers and pairing issues develop. The maximum distance between the wearable and the edge device, the necessary data rate for the wearable-to-edge device, and the necessary latency are other considerations that influence the choice of communication medium.

15.7.8 SECURITY & PRIVACY

Incorporating security into the design of wearable technology is edge computing's fundamental problem. To do this, solutions must be provided for managing, updating, and securing the wearable technology. Malicious hardware or software injections, denial-of-service attacks, various routing vulnerabilities, and physical assaults are only a few examples of security hazards. Incorporating various ML-based solutions for detecting various threats that may affect the communication network, computations, battery consumption, or storage can help protect against some of these assaults.

15.8 CONCLUSION & FUTURE SCOPE

The management of chronic conditions and more transparency between patients and clinicians will be made possible by wearable health technologies. To enhance a patient's experience of treatment and give them more control over their own health, it is essential to use tools and technology that facilitate the efficient transfer of data from patients to physicians. Future design and development of digital technology in this field will be based on ongoing research into industry best practises, trouble spots, and potential fixes for problems already present.

We have outlined the main issues and recently emerging solutions for this quickly developing sector by sharing our findings. Our work acts as a starting point for the development of a streamlined procedure to find pertinent parties in this field and offer information on the adoption of and workflows surrounding wearable health technology and EHR integration for companies across the health care sector. We hope that these findings will serve as the starting point for future research on wearable health technologies because much of this work is still in progress.

REFERENCES

[1] Ometov, Aleksandr, Viktoriia Shubina, Lucie Klus, Justyna Skibińska, Salwa Saafi, Pavel Pascacio, Laura Flueratoru et al. "A survey on wearable technology: History, state-of-the-art and current challenges." *Computer Networks* 193 (2021): 108074.

[2] Yu, Kun-Hsing, Andrew L. Beam, and Isaac S. Kohane. "Artificial intelligence in healthcare." *Nature Biomedical Engineering* 2, no. 10 (2018): 719–731.

[3] Hayano, Junichiro, Hiroaki Yamamoto, Izumi Nonaka, Makoto Komazawa, Kenichi Itao, Norihiro Ueda, Haruhito Tanaka, and Emi Yuda. "Quantitative detection of sleep apnea with wearable watch device." *PLoS One* 15, no. 11 (2020): e0237279.

[4] Delmastro, Franca, Flavio Di Martino, and Cristina Dolciotti. "Cognitive training and stress detection in mci frail older people through wearable sensors and machine learning." *IEEE Access* 8 (2020): 65573–65590.

[5] Sabry, Farida, Tamer Eltaras, Wadha Labda, Khawla Alzoubi, and Qutaibah Malluhi. "Machine Learning for Healthcare Wearable Devices: The Big Picture." *Journal of Healthcare Engineering* 2022 (2022).

[6] Beniczky, Sándor, Philippa Karoly, Ewan Nurse, Philippe Ryvlin, and Mark Cook. "Machine learning and wearable devices of the future." *Epilepsia* 62 (2021): S116–S124.

[7] Bent, Brinnae, Benjamin A. Goldstein, Warren A. Kibbe, and Jessilyn P. Dunn. "Investigating sources of inaccuracy in wearable optical heart rate sensors." *NPJ Digital Medicine* 3, no. 1 (2020): 1–9.

[8] Mateen, Bilal A., James Liley, Alastair K. Denniston, Chris C. Holmes, and Sebastian J. Vollmer. "Improving the quality of machine learning in health applications and clinical research." *Nature Machine Intelligence* 2, no. 10 (2020): 554–556.

[9] Faustino, Manuel, Jorge Calado, João Sarraipa, and Ricardo Jardim-Gonçalves. "Adaptable power consumption profiles for wearable localization devices." In *Proceedings of the SEIA'2019 Conference Proceedings*, p. 200 (2022).

[10] Baek, Sung Hoon, and Ki-Woong Park. "A Durable Hybrid RAM Disk with a Rapid Resilience for Sustainable IoT Devices." *Sensors* 20, no. 8 (2020): 2159.

[11] Zhang, Ting, Jiang Lu, Fei Hu, and Qi Hao. "Bluetooth low energy for wearable sensor-based healthcare systems." In *2014 IEEE Healthcare Innovation Conference (HIC)*, pp. 251–254. IEEE, (2014).

[12] LaBat, Karen L., and Karen S. Ryan. *Human body: A wearable product designer's guide.* CRC Press, 2019

[13] Subrahmannian, Amrutha, and Santanu Kumar Behera. "Chipless RFID Sensors for IoT-Based Healthcare Applications: A Review of State of the Art." *IEEE Transactions on Instrumentation and Measurement* (2022).

[14] Bent, Brinnae, Benjamin A. Goldstein, Warren A. Kibbe, and Jessilyn P. Dunn. "Investigating sources of inaccuracy in wearable optical heart rate sensors." *NPJ Digital Medicine* 3, no. 1 (2020): 1–9.

[15] Qaim, Waleed Bin, Aleksandr Ometov, Antonella Molinaro, Ilaria Lener, Claudia Campolo, Elena Simona Lohan, and Jari Nurmi. "Towards energy efficiency in the internet of wearable things: A systematic review." *IEEE Access* 8 (2020): 175412–175435.

[16] Saeb, Sohrab, Luca Lonini, Arun Jayaraman, David C. Mohr, and Konrad P. Kording. "The need to approximate the use-case in clinical machine learning." *Gigascience* 6, no. 5 (2017): gix019.

[17] Casilari, Eduardo, José-Antonio Santoyo-Ramón, and José-Manuel Cano-García. "Analysis of public datasets for wearable fall detection systems." *Sensors* 17, no. 7 (2017): 1513.

[18] Perez, Marco V., Kenneth W. Mahaffey, Haley Hedlin, John S. Rumsfeld, Ariadna Garcia, Todd Ferris, Vidhya Balasubramanian et al. "Large-scale assessment of a smartwatch to identify atrial fibrillation." *New England Journal of Medicine* 381, no. 20 (2019): 1909–1917.

[19] Chorba, John S., Avi M. Shapiro, Le Le, John Maidens, John Prince, Steve Pham, Mia M. Kanzawa et al. "Deep learning algorithm for automated cardiac murmur detection via a digital stethoscope platform." *Journal of the American Heart Association* 10, no. 9 (2021): e019905.

[20] Seneviratne, Suranga, Yining Hu, Tham Nguyen, Guohao Lan, Sara Khalifa, Kanchana Thilakarathna, Mahbub Hassan, and Aruna Seneviratne. "A survey of wearable devices and challenges." *IEEE Communications Surveys & Tutorials* 19, no. 4 (2017): 2573–2620.

[21] Chan, Marie, Daniel Estève, Jean-Yves Fourniols, Christophe Escriba, and Eric Campo. "Smart wearable systems: Current status and future challenges." *Artificial Intelligence in Medicine* 56, no. 3 (2012): 137–156.

[22] Siirtola, Pekka, Heli Koskimäki, Henna Mönttinen, and Juha Röning. "Using sleep time data from wearable sensors for early detection of migraine attacks." *Sensors* 18, no. 5 (2018): 1374.

[23] Meisel, Christian, Rima El Atrache, Michele Jackson, Sarah Schubach, Claire Ufongene, and Tobias Loddenkemper. "Machine learning from wristband sensor data for wearable, noninvasive seizure forecasting." *Epilepsia* 61, no. 12 (2020): 2653–2666.

[24] Hannun, A. Y. "Computer-interpreted electrocardiograms: benefits and limitations." *Nature Medicine* 25 (2019): 65–69.

[25] Kwon, Soonil, Joonki Hong, Eue-Keun Choi, Byunghwan Lee, Changhyun Baik, Euijae Lee, Eui-Rim Jeong, Bon-Kwon Koo, Seil Oh, and Yung Yi. "Detection of atrial fibrillation using a ring-type wearable device (CardioTracker) and deep learning analysis of photoplethysmography signals: prospective observational proof-of-concept study." *Journal of Medical Internet Research* 22, no. 5 (2020): e16443.

[26] Mei, Zhenning, Xiao Gu, Hongyu Chen, and Wei Chen. "Automatic atrial fibrillation detection based on heart rate variability and spectral features." *IEEE Access* 6 (2018): 53566–53575.

[27] Rashid, Nafiul, and Mohammad Abdullah Al Faruque. "Energy-efficient real-time myocardial infarction detection on wearable devices." In *2020 42nd Annual International Conference of the IEEE Engineering in Medicine & Biology Society (EMBC)*, pp. 4648–4651. IEEE, (2020).

[28] Islam, Md Zabirul, Md Milon Islam, and Amanullah Asraf. "A combined deep CNN-LSTM network for the detection of novel coronavirus (COVID-19) using X-ray images." *Informatics in Medicine Unlocked* 20 (2020): 100412.

[29] AffectNet. (n.d.). Mohammadmahoor.com. Retrieved March 13, 2023, from http://mohammadmahoor.com/affectnet/

[30] Balli, Serkan, and Ensar Arif Sağbas. "The usage of statistical learning methods on wearable devices and a case study: activity recognition on smartwatches." *Advances in statistical methodologies and their application to real problems* (2017): 259–277.

[31] Bent, Brinnae, Benjamin A. Goldstein, Warren A. Kibbe, and Jessilyn P. Dunn. "Investigating sources of inaccuracy in wearable optical heart rate sensors." *NPJ Digital Medicine* 3, no. 1 (2020): 1–9.

[32] Saeb, S. "Lonini L Jayaraman A Mohr DC Kording KP." *The Need to Approximate the Use-case in Clinical Machine Learning Gigascience* 6, no. 1 (2017): 9.

[33] Casilari, Eduardo, José-Antonio Santoyo-Ramón, and José-Manuel Cano-García. "Analysis of public datasets for wearable fall detection systems." *Sensors* 17, no. 7 (2017): 1513.

[34] Little, Max A., Gael Varoquaux, Sohrab Saeb, Luca Lonini, Arun Jayaraman, David C. Mohr, and Konrad P. Kording. "Using and understanding cross-validation strategies. Perspectives on Saeb et al." *GigaScience* 6, no. 5 (2017): 1–6.

[35] Tamburri, Damian A. "Sustainable mlops: Trends and challenges." In *2020 22nd international symposium on symbolic and numeric algorithms for scientific computing (SYNASC)*, pp. 17–23. IEEE, (2020).

[36] LaBat, Karen L., and Karen S. Ryan. *Human body: A wearable product designer's guide.* CRC Press, (2019).

[37] Zhang, Ting, Jiang Lu, Fei Hu, and Qi Hao. "Bluetooth low energy for wearable sensor-based healthcare systems." In *2014 IEEE healthcare innovation conference (HIC)*, pp. 251–254. IEEE, (2014).

[38] Balakrishna, Chitra, Elizabeth Rendon-Morales, Rodrigo Aviles-Espinosa, Henry Dore, and Zhenhua Luo. "Challenges of wearable health monitors: a case study of foetal ECG monitor." In *2019 Global IoT Summit (GIoTS)*, pp. 1–6. IEEE, (2019).

16 A Heterogeneous Medical-Imaging Social Security Analysis in Wireless Sensor Network

Prateek Singhal

Department of Computer Science & Engineering, Sagar Institute of Research Technology-Excellence, Bhopal, M.P., India

Prabhat Kumar Srivastava

Department of Computer Science & Engineering, IMS Ghaziabad, Uttar Pradesh, India

Pawan Singh

Department of Computer Science & Engineering, Amity School of Engineering and Technology, Amity University, Lucknow, Uttar Pradesh, India

CONTENTS

DOI: 10.1201/9781003333081-16

16.1   INTRODUCTION

Scholastic researchers focus on security issues in huge critical networks, similar to mix frameworks, the overall of things, cloud organizations, etc. If these networks have security issues, they'll experience an incredible monetary shortfall. Conversely, barely any scientists have considerable authority in individual security issues. Even though these occurrences cause extraordinary repercussions, they fail to cause significant misfortunes in a brief timeframe. In contrast to occurrences in mechanical organizations, the dangers of such episodes are steady and extensive. Right now, OSNs (online interpersonal organizations) have become a basic a part of human existence; a fundamental gratitude exists to acquire and share individual data. Also, administrators can employ users' own data discretionarily for a few purposes. The partner editorial manager is planning the survey of this original copy and favour it.

We have observed a drastic growth in multimedia data. Even during the current COVID-19 pandemic situation, we can clearly observe that the images are helping doctors quickly detect COVID-19 infection in patients. There are many critical applications where images play a vital role. Some of those applications include medical industry, astronomy, physics, chemistry, forensics, remote sensing, manufacturing, and defense. These applications use raw image data to extract some kind of useful information about our world. Quick extraction of valuable information from raw images is one of the challenges that academicians and professionals are facing today. This is where image processing comes into play. The primary purpose of image processing is get an enhanced image or to extract some useful information from it (Figure 16.1).

It could be deciphered in a few settings and viewpoints in controls like law, well-being science, sociologies, and PC and information science. Security assurance in various ends isn't general. The strategies in developing modern industrial networks don't appear to be reasonable for social networking. For the most part, security will be denied because of the option to be distant from everyone else and to possess independence from being impeded or interrupted. Moreover, in social networks, a particularly extravagant and huge organizational climate, homogeneity makes it difficult to ponder security assurance from just a private viewpoint; the organizational climate is where personal data is revealed. Additionally, the affirmation of security breaches of different users, like community users and normal users, changes extensively. The common strategies for ensuring users' protection in interpersonal organizations incorporate namelessness, decentralization, encryption, data security guidelines, protection setting, access control, and improving users' security consideration and security lead. The remaining four strategies depend upon the various interpersonal interaction which needs to be executed, which have beenproven to be flawed. At uncertain times, complex security settings disrupt users' experience. Studies have focused on users because of security can be effortlessly broken here. Investigatiosn are coordinated during this work. In this paper, we utilize the last methodology, which is to build up the users' security care and improve security conduct by insurance assessment to help security breaches at the foundation.

Nonetheless, we face an issue in this technique: we need to analyze the huge number of users. In accordance with the small globe opinion, more users can arrive together inside six stages. Now one user can connect with many billions of different users. With a particularly enormous and convoluted network structure, it's difficult for conventional algorithms to oblige this model successfully. An outsized number of envision accounts, android accounts, damage accounts, public accounts, and so

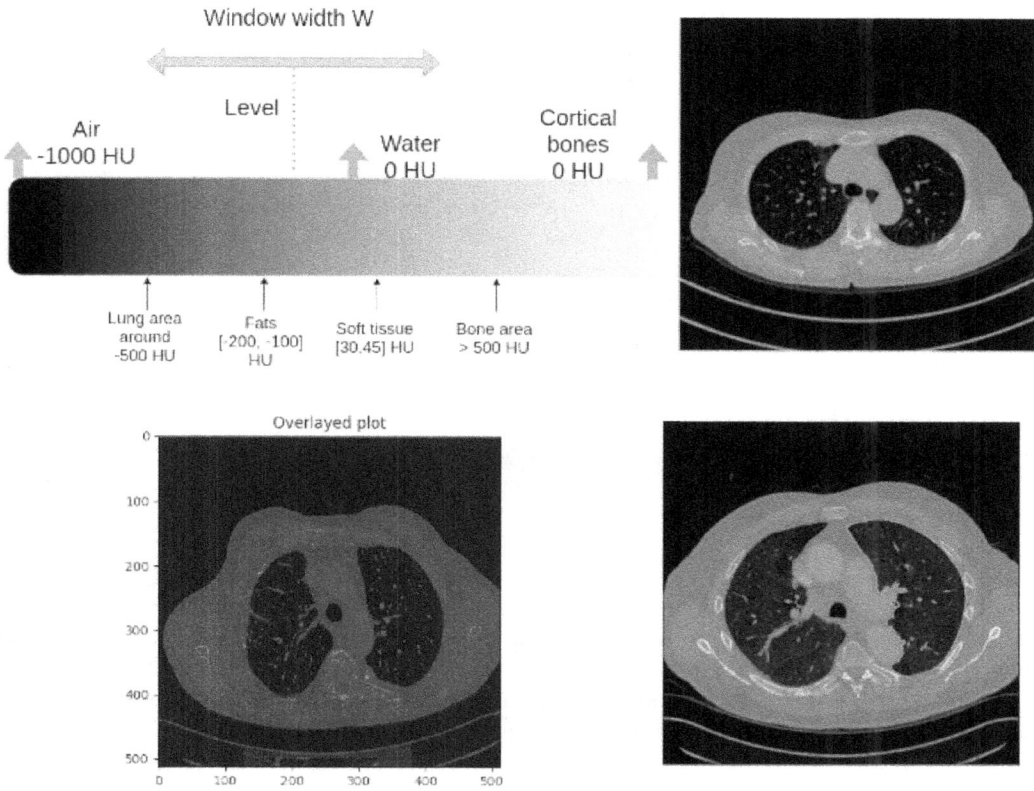

FIGURE 16.1 Medical image processing.

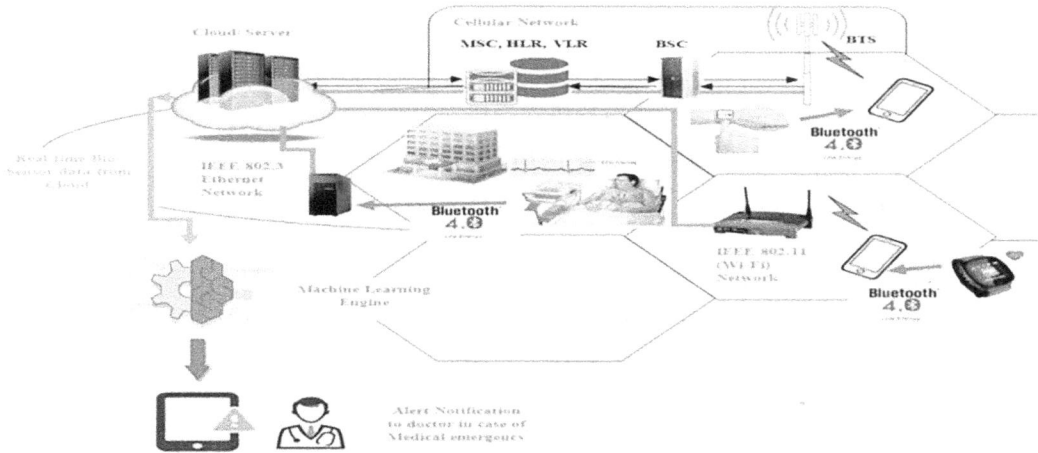

FIGURE 16.2 Heterogenous IoT framework.

on exist. These records don't influence the security of common users. In different investigations, this perception wasn't supported; they just broke down all the friends around a user (Figure 16.2).

This framework fills in asmotivation increases. If the intrusion of those users might be sensibly denied, we could simply assess the users who sway the security transparency of the goal users.

Besides, the productivity can be improved, and consequently, the accuracy of insurance measures may be significantly enhanced. During this time, exhausted users are immovably associated with the security spillage of target users. We don't want advantageousness to avoid provisions. To facilitate after effectively killing the outmoded users, we acknowledge that as yet, a couple of users have a cozy correlation with the goal abuser inside the chart arrangement, yet they cleave to information about the objective user that has misplaced its security. These users may be near the goal user; however, at this point, they're irrelevant. In the wake of end-evoking various systems, we decided to use the users' direction to loosen up this issue.

Heterogeneous networks consist of existing different Radio Access Network (RAN) technologies (e.g. WiMAX, Wi-Fi, E-UTRAN, etc.). They generally consist of multiple architectures, transmission solutions, and base stations of different energy capacity. The essential networks are used to enhance user experiences and restrict access in RAN and core-network (CN). It is possibly due to the corresponding complimentary services such as Wi-Fi: high data rates, short distance, low movement, while for UMTS: relatively low data rates, longer distance, high mobility [1]. HetNets also contribute to the intelligent routing and management of IP traffic, and also to effective load balancing and assignment of resources by not just aggregating disparate network radios but also offloading/loading selected or bulk packet-switched (ps/cs) traffic between the HetNets. In addition to other inter-technology options, 3G-WLAN has been investigated. These diverse radio interfaces can be combined in the EU and the RAN; as a consequence, multifunctional (client-based and host-based) frameworks are necessary for mobility and handover management [2–8]. Furthermore, none of the current technologies and networks of the second or third generation have the potential to provide the ubiquity of support quality of service level (QoS) needed for network coverage [2] (Figure 16.3).

Figure 16.1 It depicts the network evolution of present and future with respect to transport network plane, network layer plane, and logical network plane. The core is related to domain of future with migration and metro is a centre and related to domain with interoperability migration and other domains.

Here, as we attempt numerous strategies, we chose to utilize the users' behavior in resolving this issue. Here, in past examinations, specialists considered executing user behavior following live security; nevertheless, their utility in barring repetitive users was limited. In past assessments,

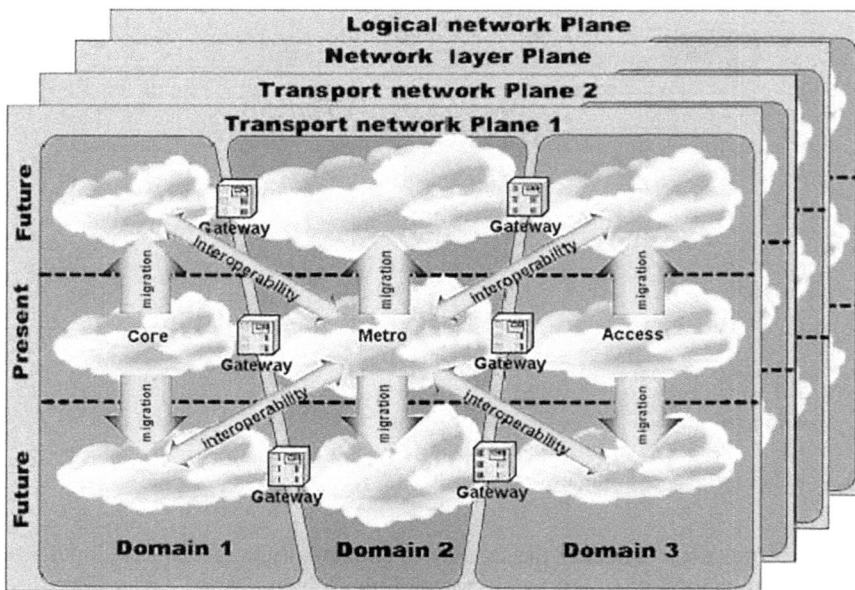

FIGURE 16.3   Network evolution.

experts considered executing user leads to live security; nevertheless, their utility in accepting unnecessary users is not worthy of mention. As such, we maintained our underlying work on individual assurance scoring systems, and we loosened up the procedure connecting individuals with everyone or any users inside the comp etc association arrangement diagram and joining the direct users to compensate for the shortcoming of past accesses. Our responsibilities during this paper are as follows:

- We propose the possibility of essential comparable structures and end the matter of advantageousness inside the traditional hub centrality situating algorithm.
- We propose direct social closeness to feature lead user conduct qualities.
- We settle the matter of reasonableness and dispose of repetitiveness with abundance users.
- We facilitate the proposed structure resemblance; direct conduct closeness and property likeness with our previous period singular insurance assessment technique; hence, we propose a more comprehensive strategy for assessing a user's security status.

Central doubt in these assessments is that all the users in web-based media all make substance, need to share the substance by making it easy to find, or talk with anticipated targets. To improve correspondence and allot resources effectively for better open organizations, government needs to grasp assorted online media content sorts and better separate occupants' web-based media practices of information sharing and dispersal. Governments should appreciate various sorts of users and their practices, and the extent of the substance types they make, and recurrence of making content less complex to arrange by others. The understanding of the user practices will have the choice to zero in some subset of user types. In this examination, we intend to perceive and arrange different sorts of online media users by user media content sorts and frequencies, and to analyze social differentiations by user sorts. We will zero in on Facebook online media to fathom the user practices in e-government settings. We present a web-based media user conduct to investigate the above requests. The user conduct perceives the web-based media users into different kinds and grants to analyse the online media-based data creation, laying out and zeroing in on practices by different user types.

Long-range interpersonal communication locales have an assortment of choices and applications that make them alluring to an expansive crowd. Facebook has made it feasible for people to meet on the web and has become ubiquitous. Facebook offers an easy method to quickly relate with companions. However, when considered, numerous issues of person-to-person communication can present, for example, reliance, protection and security issues.

In conveying these administrations, long-range interpersonal communication locales gather huge measures of sensitive data and appropriate it more rapidly and widely than user information gathers firms. Information gathering is an interesting instrument when used to help a user discover old partners or see advertisements to new user items, yet questions emerge when users theorize how much data is being gathered about themselves (Consumer Reports, 2020). How is this information being utilized? Could this data fall into unacceptable hands? Do users perceive how secure their data really is on informal organizations?

To answer these questions, this investigation is broken down into four proposals. The main proposal indicates those users who think about security as a significant factor in a long-range informal communication site; more are probably going to change their settings frequently. The subsequent proposal states users who have perceived fraud as a significant security concern are bound to change their settings at any time. The third proposal expresses that Facebook users who have left their security on a default setting are less prone to any infection or malware assault. The last proposal states that Facebook users who have their security set to a "daily schedule" setting haven't had security assaults on their profile.

There are more than 100 sites. For example, Facebook, YouTube, WhatsApp, Twitter, LinkedIn, and Instagram offer a scope of administrations for users who rely on the organizations for sharing their ideas, photographs, recordings and web journals. In any case, the fundamental

TABLE 16.1

The Best Social Networking Sites & Apps. (August 1, 2020, eBizMBA)

No.	Website/Apps	Number of Users	INFLUENCE	Monthly Visitors
1	Facebook	2,200,000,000	100%	5% Decrease (Q/Q)
2	YouTube	1,850,000,000	85%	2% Increase (Q/Q)
3	WhatsApp	1,500,000,000	20%	5% Increase (Q/Q)
4	Instagram	1,100,000,000	85%	3% Increase (Q/Q)
5	Twitter	375,000,000	90%	0% Increase (Q/Q)
6	Reddit	370,000,000	60%	1% Increase (Q/Q)
7	Pinterest	250,000,000	70%	5% Increase (Q/Q)
8	Snap Chat	110,000,000	20%	3% Increase (Q/Q)
9	Ask.fm	105,000,000	40%	12% Decrease (Q/Q)
10	Tumblr	95,000,000	50%	2% Decrease (Q/Q)
11	Flickr	90,000,000	50%	3% Decrease (Q/Q)
12	VK	85,000,000	25%	2% Increase (Q/Q)
13	LinkedIn	85,000,000	10%	2% Decrease (Q/Q)
14	Tagged	35,000,000	30%	8% Decrease (Q/Q)
15	Meetup	30,000,000	30%	12% Increase (Q/Q)

motivation behind online interpersonal organizations is sharing data. Table 16.1 exhibits the most mainstream informal communication locales as indicated by a positioning from ebizMBA (http://www.ebizmba.com).

The rest of the paper is organized as follows: the second section defines the complex structure of social media where various devices are connected through different networks. In the third section, the previous work on social media networking is explained. The fourth section explains the precise fundamentals of the graph, which helps in information flow in the social network. The fifth section provides information about the privacy and security taxonomy problems in social networks. The sixth section defines the user behavior perspective in social media network that bifurcates into analysis, characterization, recognition, and prediction. The seventh section describes types of attacks over the social media network that can mis-communicate or make an absurd file extensions that automatically download and create vulnerability. The eighth section defines user behaviors on the social network, which are based on parameters. Data preparation and representation of social media information are reflected using the analysis chart in the ninth section. At last, it concludes the quantitative and abstract techniques to research the fortunate combination between long-range social network use and risk concerns.

16.2 NETWORKS

Networks are complicated, consisting of several devices that use a variety of technologies. The technologies chosen clearly influence the properties of the whole network, and thus, the given a set of network requirements the selection of suitable technologies isn't straight forward.

The distribution of routing and labelling takes place at each hierarchical level. Including the label switches at Level 2, each LSR participates in the routing. The routing information is usually aggregated and distributed to Level N from Level N+1. In other words, all N+1 routers are presented as a simplified topology to N. There are different complexity representations, and therefore, different quantities of information are needed to describe them. Information is lost when topologies are aggregated. The routing protocol's information is therefore reduced, resulting in fewer optimal routes. The choice of how an aggregated topology is represented is therefore a compromise of the amount of routing information and the correctness of routing calculations.

16.2.1 SOCIAL NETWORKING SITE (FACEBOOK)

In person-to-person communication, Facebook is perhaps the biggest site, with 39.17 million Facebook users in India in December 2020, representing 28% of its entire people. The majority were men - 75%. People between the ages of 25 to 34 were the biggest group (14.70 million). The most striking difference among individuals occurs among people 25 to 34, where men lead by 7.30 million. The site works by getting users to interface with one another dependent on their experience or shared interests. It permits them to join packages that have equivalent tendencies. Every user seeks an online profile that contains particular information on the users, for example, their name and email address. Part of being on Facebook consolidates users postings so other users can see what they are doing or interested in. These updates show up on their mates' newsfeeds, as well as on the user's channel. This information is accessible to anybody, and viewable in the public region. Because of such a data posted, it is useful for an attacker to collect and target users dependent on the individual data they share [3,4,5].

Facebook has in the past conceded that security isn't the top feature the site offers. Redone benefits and focus on progress on Facebook depend on users' secure information [6]. Fitting associations dependent on precious data licenses relationship to zone likely users and advance their things.

Past assessments have zeroed in on the utilization examples of school understudies on Facebook and didn't analyze the security issues raised by these understudies on Facebook. In this appraisal, we incorporate the online security issues that Facebook users experience, and we propose how these issues might be moderated.

Regardless of the security outrages, the examinations, and the reports that Facebook's commitment to security is in decay, Facebook has posted an expansion in active users in its 2019 update. Most importantly, on users, Facebook currently serves 2.37 billion monthly active users, an expansion of 55 million on the past quarter [7,8].

In spite of rising concerns, and because Facebook has been around for about 15 years, utilization keeps expanding, which is an extremely large accomplishment in itself. Obviously, the larger the scale, the more Facebook's likely effect, which will keep on prompting further worries from administrative and government gatherings. However, as a business, Facebook has grown at an astonishing rate, something disparaged in most evaluations.

As should be evident from the above charts, Facebook's expansion has moved back in North American and European business areas, yet the associations had the choice to continue with its expansion in the Asia Pacific and 'Rest of the World' arrangements. That has been particularly helped by Facebook's consideration on India. Since 2018, the social network has multiplied its Indian group base to more than 300 million and looks set to continue with its development on the planet's second-most populated nation.

Since its surreptitious block-chain project has all the earmarks of being unequivocally based on Indian users, the above evaluations may even be moderate while various associations are still in a general sense subject to North American use. Facebook's development has set it in another stratosphere on this front and enabled it to get first-mover advantage in a scope of new business sectors.

Similarly significant,in its 2020 report, Facebook saw that it would in a little while be moving to another 'Gathering of Apps' utilization measure, which would join all users across Facebook, Messenger, WhatsApp, and Instagram, giving a more complete viewpoint on the association's authentic reach.

16.3 RELATED WORK

In the past protection evaluation research, analysts zeroed in on the information uncovered by users' profiles. In inventively utilized profile data to evaluate the affectability and see limits of characteristics, the user's security status was surveyed through a Bayesian model. Keeping up their examination, a more customary, considerably more numerically sensible strategy to decide user security scores in online social networks blends affectability and sets limits with IRT (item response theory); this assessment phenomenally advances the examination of affirmation appraisal. In upcoming examinations, Fang and Le Fevre masterminded an organization to give an affirmation settings wizard to users to let them control sensible profile settings. Jain and Raghuwanshi [9] masterminded a straightforward condition to discover the affectability of profile things, by then seeing the affectability and the limit of the data inside the user's profile and responding to this explanation. Xu et al. [10] found the key fragments affecting users' self-disclosure of individual data. Aghasian et al. [11] evaluated users' profiles spread on various informal organizations and got the users' security exposure status; they're the first to propose protection appraisal in different social affiliations. Malicious users in relational association stages are presumably going to show individual direct principles not equivalent to normal users, because of their goals in intensifying their own necessities and purposes (e.g. advance a particular thing or certain political points of view or theory). User direct investigation isn't only helpful in getting a start-to-finish cognizance of user objective, yet it is in like manner basic to the disclosure of toxic social bots' records in online casual networks. User lead presumably changes under different conditions. Chang [12] proposed that condition study is associated with programming administration prerequisite examination, which may empower the investigation of any change in user's necessities. Such an investigation is important to grasp the dynamic necessities of an item organization atmosphere. Zhang et al. [13] acquainted a structure with the advancement of user individual direct norm in media video proposal organizations on online casual networks. Their structure relies upon social setting and explores the changes in user need for various social conditions. Such user lead data will be jumped if we have permission to access the user's logs [14] or user's snap streams (e.g. recorded by relational association stages). The qualification in user direct is gotten, for example, by examining the image search logs of users to overview the chase objective of vacillated users [15], and this technique can support improvement of web records. Wang et al. [16] used user click stream data to fabricate a tick stream graph model to address user direct and perceive unmistakable user social affairs, and so on to distinguish poisonous records. There have also been distinctive researches that exhibit user objectives, and unusual records could similarly be settled through direct investigation and social condition in empowering the appreciation of users' dynamic lead. Liu et al. [17] constructed a novel convolution neural detail-maintained user direct, program substance and setting information to fabricate a tick model and encourage the user's gobble tendencies to enhance up chase quality. Al-Qurishi et al. [18] accumulated an outsized proportion of user information on the Twitter and YouTube, around 13 million channel activities, exploring and perceiving atypical practices that veer off basically from enormous extension subtleties through user lead in two relational associations P. Shi et al. [19].

In the current synthesis, the supervisor generally broke down affirmation concern in user information and sites [20,21]. Fundamental game-plans intertwine encoding and key spread [21] and acclimate a worker facing dark characters [18]. To help the sensibility of their answers, analysts moreover consider the liberality instead of a few assaults, for instance, sneaking around, insulting, replay, and wormhole assaults [22].

A few applications with easygoing correspondence have watched for affirmation stress by allowing users to manage their security approaches and plan security settings. Sadeh et al. [23] examined related issues in People Finder, an application that licenses users to present their locale to other people; users can refine security systems over the long haul. Emiliano et al. explored information security issues in CenceMe [20], a versatile, long awaited social correspondence application utilizing sensors. The response to the security issue is to allow users to really arrange for which sensors to use on their telephones. This prescribes that users need to disable certain sensors to perceive confirmation objectives. Access control on encoded information gives users consent to basically unscramble the blended information. The best methodology is to encode every information once and give sensible keys to users once so they can interpret supported information.

Like alluded to earlier, in PSN, thinking about the developments of user venture and trust affiliations, the interpreting key ought to be continually changed to accomplish expected security levels. Unadulterated symmetric key-based encryption and public key encryption don't appear, apparently, to be reasonable for PSN on account of either high multifaceted plan or non-capacity, especially for network-based second social exercises. Unequivocally, symmetric keys are difficult to administer in a streamed way. Information access control kept up unadulterated symmetric key encryption is tangled to help different procedures, while the overall key-based encryption plot isn't productive for multicasting/broadcasting information to a lot of users. The data proprietor ought to encode information or keys for each target beneficiary Z. Yan et al. [24].

The significant objective of OSNs is to yield substance to most remarkable users. They are use OSNs like Facebook, Twitter, and LinkedIn, to engage in standard activities [23]. In general, OSN customers share data about themselves and their lives with associates and extras. Regardless, in this scattered information, a section of the uncovered substance through the OSN are private and therefore mustn't be appropriated in any way. Constantly, customers share a couple of pieces of their way-of-life routine through notifications or the sharing of photos and records. Eventually, unprecedented OSN customers use advanced cells to require pictures and sharing trends through OSNs [25]. This data can permit noxious customers to use and attack an individual. Data recovery and information affirmation are two activities in PC programming disciplines that have various targets.

Data recovery offers frameworks for information extraction. It offers a set of procedures for a relationship for information study and settling on choices to maintain this recovered data. Information security shields data from unapproved and malicious access that uncovers, changes, assaults, or annihilates the data put in a safe spot or shared on the web. For example, specialists related with data recovery every so often don't consider security issues while masterminding answers for data recovery and the bosses [26]. On the other hand, analysts who work on information security routinely limit data-recovery strategies to shield fragile information from enemies who look for isolated data.

End-to-end message authentication using CoAP over IoT framework, a necessary authentication is required over social meda while sending or receiving a message from another [27]. The optimization of the algorithm is most important over network transmission due to quick responses [28]. Sources localize in WSN from noisy data [29]. The computational intelligence provides a great optimization over WSN in k-coverage network in social media networks [30]. A network web describes the all-over communication using one to another or via some another state also in WSN. A farmer integration monitoring system helps to get indication if any unknown activity occurs. This all has been done using various routing protocols in WSN [31–33].

- **Gap Identification with related work**
  Social media / social networking gaps that need to be focused. Gaps are:
  - Intranet versus extranet
    Social media networking brings the values to inside and outside the "organization" and uncertain, prudent, appropriate, rule-driven connection among these two worlds (social networking inside and outside the organization) can bear great profits.
  - The content here, community there
    Companies pays a lot of time and endeavour creating amazing content, yet their community interface seems to happen somewhere else, and this would be not fruitful for the community (e.g., GE's website and one of their GE Facebook pages).
  - Security and privacy
    In heterogeneous network SSL certification security must be used to protect the data breach, phishing, sybil, wormhole attacks.

16.4 FUNDAMENTALS OF SOCIAL NETWORKS IN GRAPH

The idea of graph theory is broadly utilized in social media. As a usual here, the users or individuals included are considered as the nodes or vertices. What's more, any connection between the users because of regular preferences or shared friendship is considered as edges.

16.4.1 GRAPH THEORY IN FACEBOOK

Most everyone knows about Facebook today. You can click 'like' in the event that you discover something to your liking, 'tag' your companions in different 'posts', put remarks in posts, and above all, become friends with somebody whom you know and somebody whom you don't have the foggiest idea! The idea of graph theory is utilized in Facebook [Figure 16.4] with every individual as nodes and each like, share, remark, tag as edges [34].

16.4.2 GRAPH THEORY IN TWITTER

Here the people are considered as nodes, and in the event that one individual follows another, that point is considered as the edge between the two users. Graph theory occurs in various fields: mathematical and other geometrical investigations: If we don't think about the length of the edge and vertical points of a polygon, at that point it tends to be securely expected as a graph with its vertices and edges [35]. This reality probably won't be that helpful in the investigation of polygons; however, this hypothesis is generally utilized in the investigation of surfaces and articles with higher measurement. Graph is additionally utilized in polynomial math (Figure 16.4). Figure 16.4 clearly shows the association usage of graph theory most likely on social networks, where a set or bunch with some patterns of contact or interactions between them, such as Facebook, Twitter, Instagram, LinkedIn, etc.

Figure 16.5 depicts the context of social media (such as online shopping networks, micro blogging networks, etc.), which is directly related to the users over open-source networks.

16.4.3 DESIGNING TRANSPORTATION NETWORKS

Architects and organizers utilize the idea of graphs prior to building expressways and bridges. They consider the different urban areas as nodes and the expressway associating them as edges. It is utilized locally inside the urban areas, too, for example, while developing a bus station. Here the bus station is as a node and the streets interfacing them are as edges [36]. Here the distances between the bus stations or the time taken to cross the distance are considered as a weight of the edge.

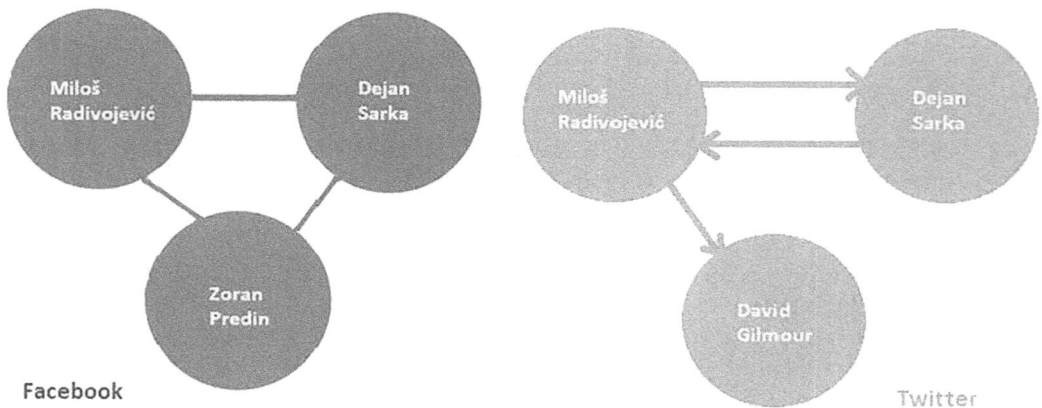

FIGURE 16.4   Graph Theory in Facebook and Twitter.

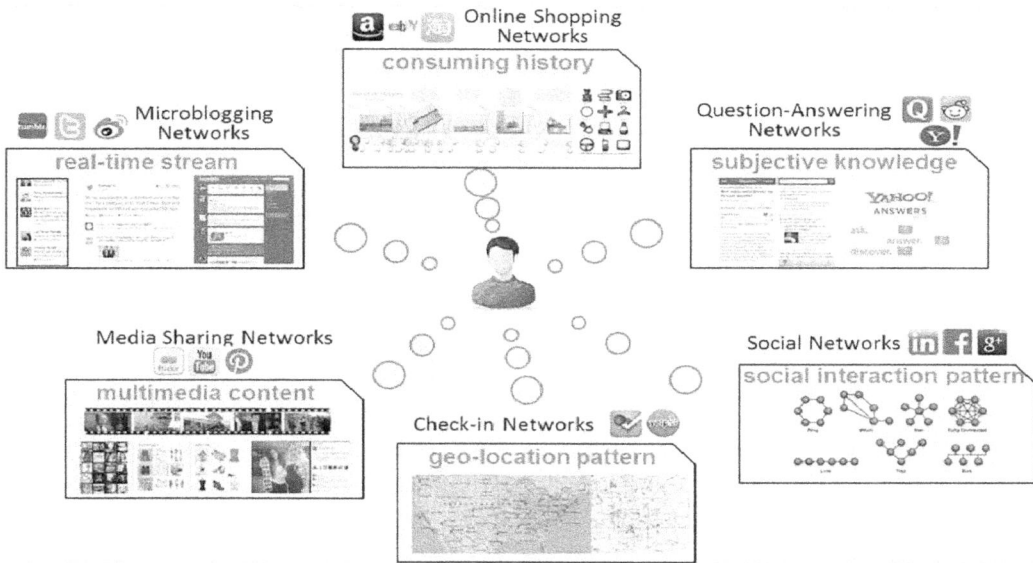

FIGURE 16.5 "Multimedia" in the context of social media: the heterogeneous data created and consumed in various OSNs.

16.4.4 Communication Networks

A PC network, whether concentrated or dispersed, represents a graph. The web-directing framework and other information and packet routing frameworks in a PC network represent a graphical structure with the different PCs or devices as nodes and the routing way between them as edges.

16.4.5 WWW

WWW is a graph diagram where various pages in the web are considered as hubs, and, if there is any hyperlink between two pages, then that is the edge between those two pages.

16.4.6 Social Network

Regardless, we need to have some ideas about the network. There are various methods of formally describing an organization based on the parameter used. The most well-known and versatile definition is taken from chart speculation; an interpersonal organization is conceptualized as a diagram, that is, a bunch of vertices (or hubs, centers) addressing social substances or objects, and a bunch of lines addressing in any event one social relations among them. An organization, nevertheless, is more than a graph since it contains additional information on the vertices and lines.

16.4.7 Brief Thought on Social Networks

When we need to represent any type of relations in the public as connections, we tend to call it a social network. The example of interdependency between every person (nodes) can be founded on various perspectives, viz. friendship, interconnection between families, basic interest, monetary trade, despise, sexual relationships, or connections of convictions, information, or renown.

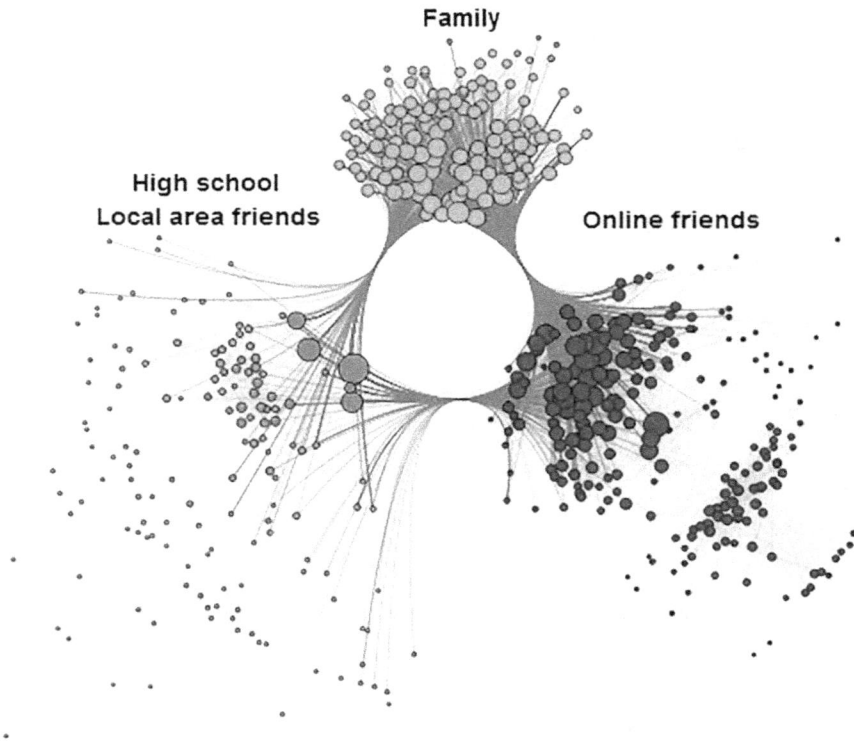

FIGURE 16.6   Network of friends.

Figure 16.6 depicts the relationship of a specific gathering of school companions. Every vertex represents to a critical individual in the friendship, and the edges indicate an association by relationship and connection of any sort that has been represented by four different colours [37]. Figure 16.7 describes the connection of heterogeneous networks with respect to routers.

16.4.8 SOCIAL AND ECONOMIC NETWORK

It comprises of a gathering of individuals associated with a type of co-operation or pattern of correspondence. For example, Facebook, Twitter, business connection among organizations and users, interrelationship between families associated with a marriage and so on.

16.4.9 DATA NETWORK

The association between data objects, for exampl, includes semantic (links between different words and images), World Wide Web (interface between different site pages; new page associating with another through hyperlinks). Measuring networks in this contextual analysis portrays the size of Facebook organizations. Not many irregular users have interacted for an entire month, and the relationship is characterized into four diverse network patterns.

16.4.10 ALL FRIENDS

This organization speaks to the summary of all allies a user has; consequently, this is the greatest among all the portrayals.

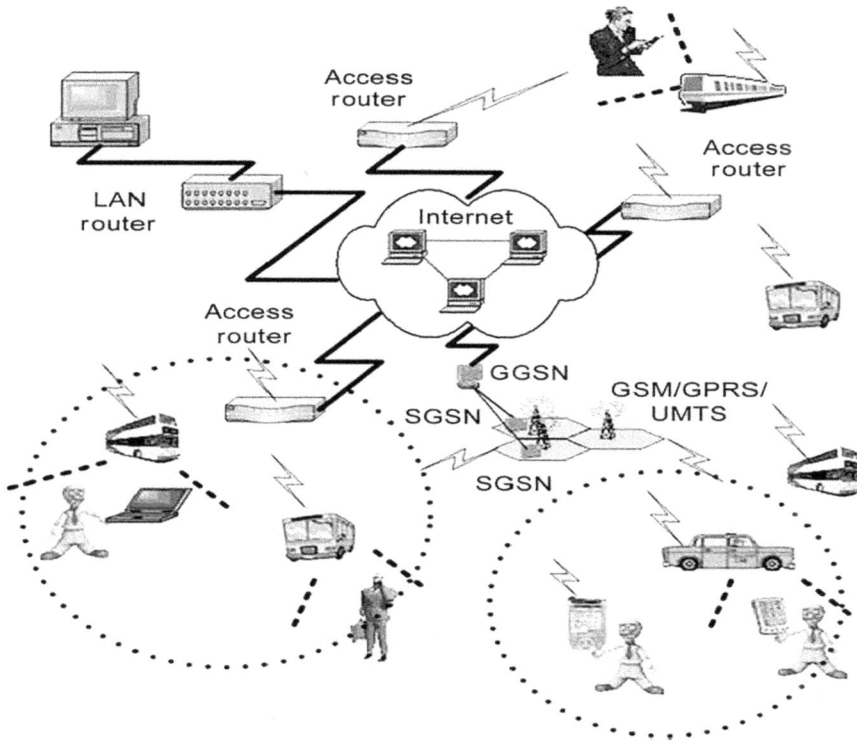

FIGURE 16.7 Heterogeneous network.

16.4.11 COMPLEMENTARY/RECIPROCAL COMMUNICATION

This portrayal shows the basic correspondence between two get-togethers, such an organization structures when there is divided exchange of information among two social occasions.

16.4.12 SINGLE DIRECTION/ONE-WAY COMMUNICATION

It contains people through whom user has granted.

16.4.13 LOOKED AFTER MAINTAINED RELATIONSHIPS

This relationship example contains people whose profile has been checked by the user more than once to take care of responsibility.

In Figure 16.8, the red line shows the quantity of proportional connections, the green line shows the single direction connections, and the blue line shows the uninvolved connections is a component of your network size. As per the Figure 16.8, more (lesser) number of people are having maintained relationships (maintained reciprocal communication) with respect to any network size.

16.5 RESEARCH METHODS

A taxonomy of privacy and security problems occurs in online social networks. Complete description of privacy and security threat in online social networks (OSN) Electronic media are a wellspring of correspondence between the information generator and end customer for online exchanges that make virtual associations through online social networks (OSN). An easygoing

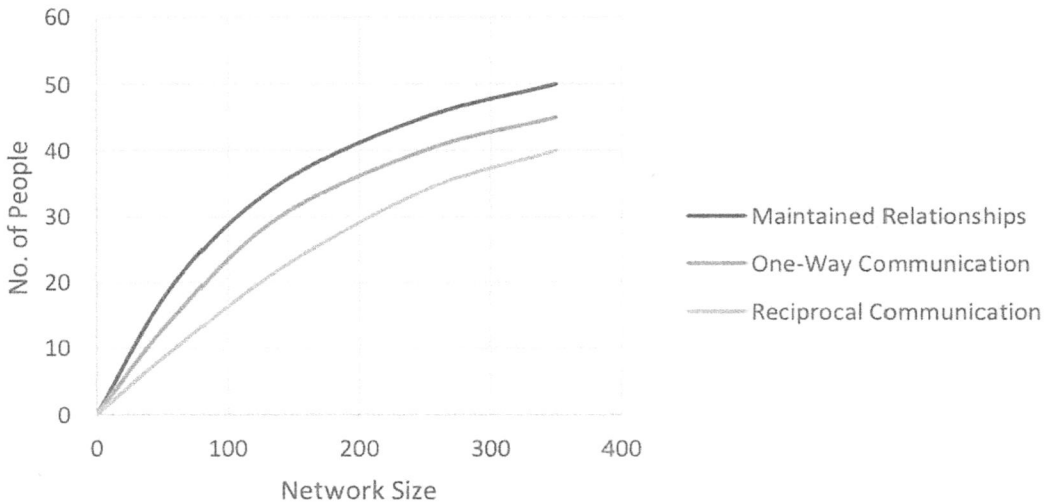

FIGURE 16.8   Active user graphical representation.

neighborhood, a social diagram reflects a relationship among customers, affiliations, and their social exercises [38]. These customers, affiliations, get-togethers, and so forth are the centers, and the relationship between the customers, affiliations, bundles are the edges of the diagram. An OSN is an online stage utilized by end customers to make easygoing organizations or relationship with others that have commensurate perspectives, interests, workouts, and more, besides genuine affiliations. Inestimable, diverse, long arrive at casual correspondence associations are accessible in the new online objections. These are the fundamental highlights of informal social-networking sites:

- Everyone existing on the web casual association social correspondence organizations is going digital by utilizing a web connection. Substances have dealt with on appropriated storing up through an assembled induction the board structure. This substance can be used from any place by utilizing an online platform for relationship, similar to online browsing.
- OSN customers need to disclose a profile for easygoing neighborhood as indicated by their pre-described stage. This profile information is in a general sense used for the register cycle to sign with the person to singular correspondence site.
- Approximately all current individual-to-individual long social correspondence associations maintains customers in developing their social relations with various customers by going through a customer's profile and comparing with others profile information.
- Individual enthralling portion of the current OSNs is to empower substances on these districts which are pre-conveyed to customer, while OSNs utilize these substances for overseeing purposes.

The essential target of OSNs is to bestow substance to most noteworthy users. Users use OSNs, for instance, Facebook, Twitter, and LinkedIn, to disseminate their typical activities. At times, OSN users share information about themselves and their exercises with relative and accomplices. Not with remaining, in these appropriated data, parts of the revealed substance through the OSN are private and likewise should not be disseminated in any way. Regularly, users share a couple of bits of their regular daily routine through notification or the sharing of photographs and accounts [39]. As of now, extraordinary OSN users use PDAs to take pictures and make accounts for sharing through OSNs. This data can have region information and some metadata introduced in it. OSN expert suppliers accumulate an extent of data about their users to offer altered administrations, yet it might be used for business purposes. Furthermore, users' data may in like manner be given to pariahs, which lead to security spillages. This information can allow pernicious users to utilize and assault the person's security. Information recuperation and data security are two creating territories in software engineering disciplines that have different targets. Information recuperation offers procedures to data extraction. It similarly offers a bunch of techniques to a relationship for data examination and making decisions subject to this recuperated information. Data security shields information from unapproved and poisonous access that discloses, changes, attacks, or obliterates the data set aside or shared on the web. For example, researchers related to information recuperation sometimes don't consider security issues while arranging answers for information recuperation and the heads. On the other hand, researchers who work on data security ordinarily limit information recuperation methodology to shield delicate data from adversaries who search for singular information [40–42].

16.6 PERSPECTIVE OF SOCIAL NETWORK USER BEHAVIOR

16.6.1 User Behavior Analysis

User behavior of social networks indicates to their inclination to accept social network services on the basics of the social impact, user requirement, and social network methodologies, along with the summation of the numerous associated activities. Traditional user behaviors in social networks augment common behaviors of information usage, content conception behaviors, and content utilization behavior. This is also the main research area on social network-based behavior analysis and modeling. For example, one can study the patterns on content writing or content utilization to determine the time of subsequent content writing or content consumption in the near future.

16.6.2 Behavior Characterization

- **Demeanor:** Positive or negative mentality toward ONS decides its utilization. A positive point toward ONS will build its utilization.
- **Weariness:** Temporary time, calming fatigue, slaughter time on ONS.
- **Usability:** Energy time should have been told and use ONS interface.
- **Feeling:** Feeling comfortable to exact assumptions and emotions on ONS.
- **Recurrence of utilization:** Usage regarding your time spent on ONS, recurrence of visits, relocation data, ofttimes change standings.
- **Delights:** Contentment and joy got from ONS use. Acquiring acknowledgment, making one's picture, superficial point of interest, social collaboration and correspondence, interfacing with loved ones, making new contacts, are the satisfactions gotten from ONS.
- **Information Control:** Data management through interface features to take care of privacy.
- **Character Traits:** Demeanour qualities fabricate users act in any case on ONS. Five qualities, in particular, extroversion, appropriateness, narcissism, neuroticism, and uprightness, are referenced widely with the use varieties in (unwinding, killing time, interfacing with loved ones, standing image, social impact, social communication), information sharing, protection, and exposure.
- **Second thoughts/Anxiety:** Regret once posting or sharing enthusiastic stuff and its outcomes in such a pressing way from the network.
- **Involvement/Enjoyment/Entertainment:** ONS use for satisfaction, recreation, delight and unwinding. It conjointly remembers inclusion for terms of what extent users are inundated in ONS that they fail to remember their environmental factors.
- **Self-Restriction/Self Attentiveness:** The degree and kind of {knowledge} revealed and uncovered by a user and utilization of security settings for one's own accommodation. Self-comprehension as far as user's information about the protection settings and strategies and the manner in which users acquire an understanding into elective user's life through ONS.

- **Poise:** Misuse ONS during a controlled way and not snared in it (not wagering on it an over the top measure of to utilize it every day).
- **Confidence:** Posting remarks on ONS increment with high confidence. Oftentimes cooperation for ahead acknowledgment and affirmation, assessment significant, valuable and expanding the feeling of certainty.
- **Self-divulgence/Self Projection:** The degree and kind of information uncovered on ONS. User's noteworthy is explained to their mindfulness and issues concerning security.
- **Self-viability:** The degree of shared data that one controls and mindfulness about protection settings and highlights.
- **Self-Presentation/Identity Organization/Self Direction:** Maintaining personalities, (for example, introducing oneself in a horny way, sharing appropriate data for keeping up impacts on others and lying to deal with or project ones' character), standing image, sharing data, (for example, pictures) with the thought of anyway others get them.
- **Social strength:** Shyness, reluctant to share related effect on revelation.
- **Social Relationship/Belonging:** Feeling a basic a piece of the group of friends, having a place.
- **Social head:** Maintaining available cooperation, more grounded ties (close loved ones), growing new relations and more fragile ties. Backing, trust, dependence, and information or information got from these connections.
- **Social Connection:** Making companions, staying in contact with ongoing companions, growing new connections, and keeping up existing relations.
- **Social Influence/Social Fetter:** Subjective standards, family or friend pressure that move or demotivate ONS use and structures a point (fortunate or unfortunate) toward ONS.
- **Accepted practices:** Norms or rules in a single group of friends can bring about one's investment and information sharing on ONS. Accepted practices affirm user conduct, love level of cooperation.
- **Social participation:** Justifying being distant from everyone else, insight of fondness, and affectability of being regarded and respectable.
- **Observation/Social Survey:** examination profiles of companions and obscure to acknowledge knowledge into their lives especially seeing someone.

Figure 16.9 represents the user behaviors attributes with flow information from one attribute to another.

16.6.3 BEHAVIOR RECOGNITION

Social media user behavior leads investigation, which is a critical territory of examination that engages different attributes of users to be considered. They study on social behavior and estimate user assumption toward explicit things that encourage businesses and enterprises to look out for the target's locales to zero in on. The assumption for client objective relies upon the joint efforts inside a site, which is huge for retargeting. Generally, e-business sites and commercial showcase networks screen user inquiries to fathom their points and practices. Besides, considering the interest and construction of pertinent documents available online to users on the friendship of the temperamental development of documents on the internet actualizes the investigation and shows the network course behavior on behalf of online users. Network removal methods could get advantageous for investigating and isolating important documents from online information; these are arranged according to network data mining, network usage, and structure mining [43]. Essentially, network records are removed for online information mining, users perusing exercises have examined by web-use mining, and the actual association organization of locales are dissected by web configuration mining. Web logging by control user webpages course in order, for instance IP address, user ID, date-time, strategy, position code and data range of the article; these are used by

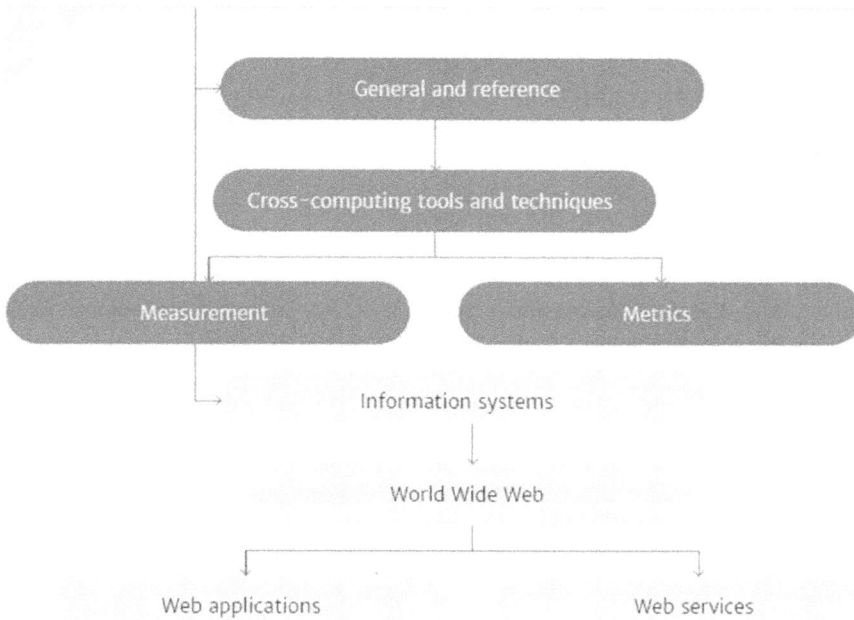

FIGURE 16.9 Characteristics user behaviors.

network information-mining to anticipate abuser behavior. The register is an assortment for user trades to invigorate each moment the user gets to locales [44]. The network data are set up by the gathering to activities, for instance, records clean-up, user classification, time duration identification, improved prototype hierarchy creation, prototype acknowledgment for recuperate to use illustration of every customer in the webpage subject to the behavior for the period of the examining, for instance, get on, visit locales, re-visitations and etc. Many delicate registering and information mining calculations have been proposed by experts to perceive accommodating examples in the user's web profile.

16.6.4 BEHAVIOR PREDICTION

As referenced already, there are highlights that can't straightforwardly be characterized as user behavior; notwithstanding, they impact of user behavior through regard ONS [45]. They characterized these highlights and depiction for each classify is given prediction on user behavior.

- **Simplicity of use:** Skill or exertion needed to work ONS & usability.
- **Gratifications:** Sentiments of joy gained from using ONS. Stream insight while using ONS, in terms of gratifications, unwinding, gluttonous, delight, and diversion.
- **Character Traits:** Individual characteristics that structure user direct on ONS and separate behavior from others activist or unfavorable demeanor for ONS that impacts its habit in terms of attitude, character qualities, colossal five sociability, reasonableness, self-importance, neuroticism, and unwavering quality.
- **Confidence:** Frequent ONS venture for gaining affirmation and certification to fabricate confidence, human being in a social context present in ONS participations and activities to facilitate make vibes of value.

- **Social impact:** Relatives, partners, companion sway to facilitate impacts ONS use. The users are ones gathering of companions that choose and influence ONS usage. This terms social effect, social shackle, relative's pressure, and acknowledged practice.
- **Lament:** Penalty of posting incorrectly substance on ONS. The ferm is regret/pressure/anxiety.
- **Feeling:** Expressing is one of them feelings on ONS successfully and straightforwardly.
- **Weariness:** By means of or sharing on ONS to unwind or alleviate exhaustion and bluntness.
- **Poise:** Ability to control ONS use and interest.
  - Simplicity of utilization decides the ability to work and utilize ONS. The ONS are not difficult to work with, and less exertion is needed to learn it. At that point, users will think about it as a persuasive factor for using it. Accordingly, convenience itself can't be classified as a behavior; in any case, it impacts ONS use.
  - Gratifications and gluttonous are named as one element since the two of them manage assumptions of delight. Users who appreciate ONS and are mollified with it are more adept to utilize it later, which prompts more prominent interest.
  - The social impact, which incorporates family, companions, friends, culture, and accepted practices, additionally affect user behavior. Relations the huge others partaking vigorously taking place ONS will be a persuasive and compelling make to utilize and take an interest taking place ONS.
  - Unhelpful occurrences related with ONS use will discourage users from dynamic cooperation, in this way impacting behavior and use in a unhelpful manner. These harmful episodes might be results of rearrangement an unseemly substance or brutal and abominable remarks.
  - Several individuals discover ONS more proper for venting their feelings than communicating them up close. This demeanour decidedly impacts their utilization and investment.
  - Several users discover ONS a valuable device for taking a break or to calm fatigue. This demeanour rouses them to utilize and take an interest on ONS at whatever point they want to destroy moment in point.
  - Self-regard is additionally a characteristic that affects user behavior. It is characterized as far as self-assessment and how high one respects oneself. Individuals having a low confidence expand their group of friends by speaking with individuals that they can't associate in the disconnected world. They attempt to deal with their low regard by regular social communications on ONS and having a broad companion list.

Starting history discussion, we can deduce that behavior can't be assessed directly. To the user in light of everything, practices are performed on ONS choosing user behavior. Besides lead, there are various segments, together with character characteristics and discussed as of now, that sway user behavior and behaviour performed on ONS [45].

Heterogeneous networks such as H-MPLS copes with e.g. optical as electrical packet switching equipment. Larger packets than their electronic counterparts are used by optical networks (whether OPS or OBS based).

16.7 TYPES OF ATTACKS

The security issue and protection concern are the significant necessities of the extensive variety interpersonal social sites. Nonetheless, there are various dead-liest attacks suffers in any person-to-person social networking sites and protecting the anticipated users from these hostile assaults have been the troublesome task of various social agent and engineers. The crucial security assaults are assembled into three classes [30].

Active Attacks: Appearance the new hubs normally & endeavouring to attach with the associated hubs and earn the permission to various hubs.

Passive Attacks: This is absolutely mysterious and imperceptible.

Security Breach: Find interface among nodes, edges and potentially distinguish the connection between them.

There are various assaults possible in online social media organizations and offered the possible response for how to manage the assaults safely.

Online Social Networking Infrastructure attacks: S-murf IP Attack, UDP Flood Attack, TCP SYN Deluge Attack.

- Use anti-virus and anti-malware software.
- Install fitting intrusion detection system.

Malware Attacks: Spy-ware, Adware, crime-product, browser ruffians, down-loader, & toolbars.

- Use of anti-virus.
- Do not go for obscure connections, applications, companions, E-mail connections etc.
- Disable cookies, sessions, ActiveX if unidentified or no counter-measures open.

Phishing Attacks: Misleading phishing (E-mail, messages), search program phishing, malware base phishing, key loggers.

- Examine the messages & E-mail with mindfulness.
- Authenticate the wellspring of the information.
- Be careful of promotions with offer.

Pernicious identical twin attacks: Collective planning attack.

- Be careful about having allies and sharing information.
- Validate the user profile and propose the information.
- Try to thoroughly understand the methodologies of having sidekicks in the individual-to-individual long-range interpersonal networking platforms.

Uniqueness extensive scam attack:

- Use complex passwords, avoid mystery key reuse.
- Destroy your E-mail or records properly.

Physical attack: Impersonation, harassment through messages.

- Need an all-around characterized long range informal social networking strategy.
- Background security and protection checks.
- Properly utilize protection settings choices options.

Cyber (Computer-generated) bullying:

- Don't perceive the messages that are proposed to damage.
- Accumulate and collection the messages while confirmations.
- Receive all threats authentically.
- Don't circulate pass on individual information to all users.

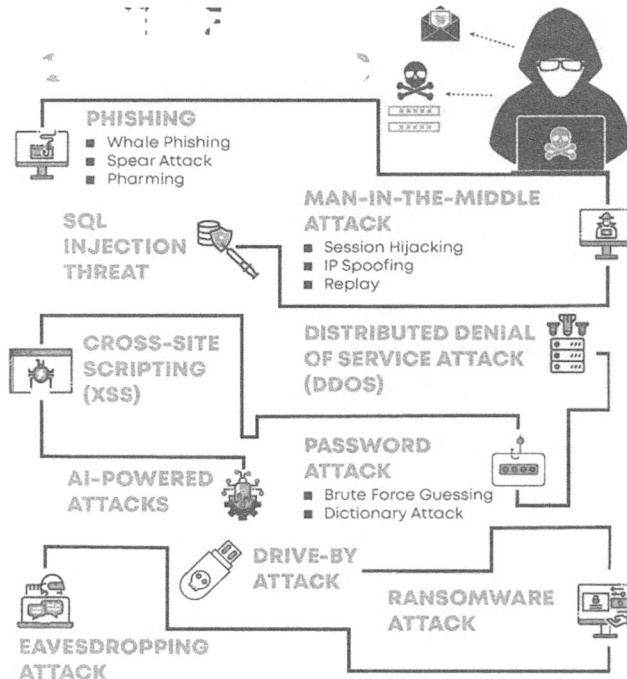

FIGURE 16.10   Types of attacks.

Figure 16.10 describe the types of attacks that are inter-related to each other in network, and we should be attenuative with our information before sharing over the network or internet.

16.8   TYPES OF USER BEHAVIOR

Alienated persons use the social media platform greatly. When various conditions were used to address a discouraging idea, we assembled critical terms and assigned them with identifiers that are more sensible to address the idea. These terms are the features used in examinations of user behavior. Identifiers are the imprints consigned by us to store up these terms. We moreover gave a minimal portrayal of all identifiers. A couple of identifiers is taken from the wording of social brain research, where suitable. The order of various user behaviors is given.

- **Social investigation:** To investigate, search, and look at exercises of elective user on ONS. ONS is that the terms of surveillance, social examination, social surfing, perusing.
- **Social relationship:** Relation with others like companions, family, and friends on ONS, creates and keep up new ties. Partner with the group of friends on ONS are considered a fundamental piece of it. Assets got from ONS bonds and associations. ONS is the platform of social association, social correspondence, social association, social alliance and social capital, which are more grounded and more vulnerable ties.
- **Recurrence of utilization:** Time spent on ONS and furthermore the degree of exercises performed on it. ONS is the terms of frequency of visits, recurrence of progress statuses.

- **Data Control:** Managing data through access the board choices on ONS and predominant the degree of information unveiled on ONS. ONS is simply the terms of confidentiality interface highlights, restriction, mindfulness, self-efficacy, self-revelation, and self-projection.
- **Self-compass reading:** Creating ideal impacts on ONS for introducing the necessary picture of one-self. ONS is that the conditions of self-introduction, personality the board, self-direction.
- **Correspondence:** Teaming up on ONS inside a similar recurrence as their ONS contacts or companions.
- **Social confidence:** Uncertainty in contributively and partaking on ONS of boldness.

16.9   RESULT AND DISCUSSION

At present, arising innovation and patterns have brought about various frameworks and stages through which social elements collaborate and speak with each other, for example, email, text messaging, telephone/mobile organizations, and above all OSNs like Facebook, Instagram, Twitter, and YouTube. These frameworks empower their users to connect and share thoughts, data, and interests through different assortments of connections they maintain. Also, OSNs permit users to publish their own data, extra sight and sound substance, and connect to different users whom they identify with. The correspondence and collaboration administrations gave by these frameworks empower to uncover the basic social networks of their users, and consequently, they speak to a novel occasion to survey and get them.

Top-to-bottom analysis of social networks structure and development can bring about a vastly improved plan of future interpersonal organization-based frameworks. Online social networks offer numerous helpful properties that reflect certifiable social networks attributes, which incorporate little world behavior, huge neighborhood bunching, and presence of colossal emphatically associated segment and arrangement of very close gatherings or networks. The wide prominence of OSNs and their basic access have become the abuse of their administrations. Other than the trouble of safeguarding user security, OSNs face the test of adapting to bother some users and their noxious exercises inside the social networks. The first normal kind of pernicious movement recognized in OSNs is spamming which includes noxious users (spammers) to communicate immaterial data inside the sort of messages, IMs, remarks, text messages and presents on as sizable measure of genuine users as could be expected under the circumstances.

Spamming is done generally with a point of advancing items, viral advertising, spreading crazes. The authentic users of an OSN diminish their trust once they are spammed. Long-range interpersonal communication alludes to gathering of individuals and associations together by means of some medium, in order to share contemplations, interests, and exercises. There are a few online informal organizations whose administrations are accessible. like Facebook, Twitter, LinkedIn, Google+ and so on. They give easy-to-use and intuitive interface to append individuals within the nation and at distant location too. There additionally are a few portable based long-range informal communication benefits of applications like WhatsApp and so on.

Facebook is the most well-known social sites on the world. With billions of users across the world, following and examining social exercises on this platform is fundamental. Here we convey an example online media report for your Facebook page and another for Facebook post administration.

In Figure 16.11, the explanation of the social media report or the usages of social media by the users are described with the relevant data. In this figure, the bifurcation of the engagement of the users in Facebook, Twitter, Instagram, YouTube, and LinkedIn is also visualized with relevant data. Number of clicks on various social media network and all are inter-related to each and form a huge heterogeneous network.

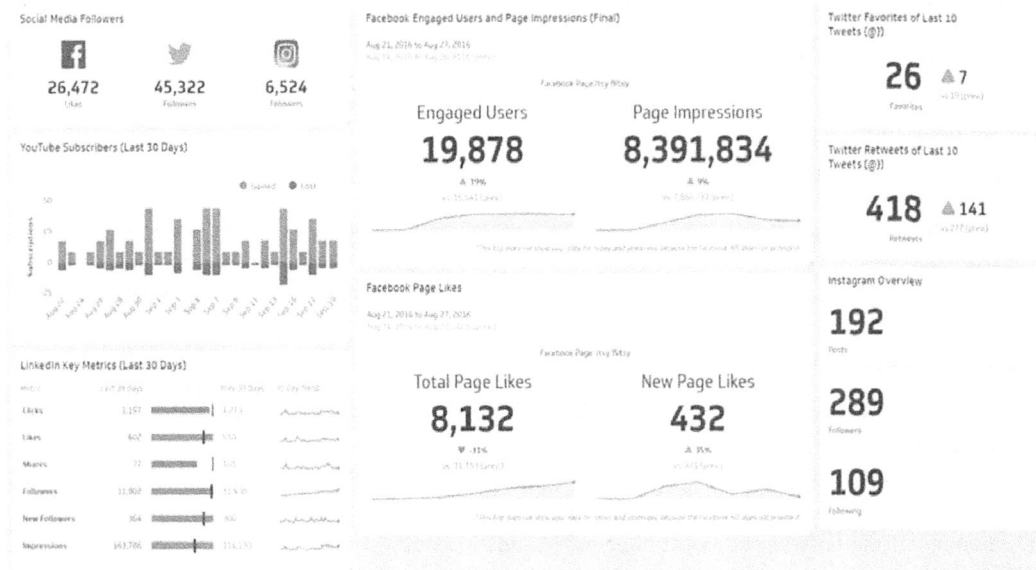

FIGURE 16.11 Social media reports.

16.10 CONCLUSION

This study concludes the heterogenous network where user activity is associated with various social media platforms such as Facebook, Instagram, etc. The user's analysis is being monitored in various aspects, such as security, which is one of the main factors. There are various factors in security to restrict the content and user. It can be protected by blocking or marking it as abused to that account, which shows unrelatable content. In social media, content is vague, but the content is shown to the user based on the user's previous activities. Information can be pictures, feeds, and most trending reels (a short video). Security and privacy measures are taken to protect the user's information by activating the two-point authentication, login notification, etc. from unsuspicious breach activity such as flooding, sybil, phishing, hacking, snitching as well as wormhole attacks. Lastly, this could lead to an improvement of the online commercial social media community.

REFERENCES

[1] Johnson, B. (2010). Privacy no longer a social norm, says Facebook founder. *The Guardian*, *11*(01).
[2] Furnell, S. M. (2010). Online identity: Giving it all away?. *Information Security Technical Report*, *15*(2), 42–46.
[3] Nyoni, P., & Velempini, M. (2018). Privacy and user awareness on Facebook. *South African Journal of Science*, *114*(5-6), 1–5.
[4] Payton, T., & Claypoole, T. (2014). *Privacy in the Age of Big Data: Recognizing Threats, Defending Your Rights, and Protecting Your Family*. Rowman & Littlefield.
[5] Singhal, P., Sharma, P., & Arora, D. (2018). An approach towards preventing iot based sybil attack based on contiki framework through cooja simulator. *International Journal of Engineering & Technology*, *7*(2.8), 261–267.
[6] Li, X., Xin, Y., Zhao, C., Yang, Y., Luo, S., & Chen, Y. (2020). Using User Behavior to Measure Privacy on Online Social Networks. *IEEE Access*, *8*, 108387–108401.
[7] Maximilien, E. M., Grandison, T., Sun, T., Richardson, D., Guo, S., & Liu, K. (2009, May). Privacy-as-a- service: Models, algorithms, and results on the facebook platform. In *Proceedings of Web* (Vol. 2).
[8] Liu, K., & Terzi, E. (2010). A framework for computing the privacy scores of users in online social networks. *ACM Transactions on Knowledge Discovery from Data (TKDD)*, *5*(1), 1–30.

[9] Fang, L., & LeFevre, K. (2010, April). Privacy wizards for social networking sites. In *Proceedings of the 19th international conference on World wide web* (pp. 351–360).

[10] S. Jain, & Raghuwanshi, S. K. (2018). Fine grained privacy measuring of user's profile over online social network. in *Intelligent Communication and Computational Technologies*. Singapore: Springer, pp. 371–379

[11] Xu, F., Michael, K., & Chen, X. (2013). Factors affecting privacy disclosure on social network sites: an integrated model. *Electronic Commerce Research, 13*(2), 151–168.

[12] Shi, P., Zhang, Z., & Choo, K. K. R. (2019). Detecting malicious social bots based on clickstream sequences. *IEEE Access, 7,* 28855–28862.

[13] Chang, C. K. (2016). Situation analytics: a foundation for a new software engineering paradigm. *Computer, 49*(1), 24–33.

[14] Zhang, Z., Sun, R., Wang, X., & Zhao, C. (2017). A situational analytic method for user behavior pattern in multimedia social networks. *IEEE Transactions on Big Data, 5*(4), 520–528.

[15] Barbon, S. Jr., Campos, G. F., Tavares, G. M., Igawa, R. A., Proença, M. L. Jr., & Guido, R. C. (2018). Detection of human, legitimate bot, and malicious bot in online social networks based on wavelets. *ACM Transactions on Multimedia Computing, Communications, and Applications (TOMM), 14*(1s), 1–17.

[16] Park, J. Y., O'Hare, N., Schifanella, R., Jaimes, A., & Chung, C. W. (2015, April). A large-scale study of user image search behavior on the web. In *Proceedings of the 33rd Annual ACM Conference on Human Factors in Computing Systems* (pp. 985–994).

[17] Wang, G., Zhang, X., Tang, S., Wilson, C., Zheng, H., & Zhao, B. Y. (2017). Clickstream user behavior models. *ACM Transactions on the Web (TWEB), 11*(4), 1–37.

[18] Liu, Y., Wang, C., Zhang, M., & Ma, S. (2017). User behavior modeling for better Web search ranking. *Frontiers of Computer Science, 11*(6), 923–936.

[19] Aghasian, E., Garg, S., Gao, L., Yu, S., & Montgomery, J. (2017). Scoring users' privacy disclosure across multiple online social networks. *IEEE Access, 5,* 13118–13130.

[20] Yan, Z., & Wang, M. (2014). Protect pervasive social networking based on two-dimensional trust levels. *IEEE Systems Journal, 11*(1), 207–218.

[21] Puttaswamy, K. P., & Zhao, B. Y. (2010, February). Preserving privacy in location-based mobile social applications. In *Proceedings of the Eleventh Workshop on Mobile Computing Systems & Applications* (pp. 1–6).

[22] Beach, A., Gartrell, M., & Han, R. (2009, August). Solutions to security and privacy issues in mobile social networking. In *2009 International Conference on Computational Science and Engineering* (Vol. 4, pp. 1036–1042). IEEE.

[23] Singhal, P., Sharma, P., & Rizvi, S. (2019). Thwarting Sybil Attack by CAM Method in WSN using Cooja Simulator Framework. *International Journal of Engineering & Technology, 8*(1.5), 116–125.

[24] Al-Qurishi, M., Hossain, M. S., Alrubaian, M., Rahman, S. M. M., & Alamri, A. (2017). Leveraging analysis of user behavior to identify malicious activities in large-scale social networks. *IEEE Transactions on Industrial Informatics, 14*(2), 799–813.

[25] Sadeh, N., Hong, J., Cranor, L., Fette, I., Kelley, P., Prabaker, M., & Rao, J. (2009). Understanding and capturing people's privacy policies in a mobile social networking application. *Personal and Ubiquitous Computing, 13*(6), 401–412.

[26] Miluzzo, E., Lane, N. D., Fodor, K., Peterson, R., Lu, H., Musolesi, M., ... & Campbell, A. T. (2008, November). Sensing meets mobile social networks: the design, implementation and evaluation of the cenceme application. In *Proceedings of the 6th ACM Conference on Embedded Network Sensor Systems* (pp. 337–350).

[27] Singhal, P., Sharma, P., & Hazela, B. (2019). End-to-end message authentication using CoAP over IoT. In *International Conference on Innovative Computing and Communications* (pp. 279–288). Singapore: Springer.

[28] Kandris, D., Alexandridis, A., Dagiuklas, T., Panaousis, E., & Vergados, D. D. (2020). Multiobjective Optimization Algorithms for Wireless Sensor Networks. *Wireless Communications and Mobile Computing, 2020.*

[29] Hussain, A. (2020). Decentralized Source Localization Using Wireless Sensor Networks from Noisy Data. *arXiv preprint arXiv:2009.01062.*

[30] Tarnaris, K., Preka, I., Kandris, D., & Alexandridis, A. (2020). Coverage and k-coverage optimization in wireless sensor networks using computational intelligence methods: a comparative study. *Electronics, 9*(4), 675.

[31] Abd Rahman, A. H., Sulaiman, R., Sani, N. S., Adam, A., & Amini, R. (2019). Evaluation of Peer Robot Communications using CryptoROS. *Evaluation*, *10*(7).

[32] Dutta, P. K., Vinayak, A., & Kumari, S. Farmers Assistant Innovation and Resolution Web Server based plant monitoring for smart Irrigation.

[33] Nakas, C., Kandris, D., & Visvardis, G. (2020). Energy efficient routing in wireless sensor networks: a comprehensive survey. *Algorithms*, *13*(3), 72.

[34] Yan, Z., Zhang, P., & Vasilakos, A. V. (2014). A survey on trust management for Internet of Things. *Journal of network and computer applications*, *42*, 120–134.

[35] Nyoni, P., & Velempini, M. (2018). Privacy and user awareness on Facebook. *South African Journal of Science*, *114*(5-6), 1–5.

[36] Balduzzi, M., Platzer, C., Holz, T., Kirda, E., Balzarotti, D., & Kruegel, C. (2010, September). Abusing social networks for automated user profiling. In *International Workshop on Recent Advances in Intrusion Detection* (pp. 422–441). Berlin, Heidelberg: Springer.

[37] Digital Insights. Social media statistics for 2014 [webpage on the Internet]. c2014 [cited 2016 Apr 14]. http://www.adweek.com/socialtimes/files/2014/06/social-media-statistics-2014.htm

[38] Social Bakers. Africa Facebook users infographic [webpage on the Internet]. c2013 [cited 2016 Nov 20]. Available from: http://www.socialbakers.com/africa-facebook-users-infographic.jpg

[39] Erikson, E. H. (1993). *Childhood and society*. WW Norton & Company.

[40] Facebook. Accessed: Aug. 16, 2016. [Online]. Available: https://zhtw.facebook.com/

[41] Norouzizadeh Dezfouli, F., Dehghantanha, A., Eterovic-Soric, B., & Choo, K. K. R. (2016). Investigating Social Networking applications on smartphones detecting Facebook, Twitter, LinkedIn and Google+ artefacts on Android and iOS platforms. *Australian Journal of Forensic Sciences*, *48*(4), 469–488.

[42] Li, C. T., Wu, T. Y., & Chen, C. M. (2018). A provably secure group key agreement scheme with privacy preservation for online social networks using extended chaotic maps. *IEEE Access*, *6*, 66742–66753.

[43] Kandris, D., Nakas, C., Vomvas, D., & Koulouras, G. (2020). Applications of wireless sensor networks: an up-to-date survey. *Applied System Innovation*, *3*(1), 14.

[44] Numan, M., Subhan, F., Khan, W. Z., Hakak, S., Haider, S., Reddy, G. T., … & Alazab, M. (2020). A systematic review on clone node detection in static wireless sensor networks. *IEEE Access*, *8*, 65450–65461.

[45] Patel, H., Singh Rajput, D., Thippa Reddy, G., Iwendi, C., Kashif Bashir, A., & Jo, O. (2020). A review on classification of imbalanced data for wireless sensor networks. *International Journal of Distributed Sensor Networks*, *16*(4), 1550147720916404.

17 Wearable Technology

Concepts, Classification and Applications

Vandana Dubey and Priti Kumari
Ashoka Institute of Technology and Management, Varanasi,
Uttar Pradesh, India

O. P. Singh
Amity School of Engineering & Technology, Amity University, Lucknow,
Uttar Pradesh, India

G. R. Mishra
Dr. Ram Manohar Lohia Avadh University, Faizabad, Uttar Pradesh, India

CONTENTS

DOI: 10.1201/9781003333081-17

17.1   INTRODUCTION

Wearable technology refers to the systems worn by persons for any particular application. These devices are equipped with some desired properties [1–9]. The capabilities for sensing parameters, computational ability, and response techniques decide the cost, demand, and utilization of these wearable technology systems. Some examples of these wearable devices are shown in Figure 17.1 below.

Despite the fact that many of us are awestruck by the most recent development in wearable technology, the idea of wearable "devices" has actually been around for millennia. Here is a brief chronology of wearable technology's development [10,12–21]:

History of Wearable Technology

- Peter Henlein, a clockmaker from Germany, invented the "Pomander" in the 1500s, the first "smartwatch."
- Chinese inventors created the first working abacus ring in 1644.
- Dr. Julius Neubronner invented the "pigeon-cam," which was attached to pigeons, in 1908. It had a pneumatic system to regulate the amount of time before a picture was shot.
- The "Stereophonic Television Head-Mounted Display" was created and patented by cinematographer Morton Heilig in 1960. He holds the title of "Father of virtual reality."
- Year 1964 saw the creation of the first shoe-sized wearable computer by Edward Thorp.
- In 1975, Pulsar introduced the first "wristwatch calculator."
- Sony introduced the Walkman in 1979, the first portable cassette tape player.

(a)

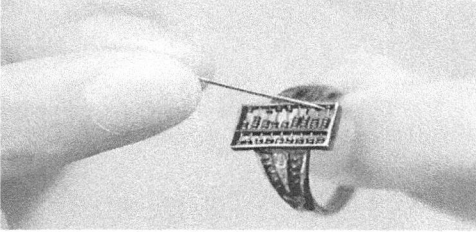

(b)

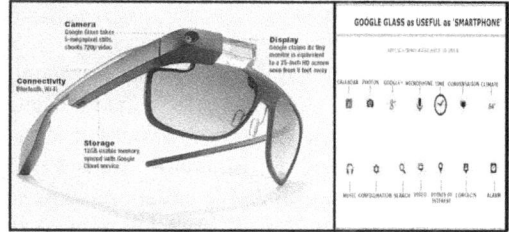

(c)

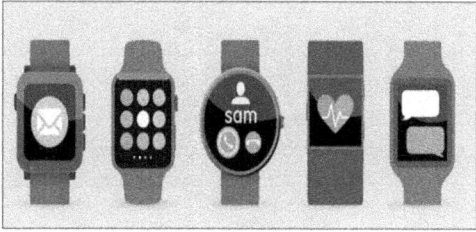

(d)

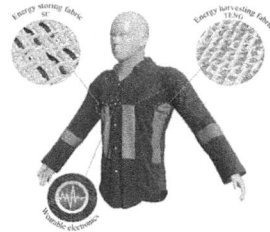

(e)

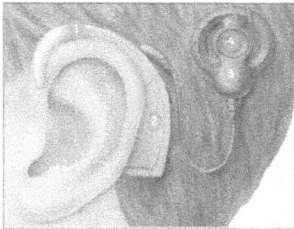

(f)

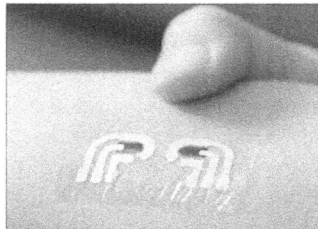

(g)

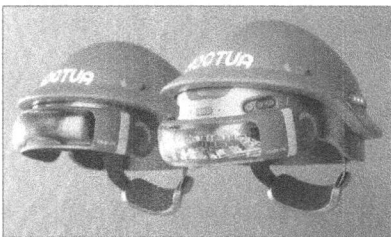

(h)

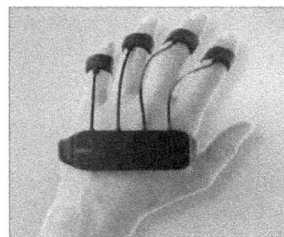

(i)

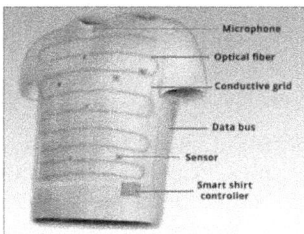

(j)

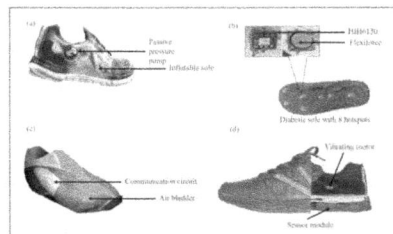

- In 1998, Steve Mann created a GNU/Linux Wristwatch Videophone prototype that was fully functional.
- The mBracelet was created by Studio 5050 in 1999. It might be used as a fashion piece and could computerize financial transactions with ATMs.
- The Levi ICD + jacket, which "had a changeable wiring harness linking a range of portable electronic devices carried by young professional individuals," was first introduced in 2000.
- Nokia unveiled the Bluetooth headset in the year 2002.
- In 2006, Nike and Apple collaborated to develop the Nike+iPod Sport Kit, which includes a smart shoe, a clip-on receiver, and iPod Nano software.
- Later, 2008 saw the release of the Fitbit Classic Wristband, an activity and sleep tracker.
- Google Glass, an optical head-mounted screen display that resembles a pair of spectacles, was introduced in 2012.
- Tommy Hilfiger debuted solar-powered coats in 2014.

Later, heavy prototypes of this particular technology evolved into more compact, lightweight, and transportable final products. It is clear that the development of wearable technology was driven by the need to offer users the portability and, ultimately, hands-free access to computers and other electronic devices.

This chapter discusses some fundamental terms related to this technology that builds the ground of awareness for the study. This discussion is followed by major qualities desired in a good wearable device. Further, the categorisation of wearable technology devices can be done on different grounds. This chapter also covers the classification of wearable devices on different grounds. Furthermore, future applications of wearable devices are discussed in brief. For future work attention, some selected key areas are focussed upon, such as accuracy, storage and performance, and possible solution for these issues has been also suggested.

This chapter is organised in a total of seven sections. Section 17.1 gives a brief introduction of wearable technology to build the basic awareness about the area of discussion, followed by section 17.2, about the basic concept of the technology in brief. After that, section 17.3 gives the classification of wearable devices, and future applications domains are discussed in section 17.4. Further, advantages and disadvantages of wearable technology devices are discussed in section 17.5. After that, proposed approaches are presented for key issues of wearable technology in section 17.6, and the chapter is finally concluded in section 17.6.

17.2   FUNDAMENTAL CONCEPT OF WEARABLE TECHNOLOGY

Wearable technology or devices are systems worn by users with a particular aim [11,22–30]. These devices are considered to be equipped with efficient hardware and software parts that coordinate walk-in Singh to provide almost real-time processing and desired form of results in the targeted or

FIGURE 17.1 Examples of Wearable Technology Devices. (a): Abacus Ring: An Early Wearable Computing Device [10]. (b): Google Glass and its Applications [10]. (c): Smart Watches. (d): Smart Textile [11]. (e): Cochlear Implant. (f): Tattoo Sensor as Needleless Glucose Monitor for Diabetes Patients. (g): Smart Helmets. (h): Gesture Control Smart Gloves. (i): Smart Shirt. (j): Smart Shoes.

Sources: https://electricalfundablog.com/wearable-computing-devices-technology/; https://electricalfundablog.com/wearable-computing-devices-technology/; https://xd.adobe.com/ideas/principles/app-design/designing-for-wearables-11-things-to-keep-in-mind/; https://onlinelibrary.wiley.com/doi/10.1002/adma.201504403; https://commons.wikimedia.org/wiki/File:Cochlear-implant-external-part.jpg; https://jacobsschool.ucsd.edu/news/release/2529; https://www.yankodesign.com/2019/03/04/; https://www.analyticsinsight.net/things-about-gesture-control-devices-you-should-not-miss/; https://nazoharoon.wordpress.com/2017/12/27/georgia-tech-wearable-motherboard-gtwm-smart-shirt/; https://svv-research-data.s3.ap-south-1.amazonaws.com/paper_161001_1600529865.pdf

defined issue. This sections details about some key terms related to wearable technology and fundamental properties of wearable devices.

17.2.1 Key Terms Used in Wearable Technology

Some key terminologies used in wearable technology are discussed as follows:

17.2.1.1 User

Any human (or living organisms) or machine that is communicating and interacting wearable devices for the purpose of receiving the signals and also providing required actions.

17.2.1.2 Wearer

Any human (or living organism) on which the device is attached. The location of device on the surface depends on the type of the device, as well as application area. Wearables (i.e. wearable devices) basically observe and sends the defined parameter of the wearer.

17.2.1.3 Wearable Devices

These are systems, worn by the wearer, having capabilities of sensing, storing, and communicating. Moreover, these devices may or may not have the ability to control, process, and display remote applications.

17.2.1.4 Processing Module

These systems may or may not reside inside the wearables. These devices process the sensed parameters by the wearables and produce computed results. Now, according to these results communicated to wearable devices, the display or actions can be generated accordingly.

Figure 17.2 clearly shows the interaction between these entities of wearable technology systems.

17.2.2 Fundamental Properties of Wearable Technology Devices

Furthermore, wearable technology must have some properties to make it 'in demand'. These properties are shown in Figure 17.3 in short and discussed as follows in detail.

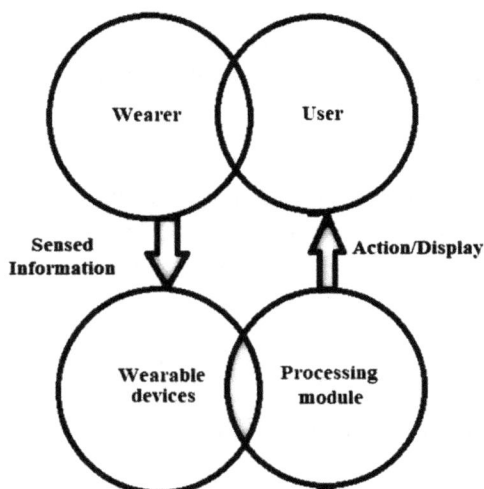

FIGURE 17.2 Interaction among fundamental entities of wearable technology systems.

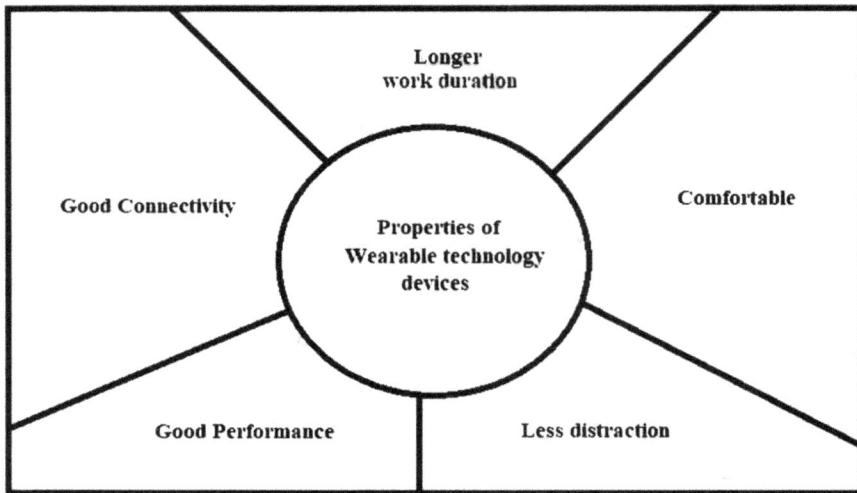

FIGURE 17.3   Properties of wearable technology.

17.2.2.1   Longer Work Duration

Good wearable devices are required to work on low power, so that once charged, this may work for longer. Moreover, as these devices are expected to be working 24 × 7, power-saving efficiency is required, which necessitates instant waking up and background processing.

17.2.2.2   Comfortable

Wearable devices must be hands-free and comfortable to wear. Their actions or working should involve minimal interaction by the wearer or user. Moreover, these devices must not interfere with the movement of any part of the body.

17.2.2.3   Less Distraction

The design, colour, material, and sound, etc., of wearable devices must be such that it doesn't grab the attention of anybody during the operation or in idle condition. So, not only appearance, but events of communication must also be less disturbing to the environment.

17.2.2.4   Good Performance

The wearable technology devices must be able to accurately sense and observe the required parameter, process, and provide optimum result for action very fast. The speed of response and accuracy of these wearable devices are among the key areas of research.

17.2.2.5   Good Connectivity

These devices are required to be connected to some other systems for advanced calculations for reactions. The network supported by wearable devices decides the speed, range, and security, etc., of the application. So, depending upon the severity or criticality of the usage, the connectivity standard is decided.

Apart from these major five properties, there are some other parameters also that may be considered, such as cost, development platform, etc.

17.3   CLASSIFICATION OF WEARABLE TECHNOLOGY DEVICES

Although the demand and application of wearables have increased tremendously over the past few years, due to the pandemic, this technology has already been in use since the 15th century [31–39].

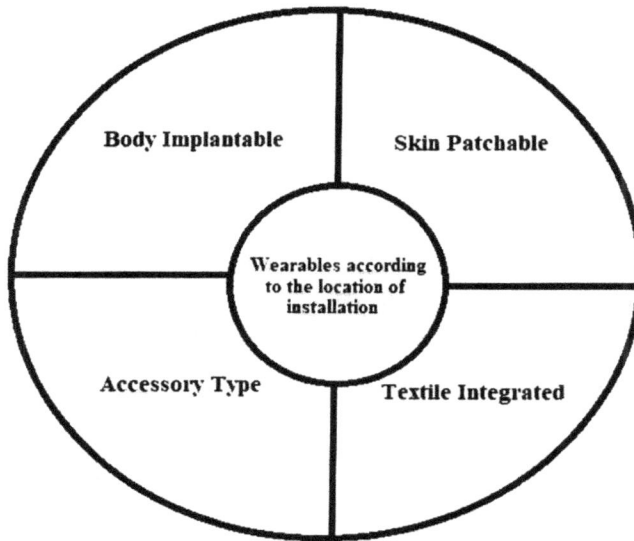

FIGURE 17.4 Wearables according to the location of installation.

To classify wearable devices, we may follow different approaches. Here, in this section, the classification is performed first on the location of installation and then on the application area of the wearables. These classifications are discussed as follows:

17.3.1 CLASSIFICATION ACCORDING TO THE LOCATION OF INSTALLATION

As shown in Figure 17.4 below, according to the place of installation, wearables may be categorized in four categories, namely body implantable, skin patchable, textile integrated, and accessory type devices.

17.3.1.1 Body-Implantable Wearable Devices

These devices are implanted temporarily on the body parts of the wearer, such as on the ear, hair, eyes, etc. Basically, these devices are lightweight, so that it is comfortable to wear them. Moreover, self-sustainability and safety to the human body are additional features required in this category. Some examples of these devices are cochlear implants, neuro prosthetics, and insulin implants, etc.

17.3.1.2 Skin Patchable Wearable Devices

As skin covers almost the full body of the living organisms, these types of wearables provide a large scope of sensory area. Moreover, apart from sensing cardiovascular and neuro-muscular events, these devices may also perform analysis and observation of skin secretions. Smart-skins and smart-tattoo-based wearables fall into this category, along with healing chips and cyber pills. Characteristics of these devices includes being ultra-thin, stretchable, and comfortable to skin, etc.

17.3.1.3 Textile-Integrated Wearable Devices

Earlier textiles and clothes were assumed to be required for covering the body, providing protection from environmental parameters and serving as art, but now, with the integration of wearables, the approach has been diverted to some extent. Now, e-textiles containing wearables have the ability to sense and respond to body parameters according to the application. Properties of these smart fabrics are flexibility and integration of various electronic systems, etc.

17.3.1.4   Accessory Type Wearable Devices

These wearables are worn on the wearer's body as an accessory that can perform a set of observation and provide the results. These devices are low power consuming and comfortable to the wearer's body. Nowadays, these devices are very high in demand and usage due to the affordable prices, comfort, and application domain. Some examples of these devices are smart watches, fitness bands, smart jewellery, and smart glasses, etc.

17.3.2   CLASSIFICATION ACCORDING TO THE APPLICATION

Nowadays, wearables are utilized to improve almost all domains of life. Basically, according to the target domain, we may classify these devices in five major categories, as shown in Figure 17.5 below.

17.3.2.1   Wearable Devices for Healthcare

In this area, generally, devices are used to diagnose and monitor body parameters of the wearer. Moreover, treatment procedures, such as medication and any other operative function, may also be included in this category. As this category of devices concerns health issues, so precision and accuracy are the key requirements in the observation, communication, and action of the wearables. Some examples of these devices are wearable ECG monitors, wearable blood pressure monitors, and wearable biosensors, etc.

17.3.2.2   Wearable Devices for Sports and Fitness

The training as well as practice or performance of individuals in any kind of sports, fitness, or well-being activity can be assisted and improved with the use of wearables. Several types of wearable fitness watches, glasses, helmets, and fabrics fall under this category. These devices measure and observe life parameters during the session, and accordingly, further actions may be taken to improve the overall performance of the sportsperson or the trainer. These variables provide better monitoring of life parameters with great convenience and no obstructions in the activities.

17.3.2.3   Wearable Devices in Workplace

There are some workplaces where safety and security of individuals are required to be monitored and assured using wearable devices, such as the case of firefighters, paramedics, police,

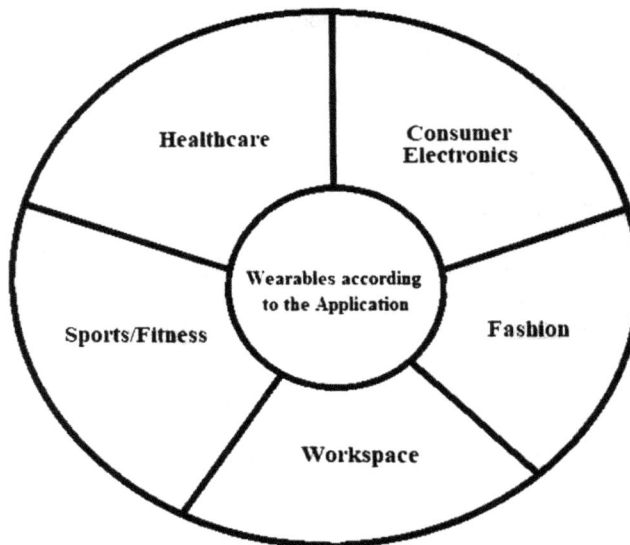

FIGURE 17.5   Classification of wearables based on application.

astronauts, etc. These personnel's safety parameters can be observed and used accordingly to avoid any type of loss. Moreover, employee safety and security can be assured at other places with these wearables. E-textiles and health-monitoring wearables are generally used for this category of applications.

17.3.2.4 Wearable Devices for Fashion

Wearables have also interfered in the fashion industry in terms of choices and usage. Now, we may think of clothes with real-time colour variation according to the emotion of the wearer. Further, this colour change may also be associated with the help parameter of the wearer. Basically, wearables in fabrics have electro sensors that are used to sense, monitor, and control (up to some extent) the body functions, parameters, and environment factors etc. One of the examples of this category is Firefly dress, which displays light with the movement of wearer.

17.3.2.5 Consumer Electronics

This category of wearables is basically applied in entertainment, communication, and work-related tasks. Smart watches, smart glasses, cameras, and headphones, etc., fall under this category. Usually, these wearables provide entertainment facilities like music, photo, video, etc., communication facilities like sending and receiving calls and texts and other work-related utilities.

So, here we have categorized wearables according to two approaches only, although there can be various other approaches to perform the classification.

17.4 FUTURE APPLICATIONS OF WEARABLE TECHNOLOGY DEVICES

Currently, major focus of electronic manufacturing and design entities are toward efficient wearable devices, due to the high demand in almost all significant domains of life [40–50]. The range of wearables available in the market is basically motivating research and designers to work on enhanced features and application integration with high optimization of parameters. This optimization of parameters makes wearable devices approachable, affordable, and applicable in major sections of interest. As shown in Figure 17.6 below, some application areas of these devices are discussed as follows:

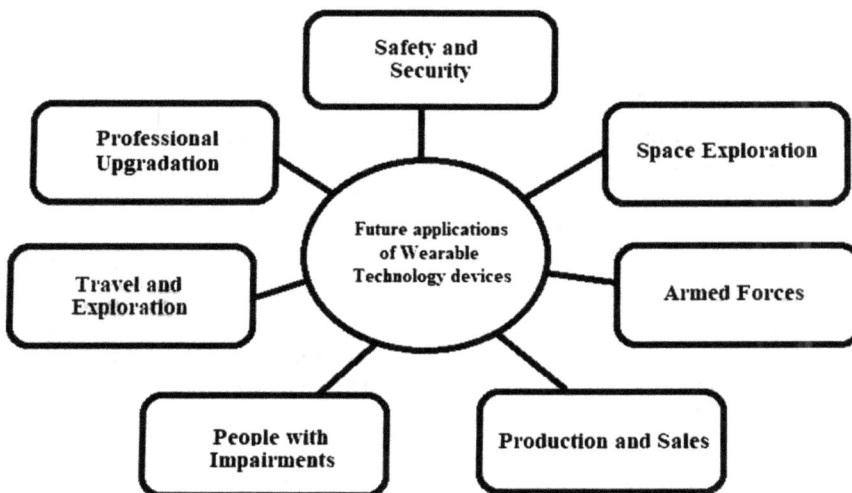

FIGURE 17.6 Future applications of wearable technology devices.

17.4.1 Safety and Security

In this application domain, wearable devices are required to have a good quality of sensors. The sensors will sense any malicious activity in the surrounding and communicate to the respective wearer or user regarding probable traffic issue, attack, or health issue, etc.

In the traffic scenario, wearable smart glasses can inform about the disturbance in either driver's physical condition or any obstruction on road traffic so that concerned users or authorities may take action to avoid any harm. Further, at the entrance of any building, institution, or section where security checks are required, wearable devices equipped personnel may speed up the process of entry with greater accuracy.

Furthermore, wearable devices with biosensors senses health parameters of wearer and generate required display or communicate to avoid any adverse event.

17.4.2 Professional Upgradation

Wearable technology can be very actively and efficiently utilized for professional activities upgradation. Like, communication and recording of any idea in wearer's mind or talk will be done in the quick span of time. Moreover, scheduling of meetings among persons at different locations and movement may be possible in a convenient manner with the help of wearable devices.

Furthermore, during discussion, wearables may sense, observe, analyse, and finally produce a cumulative report or agenda for the particular issue based on the verbal and nonverbal inputs from the participants. Moreover, wearable devices may also be included to improve the virtual assistance process for efficient planning, collection, and monitoring, etc.

17.4.3 Travel and Exploration

Augmented and virtual reality-enabled wearables are also applied in this area, apart from gaming and entertainment. With the help of these wearables, visitors may virtually see and feel any location, city, mountains, etc., without actually visiting there. People also can see the hotel rooms, restaurants, or foods also from remote locations.

This application of wearable devices actually helps pre-plan the schedule of vacations. Wearables also assist to send and receive calls, take pictures, schedule time slots for different activities during leisure time, and so on.

17.4.4 People with Impairments

Wearable devices found a white scope in this area. People who are enabled with these wearables can overcome their limitation of activities with promising technology. For example, any blind person wearing smart glasses can be sent the environment and people or things nearby to them. This awareness will increase their comfort level as well as safety and security during movement. Moreover, they can actively participate in major activities in the surroundings. People with hearing loss may improve their understanding of the world with the help of smart hearing aids. Moreover, their understanding, response, safety, and security also improves with the involvement of wearables as these machines basically enable these people to hear or understand outside sound up to some extent of clarity. Also, for people who are not able to move, their mind-waves or thoughts can be sensed, analysed, and understandable results are generated utilizing efficient wearable devices.

17.4.5 Production and Sales

In the process of production, workers equipped with smart wearable devices may work quickly with ease as these devices may assist workers in locating goods, process upgrading, information or suitability of the type or structure of materials etc. Moreover, worker's health and intelligence can also be monitored continuously or at intervals. The application of wearable devices improves the overall production of the organisation.

Moreover, during the process of sales, people can know or experience the product without touching it, such as clothes, accessories, footwears, glasses, etc. This ease of trial lets buyers make decisions comfortably as they can feel the appearance of self in that product without actually wearing it. Smart glasses or helmets are among the wearables that can be widely used to improve the sales of the product.

17.4.6 ARMED FORCES

Army personnel are required to work very hard, starting from the time of training until actual performance on the field. Wearable technology devices can be utilized to assist these people for their health-related issues, as well as safety and security parameters. Wearables, like watches, patches, or chips, etc., can be used to measure the physical and biological parameters of the person to calculate the level of fitness at the moment. Moreover, in the field, the current location, any injury, or any message can be communicated to the concerned with ease. Here, skin patches, chips, watches, smart glasses, and smart helmets with enable technology can be used for better results.

17.4.7 SPACE EXPLORATION

Astronaut or space personnel are required to be safe during their mission. Wearable technology devices monitor the health, emotion, or thoughts of these persons in space. After communicating the current situation of parameter, these devices also provide the required reactions through displays, commands, or actions.

Although we have discussed only seven future application domains of wearable technology in this chapter, the list is endless.

17.5 ADVANTAGES AND DISADVANTAGES OF WEARABLE TECHNOLOGY DEVICES

Wearable technology has become an inseparable part of individuals in leading a comfortable, safe, and progressive life. With the integration of various established, as well as disruptive technology in this domain, the wearable technology has attracted attention by wearers and researchers in last few decades. As each technology has its own pros and cons related to working and application, wearable technology devices also possess some of these issues [51–58]. Moreover, research and development works are already going on to reduce limitations of these devices in the future. Following subsections discuss some advantage and disadvantages of wearable technology, in short:

17.5.1 ADVANTAGES OF WEARABLE TECHNOLOGY DEVICES

Figure 17.7 shows some of the advantages of wearable technology devices. These advantages are discussed as follows:

17.5.1.1 Increased Productivity

With proper application wearable technology, wearers are able to efficiently solve some selective problems more quickly. This assistance provided by wearable devices actually increase the productivity of employees.

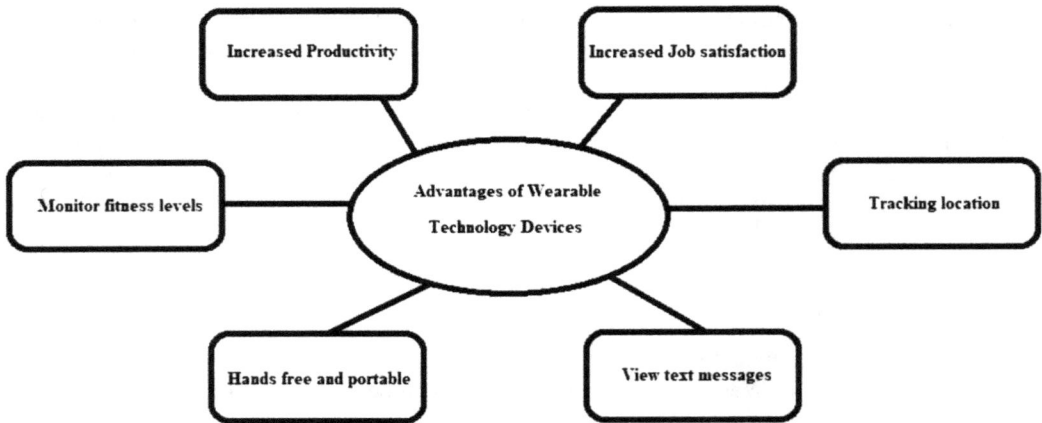

FIGURE 17.7   Advantages of Wearable technology devices.

17.5.1.2   Increased Job Satisfaction

As discussed in the previous point, wearable devices help individuals to improve their efficiency and productivity; this in turn increases the level of job satisfaction at the same time.

17.5.1.3   Tracking Location

Many wearable technology devices are enabled with the facility of tracking the location with GPS. Moreover, connectivity to a network is also required to find any targeted location by the wearer.

17.5.1.4   View Text Messages

With the help of wearable technology devices, wearers need not to reach to their phone or laptop to send and receive messages. These devices provide the facility to view text messages more quickly.

17.5.1.5   Hands Free and Portable

Most of the wearable technology devices have the ability of working in hands-free and portable mode. This facility eliminates the need of the wearers to take devices out of their pocket.

17.5.1.6   Monitor Fitness Levels

This is one of the main advantages and most demanded features in wearable technology devices today. With the inclusion of required components, wearable devices very easily and efficiently provide the facility of regularly monitoring an individual's fitness levels.

17.5.2   Disadvantages of Wearable Technology Devices

Figure 17.8, shows some of the disadvantages of wearable technology devices. These disadvantages are discussed as follows:

17.5.2.1   Short Battery Life

Depending upon the type of technology used and application of the wearable devices, power requirements vary. Generally, these devices have a fairly short battery life.

17.5.2.2   Repeated Removal and Charging Process

Wearables are required to be removed from the wearer's body occasionally for different reasons, such as cleaning, battery charging, or sync processing, etc.

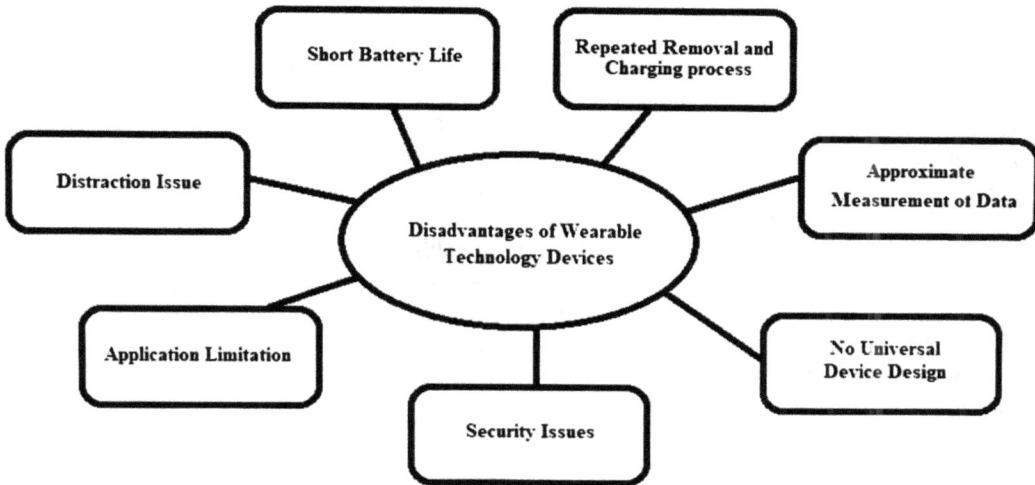

FIGURE 17.8 Disadvantages of wearable technology devices.

17.5.2.3 Approximate Measurement of Data

Sometimes wearables may produce approximate value of intended measured data due to environment factors or internal component limitations. This may lead to erroneous results and actions in critical applications.

17.5.2.4 No Universal Device Design

Generally, wearable devices must be connected to other complex devices for required advance display, calculation, or actions. So, wearable devices are lacking in universal device design in which all processing and response-generating modules are included.

17.5.2.5 Security Issues

As wearable devices are connected to the internet most of the time, it leads to the increase in vulnerability of the system. The information attached to these devices are prone attacks.

17.5.2.6 Application Limitation

As wearable devices are compact in size and design, their application domains are very limited. Their technology and components are the deciding factors for the usefulness of the wearable devices.

17.5.2.7 Distraction Issue

Many times, wearables generate sound for notifications or the screen illuminates. These events seek the attention of the wearer as well as the surrounding. These disturbances, caused by the devices due to appearance or notifications, hamper the level of concentration while doing any task.

17.6 PROPOSED SOLUTION FOR SELECTED ISSUES·IN WEARABLE TECHNOLOGY

As discussed in earlier sections, there are some limitations of wearable technology. Here, in this section, we proposed possible approaches for some selected issues of wearables, such as analysis, storage, and security of data involved for efficient performance. These proposals are as follows:

17.6.1 PROPOSAL 1 (ANALYSIS)

For continuous monitoring of the human activities, wearable devices include different types of signals, such as bimetric temperature optical sensor and so on. However, the reading of some of these sensors are not as accurate as stationary devices. Today, these devices are considered a big source of data. From the data, it is possible to extract features, and further machine-learning algorithms can be applied to detect and learn useful patterns. It is also possible to perform analysis on data, which is generated by wearable devices.

In future proposed work, we may consider the healthcare data and apply machine-learning algorithms to measure the accuracy of data. As shown in Figure 17.9, steps to create this machine-learning model contain downloading of datasets, performing data-cleaning steps, finding useful features, and then applying various machine-learning algorithms to measure and analyze the beneficial patterns of the data.

17.6.2 PROPOSAL 2 (STORAGE)

Today, huge amount of data is being generated by wearable devices. As shown in Figure 17.10, saving all the data in the fog node is not a wise idea as it consumes much energy and produces high latency values.

Therefore, in future it is possible to work with fog node to cache only popular or important content. Moreover, there is is requirement to select appropriate fog node as a cache node having good storage capacity, where is important content can be placed, as shown in Figure 17.11.

17.6.3 PROPOSAL 3 (SECURITY)

In today's scenario, wearable devices are collecting huge amounts of personal data. But due to the security vulnerability, authentication and privacy issues, wearable devices are one of the noticeable areas for attacks. However, in the future, it is possible to use blockchain technology with wearable devices because, with the help of integration of blockchain concept in wearables, there will be improvement in the security of transmission. This integration of blockchain technology enables users to access and utilize secure data with improved confidence. In future, using blockchain, it is possible to secure health data transmission, which is generated by wearable devices. Figure 17.12 demonstrates the use of blockchain while sharing health-related data.

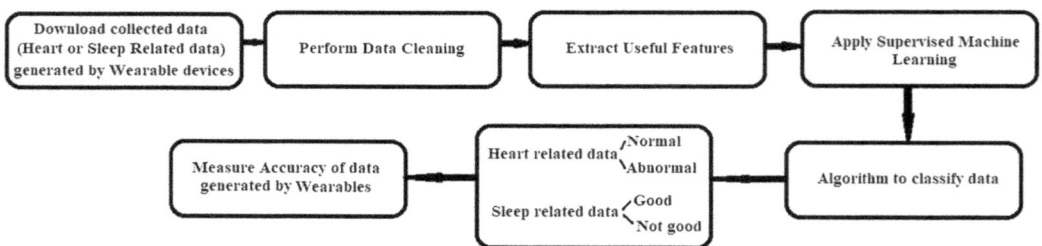

FIGURE 17.9 Proposed algorithm for efficient wearables.

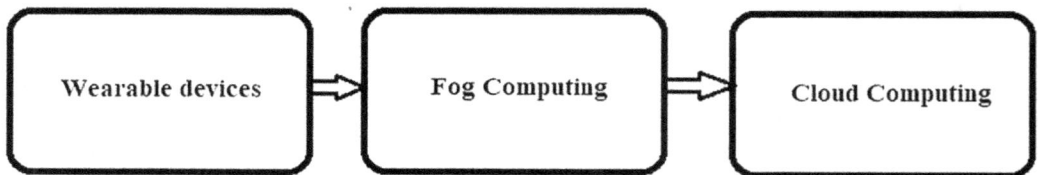

FIGURE 17.10 Storage concept in wearable technology.

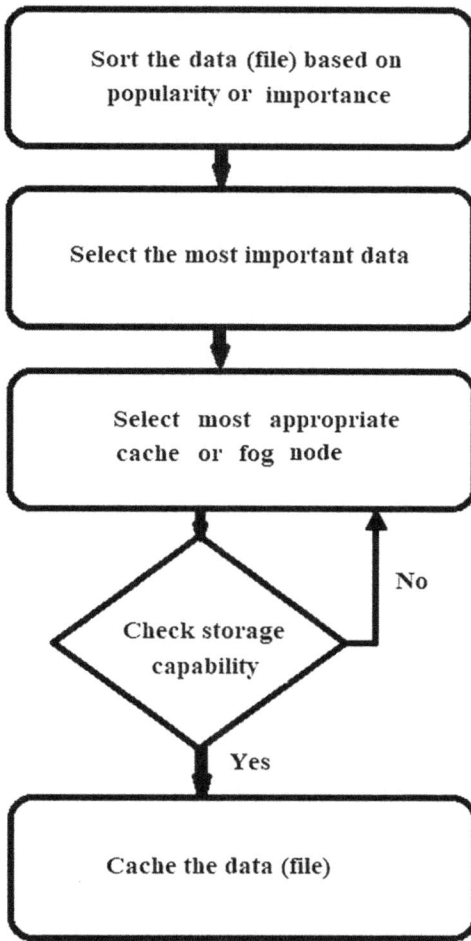

FIGURE 17.11   Proposed approach for storage in wearable technology.

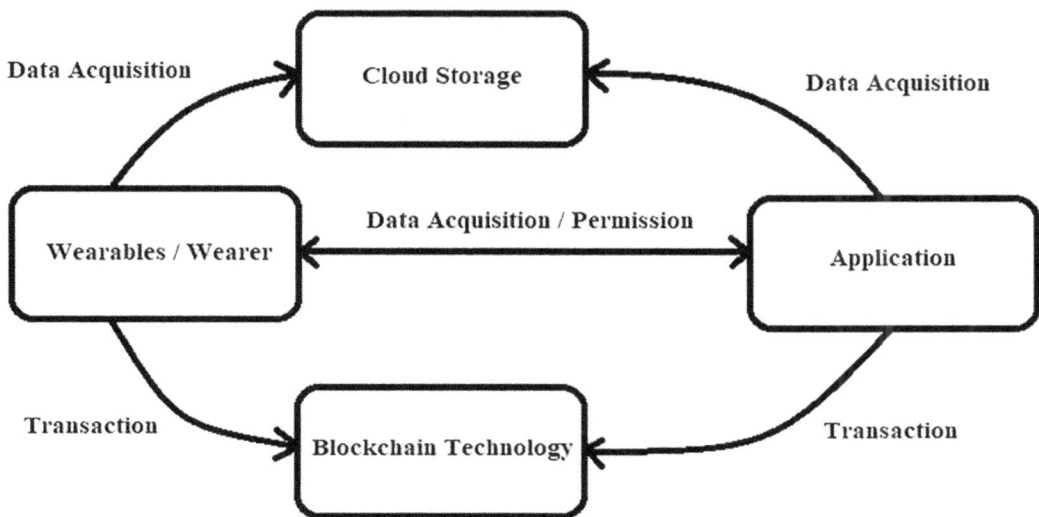

FIGURE 17.12   Proposed approach for blockchain integration for enhanced security.

17.7 CONCLUSION

Wearable technology has actually upgraded the level of comfort in our life. It has reduced the stress level by better connectivity, efficiency, security, performance, and optimization. Although wearable technology came into existence in the 15th century, its application has experienced a boom in the 21st century because of the pandemic. Here, in this chapter, some fundamental concepts of this technology have been discussed, such as history, key terms, and properties of wearable technology. After that, classification of wearables has been presented in two domains, categorization based on location of installation and then based on application areas. After that, future applications of wearable technology, along with advantages and disadvantages of wearable devices, are discussed in detail. This chapter basically provides a brief discussion about the awareness of wearable technology and its prospect future. Furthermore, it can be observed that this technology is having very wide utilization and integration in almost all domains of concerned with the rise of technology. Here, few approaches are proposed for some selected key issues of wearable technology which opens the doors of future work domains.

REFERENCES

[1] P. F. Binkley, "Predicting the Potential of Wearable Technology", *IEEE Engineering in Medicine and Biology Magazine*, pp. 23–27, May/June 2003.

[2] M. Kurwa, A. Mohammed, W. Liu, "Wearable Technology, Fashioning the Future", *Flextronics*, 2008.

[3] M. Ghahremani Honarvar, M. Latifi, "Overview of wearable electronics and smart textiles", *The Journal of the Textile Institute*, Vol. 108(4), pp. 631–652, 2017.

[4] M. Malmivaara, "The emergence of wearable computing", In: *Smart clothes and wearable technology*, McCann, J. & Bryson, D. (eds.). Cambridge, England: Woodhead publishing Ltd, pp. 3–24, 2009.

[5] E. Ackerman, "Google Gets in Your Face-Google Glass offers a Slightly Augmented Version of Reality", *Spectrum IEEE*, pp. 26–29, 2013.

[6] P. Bonato, "Advances in wearable technology and applications in physical medicine and rehabilitation", *Journal of Neuroengineering and Rehabilitation*, Vol. 2(1), pp. 1–4, 2005.

[7] P. Bonato, "Advances in wearable technology and its medical applications", 32nd Annual International Conference of the IEEE Engineering in Medicine and Biology Society, Vol. 2010, pp. 2021–2024, 2010.

[8] M. Çicek, "Wearable Technologies and Its Future Applications", *International Journal of Electrical, Electronics and Data Communication*, Vol. 3(4), pp. 45–50, April-2015.

[9] S. Brady, D. Diamond, B. Carson, D. O'Gorman, N. Moyna, "Combining wireless with wearable technology for the development of on-body networks", International Workshop on Wearable and Implantable Body Sensor Networks (BSN'06), IEEE, pp. 31–36, 2006

[10] Matthew J. Zieniewicz, Douglas C. Johnson, Douglas C. Wong, John D. Flatt, "The Evolution of Army Wearable Computers", *IEEE Pervasive Computing*, Vol. 1(4), pp. 30–40, October, 2020.

[11] Pragati Chaplot Jain, "Five Features to look for in wearable Devices", Sci-Tech, The Hindu, November, 2021. https://www.thehindu.com/sci-tech//article60042752.ece

[12] L. M. Baumann, "The Story of Wearable Technology: A Framing Analysis", Thesis submitted to Virginia Polytechnic Institute and State University, June 20, 2016.

[13] V. Ometov, L. Shubina, J. Klus, S. Skibińska, P. Saafi, L. Pascacio, D. Q. Flueratoru, N. Gaibor, O. Chukhno, A. A. Chukhno, "A survey on wearable technology: History, state-of-the-art and current challenges", *Computer Networks*, Vol. 193, July, 2021.

[14] S. Seneviratne, Y. Hu, T. Nguyen, G. Lan, S. Khalifa, K. Thilakarathna, M. Hassan, A. Seneviratne, "A Survey of Wearable Devices and Challenges", *IEEE Communications Surveys & Tutorials*, Vol. 19 (4), pp. 2573–2620, 2017.

[15] Y. Xue, "A Review on Intelligent Wearables: Uses and Risks", *Human Behavior and Emerging Technologies*, Vol. 1 (4), pp. 287–294, 2019.

[16] N. Niknejad, W. B. Ismail, A. Mardani, H. Liao, I. Ghani, "A Comprehensive Overview of Smart Wearables: The State of the Art Literature, Recent Advances, and Future Challenges", *Engineering Applications of Artificial Intelligence*, Vol. 90, Article 103529, 2020.

[17] P. J. Soh, G. A. Vandenbosch, M. Mercuri, D. M. P. Schreurs, "Wearable Wireless Health Monitoring: Current Developments", *IEEE Microwave Magazine*, Vol. 16 (4), pp. 55–70, 2015.

[18] B. Rhodes, "A Brief History of Wearable Computing", *MIT*, 2019, https://www.media.mit.edu/wearables/lizzy/timeline.html

[19] E. O. Thorp, "The Invention of the First Wearable Computer", Digest of Papers, Second International Symposium on Wearable Computers (Cat. No. 98EX215), IEEE, pp. 4–8, 1998.

[20] S. D. Guler, M. Gannon, K. Sicchio, "A Brief History of Wearables", *Crafting Wearables*, Springer, pp. 3–10, 2016.

[21] O. Amft, P. Lukowicz, "From Backpacks to Smartphones: Past, Present, and Future of Wearable Computers", *IEEE Pervasive Computing*, Vol. 8 (3), pp. 8–13, 2009.

[22] M. Lawo, O. Herzog, P. Lukowicz, H. Witt, "Using wearable computing solutions in real-world applications", *CHI'08 extended abstracts on human factors computing systems*, Florence, Italy: ACM, pp. 3687–3692, 2008.

[23] D. Curone, E. L. Secco, A. Tognetti, G. Loriga, G. Dudnik, M. Risatti, R. Whyte, A. Bonfiglio, G. Magenes, "Smart garments for emergency operators: the ProeTEX project", *IEEE Transactions on Information Technology in Biomedicine*, Vol. 14(3), pp. 694–701, 2010.

[24] J. Fortmann, M. Heiko, S. Boll, W. Heuten, "Illumee: Aesthetic Light Bracelet as a Wearable Information Display for Everyday Life", *UbiComp 2013*, pp. 393–396, 2013.

[25] H. Hartmann, T. Trew, J. Bosch, "The changing industry structure of software development for consumer electronics and its consequences for software architectures", *Journal of Systems and Software*, Vol. 85(1), pp. 178–192, 2012.

[26] G. Kortuem, Z. Segall, M. Bauer, "Contextaware, adaptive wearable computers as remote interfaces to 'intelligent' environments", *2012 16th International Symposium on Wearable Computers*, IEEE Computer Society, pp. 58, 2012.

[27] J. McCann, D. Bryson, "Smart Clothes and Wearable Technology", 1st ed., Oxford: Woodhead Publishing Limited, pp. 1–445, 2009.

[28] R. Paradiso, G. Loriga, N. Taccini, "A wearable health care system based on knitted integrated sensors", *IEEE Transactions on Information Technology in Biomedicine*, Vol. 9(3), pp. 337–344, 2005.

[29] S. Park, S. Jayaraman, "Enhancing the quality of life through wearable technology", *IEEE Engineering in Medicine and Biology Magazine*, Vol. 22(3), pp. 41–48, 2003.

[30] O. J. Muensterer, M. Lacher, C. Zoeller, M. Bronstein, J. Kübler, "Google Glass in pediatric surgery: An exploratory study", *International Journal of Surgery*, Vol. 12(4), pp. 281–289. 2014.

[31] A. Salman, "Wearable Computing Devices – Technology Features, Working and Evolution History", Electricalfundablog. https://electricalfundablog.com/wearable-computing-devices-technology/

[32] J. Nugroho, "A Conceptual Framework for Designing Wearable Technology", University of Technology Sydney, 2013.

[33] P. I. Okwu, I. N. Onyeje, "Ubiquitous Embedded Systems Revolution: Applications and Emerging Trends", *International Journal of Engineering Research and Applications*, Vol. 3(4), pp. 610–616, 2013.

[34] J. J. Rutherford, "Wearable Technology: Health-Care Solutions for a Growing Global Population", *IEEE Engineering in Medicine and Biology Magazine*, pp. 19–24, May/June 2010.

[35] D. Sanganee, "The effects of wearable computing and augmented reality on performing everyday tasks", *Research Topics in HCI*, pp. 1–15, 2013.

[36] X. Pu, L. Li, M. Liu, C. Jiang, C. Du, Z. Zhao, W. Hu, Z. L. Wang, "Wearable Self-Charging Power Textile Based on Flexible Yarn Supercapacitors and Fabric Nanogenerators", *Advanced Materials*, November 2015.

[37] X. Tao, "Wearable Electronics and Photonics", Cambridge: Woodhead Publishing Limited, 1st ed. pp. 1–244, 2005.

[38] H. P. Profita, "Social Acceptability of Wearable Technology Use in Public: An Exploration of the Societal Perceptions of A Gesture-Based Mobile Textile Interface", Georgia Institute of Technology, 2011.

[39] K. Watier, "Marketing Wearable Computers to Consumers: An Examination of Early Adopter Consumers' Feelings and Attitudes toward Wearable Computers", Georgetown University, 2003.

[40] LiveScience.com. 'Will Wearable Tech Bring Humanity A 'Sixth Sense?''. N. p., 2014. Web. 20 May. 2014. http://www.livescience.com/42490-wearable-biosensortechnology.html

[41] U. Anliker, J. A. Ward, P. Lukowicz, G. Troster, F. Dolveck, M. Baer, F. Keita, E. B. Schenker, F. Catarsi, L. Coluccini, A. Belardinelli, "AMON: a wearable multiparameter medical monitoring and alert system", *IEEE Transactions on Information Technology in Biomedicine*, Vol. 8(4), pp. 415–427, 2004.

[42] Samsung.com. 'Samsung Gear'. N. p., 2014. Web. 20 May, 2014. http://www.samsung.com/global/microsite/gear/gear2_features.html

[43] M. Di Rienzo, F. Rizzo, G. Parati, G. Brambilla, M. Ferrantini, P. Castiglioni, "MagIC system: a new textile-based wearable device for biological signal monitoring. Applicability in daily life and clinical setting", Annual international conference of the IEEE engineering in medicine and biology society, Shanghai, China. IEEE, pp. 7167–7169, 2005.

[44] S. Wilson, R. Laing, "Wearable Technology: Present and Future", Conference paper, 2018.

[45] U. Gollner, T. Bieling, G. Joost, "Mobile Lorm Glove: introducing a communication device for deaf-blind people", 6th international conference on tangible, embedded and embodied interaction, 2012 Kingston, Ontario, Canada. ACM, pp. 127–130, 2012.

[46] Rinkworks.com. 'Things People Said: Bad Predictions'. N. p., 2014. Web. 20 May, 2014. http://www.rinkworks.com/said/predictions.shtml

[47] M. Chan, D. Estève, J. Y. Fourniols, C. Escriba, E. Campo, "Smart wearable systems: current status and future challenges", *Artificial Intelligence in Medicine*, Vol. 56(3), pp. 137–156, 2012.

[48] S. Scataglini, G. Andreoni, J. Gallant, "A review of smart clothing in military", Workshop on wearable systems and applications, Florence, Italy. ACM, pp. 53–54, 2015.

[49] L. E. Dunne, "The Design of Wearable Technology: Addressing the Human-Device Interface through Functional Apparel Design", Cornell University, 2004.

[50] K. A. Popat, P. Sharma, "Wearable Computer Applications A Future Perspective", *International Journal of Engineering and Innovative Technology*, Vol. 3(1), pp. 213–217, 2013.

[51] Fred Coon, "Wearable Technology in the Workplace: Pros and Cons". https://stewartcoopercoon.com/wearable-technology-in-the-workplace-pros-and-cons/

[52] S. Duval, H. Hashizume, "Questions to Improve Quality of Life with Wearables: Humans, Technology, and the World," in 2006 International Conference on Hybrid Information Technology, Vol. 1, pp. 227–236, 2006.

[53] J. Lee, D. Kim, H. Y. Ryoo, B. S. Shin, "Sustainable Wearables: Wearable Technology for Enhancing the Quality of Human Life", *Sustainability* (8:5), p. 466, 2016.

[54] R. W. Picard, J. Healey, "Affective wearables", Vol. 1(4), pp. 231–240, Dec. 1997.

[55] A. Godfrey, V. Hetherington, H. Shum, P. Bonato, N. H. Lovell, S. Stuart, "From A to Z: Wearable technology explained", *Maturitas*, Vol. 113, pp. 40–47, 2018.

[56] T. Page, "A forecast of the adoption of wearable technology", *International Journal of Technology Diffusion*, Vol. 6 (2), pp. 12–29, 2015.

[57] P. Bush, "The craft of wearable wellbeing", Proceedings of the Third European Conference on Design4Health, Sheffield (2015), pp. 1–9, 13–16 July 2015.

[58] C. Wang, X. Guo, Y. Wang, Y. Chen, B. Liu, "Friend or foe? Your wearable devices reveal your personal pin", In Proceedings of the 11th ACM on Asia Conference on Computer and Communications Security, pp. 189–200, May, 2016.

18 Analysis of Cardiac Dynamics and Assessment of Arrhythmia by Classifying Heartbeat Using Electrocardiogram

Jayanthi Ganapathy
Sri Ramachandra Institute of Higher Education and Research, Chennai, India

Aunu Singhal
SRM Institute of Science and Technology, Delhi NCR Campus, Ghaziabad, Uttar Pradesh, India

Medha Raghavendra Prasad, Cheekireddy Dhamini, and Rishikesh Swaminathan
Sri Ramachandra Institute of Higher Education and Research, Chennai, India

CONTENTS

DOI: 10.1201/9781003333081-18

18.1 INTRODUCTION

Classification essentially takes a given set of data points and predicts which class the item belongs to. These classes are often referred to as targets or labels or even categories. The simplest example of classification is spam detection in electronic mail. It's an example of a binary classification where there are only two targets, namely, spam and not spam. The classifier understands how the given input variables are related to a particular class with the help of training data. Training the classifier is done by using the datasets that are already labelled and tested with a sample that is not seen by the machine (Jason Brownlee, 2020a, 2020b, 2020c). The machine-learning concepts of artificial intelligence were recently established in medical diagnosis. One such diagnosis investigated in this chapter is classification of arrhythmia. The source of data for this investigation is the MIT-BIH dataset acquired from Kaggle, consisting of ECG signals of 45 patients among which 19 were female of the age group 23–89 and 26 were male of the age group of 32–89. Initially, the ECG signals contained 17 classes out of which 15 classes were different types of vascular diseases. Pacemaker rhythm and normal sinus rhythm were among the remaining classes. These 17 classes were broadly classified into five classes, namely, supraventricular ectopic beats, non-ectopic beats, fusion beats, ventricular ectopic beats, and unknown beats. 360 Hertz was the frequency at which the ECG signals were recorded. Data was available in '.csv' format in Kaggle and was already pre-processed (Alfaras Miquel et al., 2019; Elgendi M, 2016).

The PTB-DB dataset consists of 549 ECG signal records from a total of 290 subjects whose age range was from 17 to 87. It consists of 209 men and 81 women whose mean age was 57.2 and 55.5, respectively. There are nine different classes: myocardial infarction, cardiomyopathy, myocarditis, miscellaneous, healthy controls, dysrhythmia, bundle-branch block, valvular heart disease, and myocardial hypertrophy. All these classes were broadly classified into two final classes, namely, normal and abnormal beats. Data was collected from Kaggle in '.csv' format, and pre-processing was already performed (Moody, 2001).

18.1.1 TYPES OF ARRHYTHMIAS

Arrhythmias can be broadly classified into four types: tachycardia, bradycardia, supraventricular, and ventricular arrhythmias. Tachycardia is when the heart rate is more than 100 beats per minute. When the heart rate is less than 60 beats per minute, it is called bradycardia, where the heart cannot pump enough blood to our body. Tachycardia in the atria is called supraventricular tachycardia. Tachycardia in the ventricles with rapid and regular contractions is called ventricular arrhythmia. The body does not receive enough blood because the ventricles contract before filling with blood completely. Depending on the type of arrhythmia, there are different treatments, such as lifestyles changes like exercising and quitting smoking, heart-related medications, or even machinea such as a defibrillator or a pacemaker that helps that heart to maintain a normal rhythm (Maciejewski M, 2017; Padmavathi 2015; Weimann, 2021).

18.1.1.1 ECG (Electrocardiogram) and the Different Types of Arrhythmic Heartbeats

A heartbeat is a result of the heart's electrical system. Each and every beat of the heart can be visualised with the help of ECG, which is a medical device that is used to monitor the heart's electrical activities. By analysing the pattern of electrical signals of each and every heartbeat, it is possible to detect heart abnormalities. The different types of heartbeats included in this project are supraventricular ectopic beats, ventricular ectopic beats, non-ectopic beats, fusion beats, and unknown beats. The type of heartbeats investigated in this study are shown in Table 18.1.

18.2 IMPLEMENTATION

The initial study started with the MIT-BIH arrhythmia dataset, which contained ECG signal waveforms in the form of a matrix. This dataset was used to classify different types of heartbeats in arrhythmia. And the PTB-DB dataset was used to make a general analysis on the different types of

TABLE 18.1
Type of Heart Beats

AAMI Heartbeat Class	N	S	V	F	Q
Description	Any heartbeat not in the S,V, F or Q class	Supraventricular ectopic beats	Ventricular ectopic beats	Fusion beat	Unknown beat
MIT-BIH heartbeat type	Normal beat (NOR)	Atrial premature beat (AP)	Premature ventricular contraction (PVC)	Fusion of ventricular and normal beat (IVN)	Packed beat (P)
	Left bundle branch block beat (LBBB)	Aberrated atrial premature beat (aAP)	Ventricular escape beat (VE)		Fusion of paced and normal beat (fPN)
	Right bundle branch block beat (RBBB)	Nodal premature beat (NP)			Unclassified beat
	Atrial escape beats (AE)	Supraventricular Beat (SP)			
	Nodal escape beat				

heartbeats. Both the datasets are originally available in Physionet. Additionally, both the datasets were pre-processed.

Once the datasets were obtained, a visual and descriptive analysis was performed on both of them. Later, a machine-learning classification model was built to assess the heart rhythm. KNN, SVM, and Random Forest were the models used in this project. All the models were evaluated based on different evaluation metrics, such as precision, recall, sensitivity, specificity, and f1 measure. Ada boosters and XGBoost were added with Random Forest Classifier to see if there would be any increase in the model's accuracy.

Neural network models, homogenous ANN and CNN, were also implemented. Few neural network assembling models like model capacity, stack ensemble, and ANN averaging were implemented to obtain the higher accuracy and to overcome over fitting and under fitting of the model.

All of these models were implemented on both MIT-BIH arrhythmia and PTB-DB datasets, both individually and combined. Model averaging one of the neural ensemble reduces variance in a final neural network model. The problem contains both multiclass classification and binary class problems, so softmax and sigmoid activation functions were used, respectively, in the output layer and categorical cross-entropy loss function to optimize the model and the efficient Adam flavour of stochastic gradient descent.

Model capacity was an MLP model with a single hidden layer that uses rectified linear activation function and the random weight initialization method. The output layer will use the softmax activation (multiclass) function to predict a probability for each target class. The number of nodes in the hidden layer will be provided via an argument called n nodes. The model will be optimized using stochastic gradient descent with a modest learning rate of 0.01 with a high momentum of 0.9, and a categorical cross-entropy loss function will be used, suitable for multiclass classification and binary cross entropy for binary class classification. Figure 18.1 shows the learning curve for five nodes with respect to loss. Similarly, Figure 18.2 shows the model's learning curve.

Stack ensemble is another neural ensemble model. The problem is a multiclass classification problem, and the model is fitted using a softmax activation function on the output layer. The model will expect samples with two input variables. The model then has a single hidden layer with 25 nodes and a rectified linear activation function, then an output layer with three nodes to predict the probability of each of the three classes and a softmax activation function. Because the problem is multiclass, categorical cross-entropy loss function is used to optimize the model and the efficient Adam flavour of stochastic gradient descent. The accuracy and other different evaluation metrics for all the models are shown in Table 18.2.

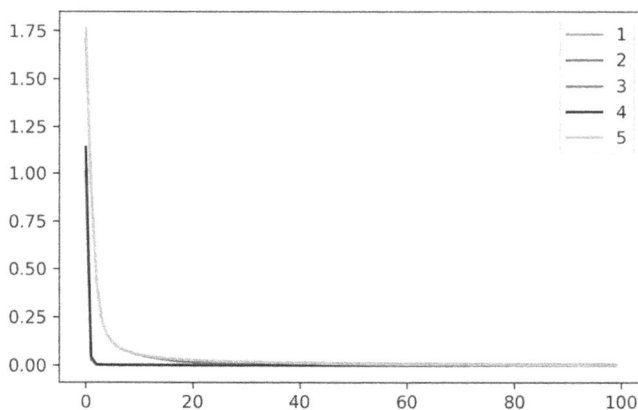

FIGURE 18.1 Modal capacity of MIT-BIH dataset with 5 number of epochs.

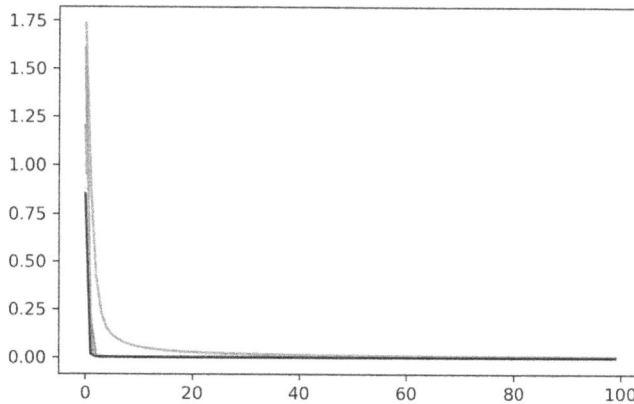

FIGURE 18.2   Modal capacity for the dataset MIT-BIH dataset with 10 number of epochs.

The accuracy and loss curve have been plotted for MIT-BIH and PTB-DB combined dataset. These curves can be very helpful as they determine the behaviour of any machine-learning model. The accuracy and loss curves for PTB-DB dataset has been shown below.

In the Figures 18.3 and 18.4, both validation and training accuracies are increasing, which means that the still capable of learning by increasing the number of epochs. The training loss is decreasing. Hence, it can be inferred that it has a good learning rate, and the gap between the training and validation loss is small, which makes our model a good one.

In the Figures 18.5 and 18.6, since the validation accuracy is below training accuracy, the model is slightly over-fitted as it is not that significant. Training loss shows improvement in learning, but there is a large gap between the validation loss and accuracy loss because of a class imbalance issue. Hence, noise was added to the ECG signals to get high accuracy.

In Figure 18.7 and Figure 18.8, both training and validation loss are a flat line. This indicates that our model is underfit and has the capability to learn more. Since the gap between the validation and training loss is very high, training dataset does not provide sufficient data to learn the problem.

Since the training accuracy is higher than validation accuracy, the model is over fitted.

TABLE 18.2
Accuracy of All the Models

Models	MIT-BIH	PTB-DB	MIT-BIH AND PTB-DB COMBINED
KNN	84.39%	91.14%	84.31%
SVM	83.98%	82.71%	90.63%
RANDOM FOREST	90.81%	95.95%	95.27%
VOTING CLASSIFIER	90.64%	93.84%	90.87%
ADA BOOST	58.57%	87.32%	47.15%
XG BOOST	93.54%	99.32%	99.42%
ANN	84.81%	94.78%	84.28%
CNN	98.78%	98.96%	99.04%
MODEL AVERAGING	76.8%	76.7%	76.9%
STACK ENSEMBLING	Train accuracy: 81.0% Test accuracy: 80.8%.	Train accuracy: 83.0% Test accuracy: 81.4%	Train accuracy: 86.0% Test accuracy: 81.5%

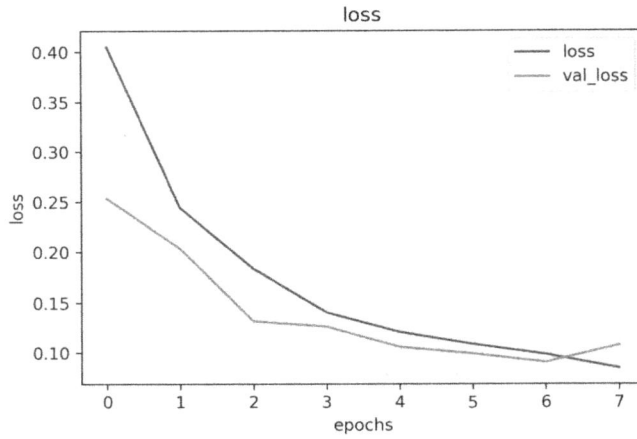

FIGURE 18.3   Accuracy and validation loss graph for PTBDB dataset.

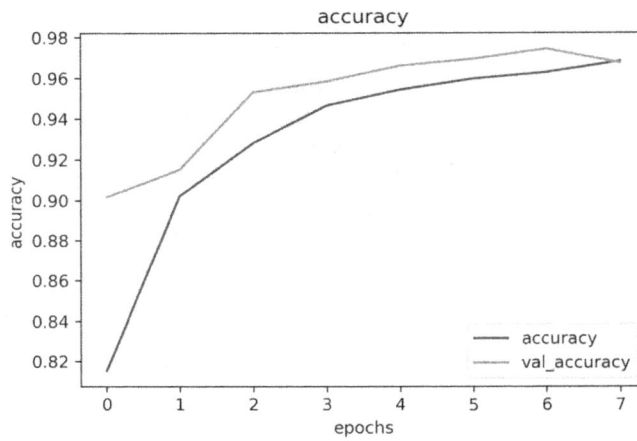

FIGURE 18.4   Accuracy and validation accuracy graph for PTBDB dataset.

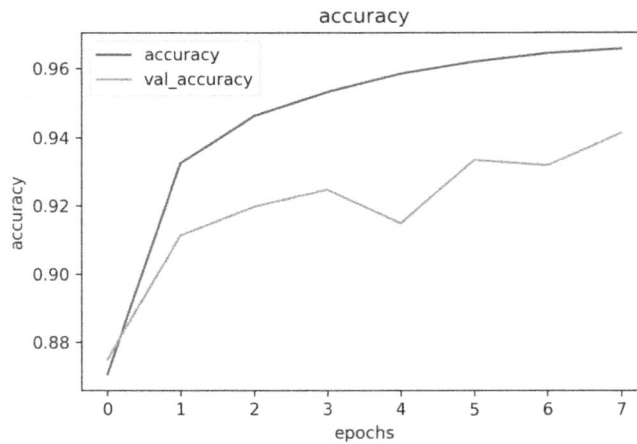

FIGURE 18.5   Accuracy and validation accuracy graph for MIT-BIH dataset.

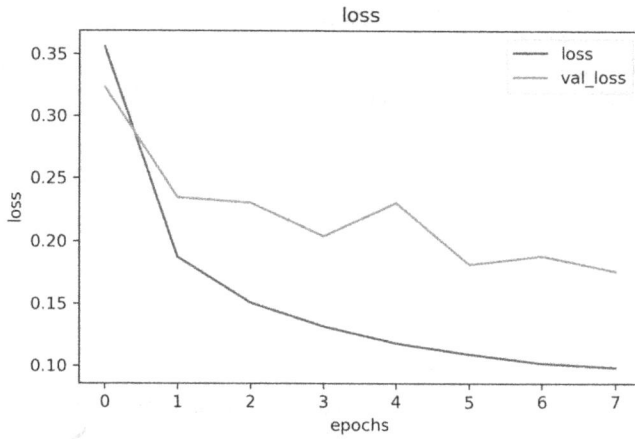

FIGURE 18.6 Accuracy and validation loss graph for MIT-BIH dataset.

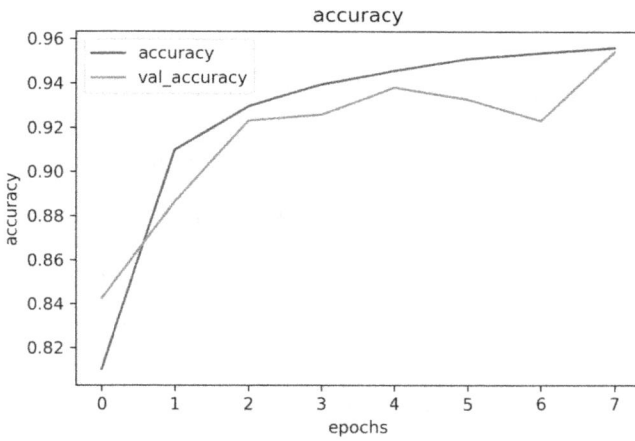

FIGURE 18.7 Accuracy and validation accuracy for MIT-BIH + PTBDB dataset.

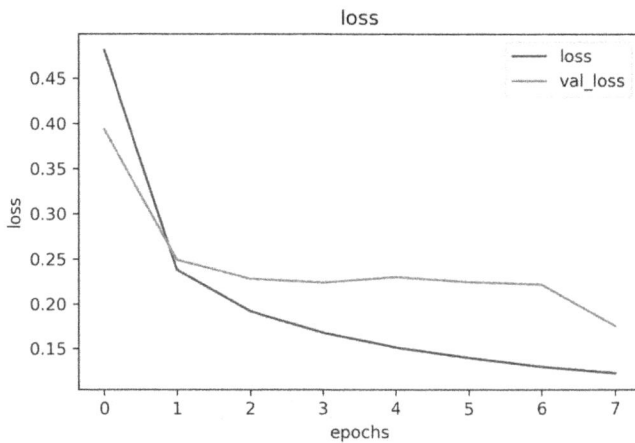

FIGURE 18.8 Loss and validation loss for MIT-BIH + PTBDB dataset.

18.3   VISUALIZATION AND DEPLOYING

After building the machine-learning and deep-learning models, Streamlit has been used to integrate the model, as a result creating a dashboard with a efficient UI/UX. This dashboard gives us the following:

- Dataset visualization
- About the dataset
- Information about the model
- Metrics from the model
- Heat map of the dataset

18.3.1   STREAMLIT

Open-source app framework is used to create web apps for data science and machine-learning web apps, which are compatible using Python. It comes with a well-designed UI/UX, which makes it easier for the developer to create a web app in a short time. Streamlit makes it easy to work on debugging and viewing the result in the web app.

18.3.2   CONTENTS OF THE DASHBOARD

18.3.2.1   Dataset Visualization

The dashboard contains the visualization for the datasets MITBIH and PTBDB. This section of the dashboard gives the better understanding of the classes present in the datasets. All the classes are explained and given a graph format.

From the given dataset, supraventricular ectopic beats have nearly 65000 datapoints, whereas unknown beats, abnormal beats, normal beats, ventricular beats, fusion beats, and non-ectopic beats have very a smaller number of data points, i.e., less than 10000, which leads to the unbalanced issue.

18.3.3   ABOUT THE DATASET

The dashboard displays exploratory data analysis that was done to understand the data, such as the shape, number of null values, number of classes, the ECG signal of different types of beats, and so on. There are mainly seven different classes present in the dataset, five classes from the MIT-BIH dataset and two classes from PTBDB dataset. Figures 18.9 through 18.15 show the ECG signals of different classes in 180 ms.

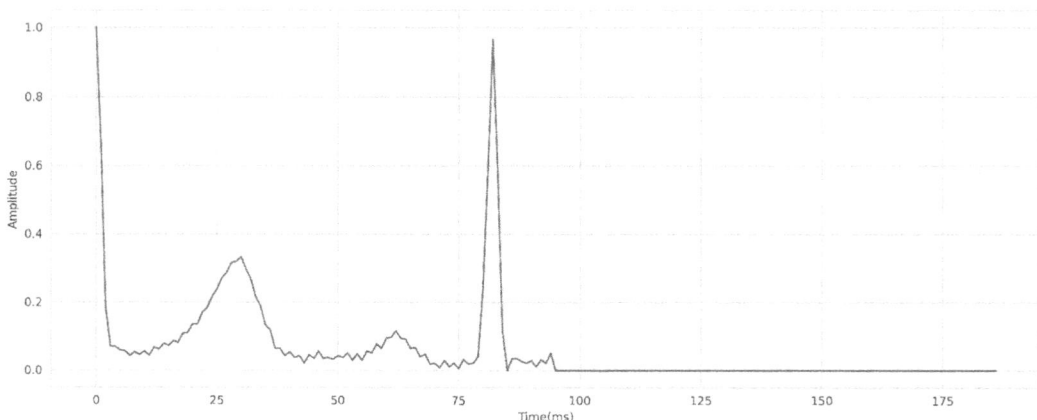

FIGURE 18.9   Ventricular ectopic beat.

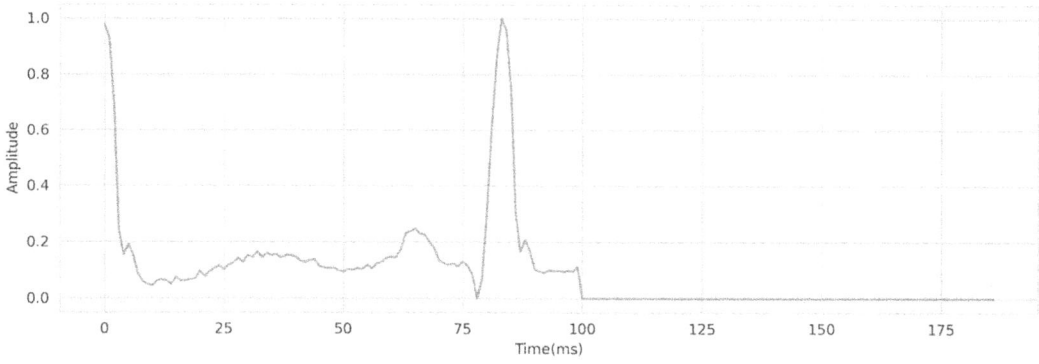

FIGURE 18.10   Non-ectopic beats.

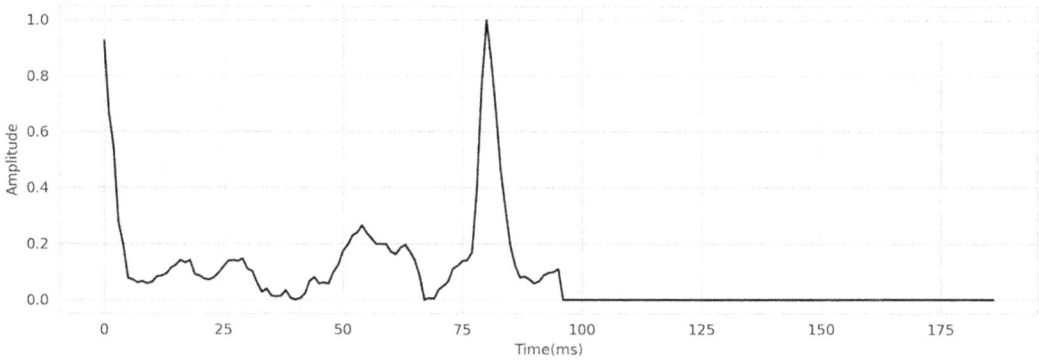

FIGURE 18.11   Fusion beats.

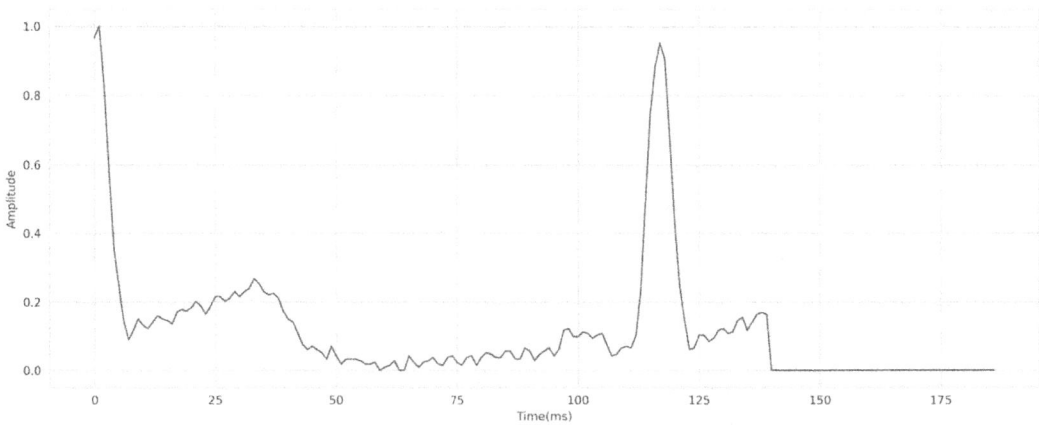

FIGURE 18.12   Unknown beat.

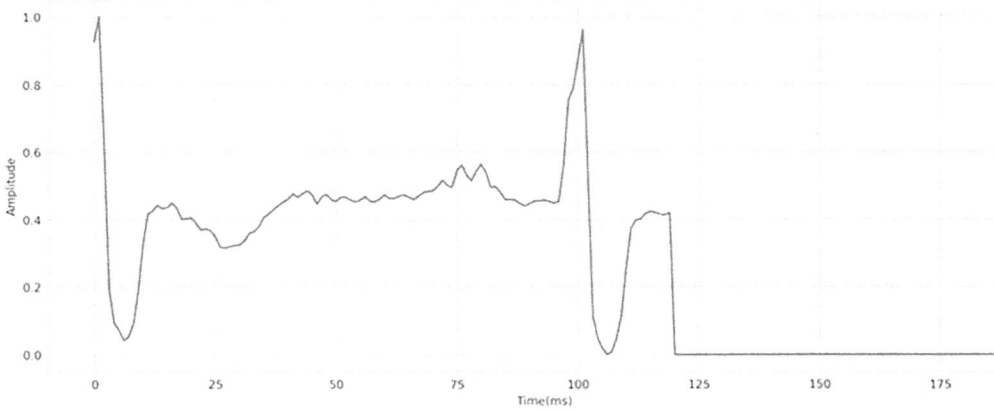

FIGURE 18.13   Abnormal beat.

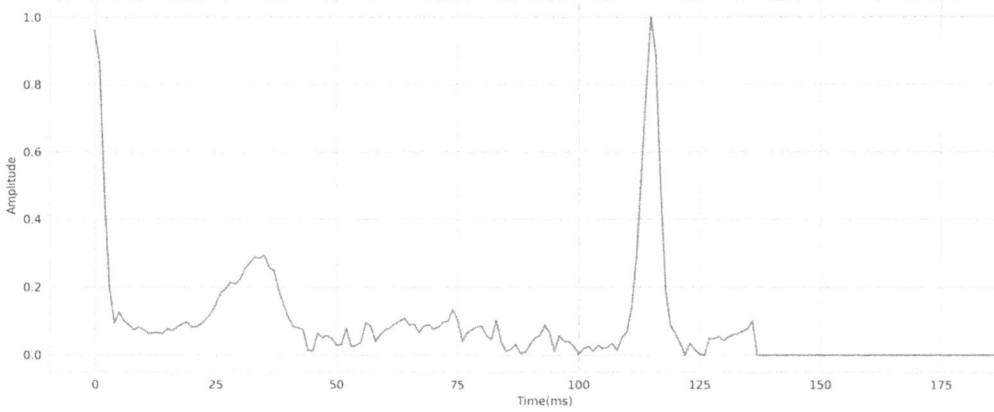

FIGURE 18.14   Normal beat.

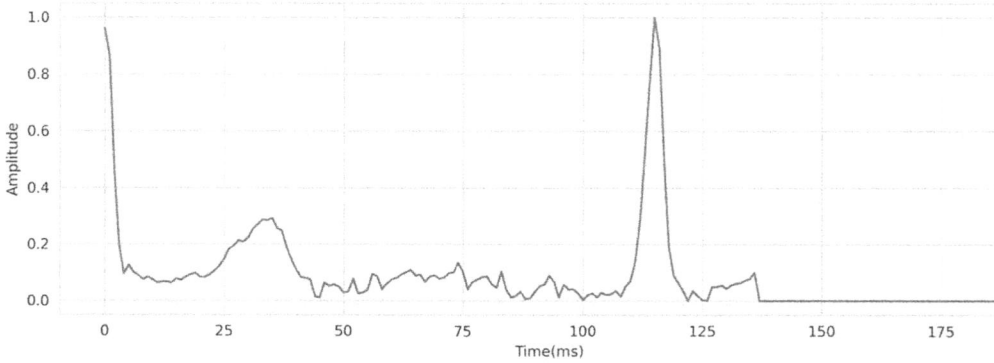

FIGURE 18.15   Supraventricular ectopic beats.

18.3.4   Information about the Model

As for the model, it displays the name of the algorithm that has been used. The accuracy score of the classification tells the user how accurate they will be using the current model. It also displays the confusion matrix, which tells the user about the classification with respect to the number of classes present. Finally, the classification report displays the metrics from the model. Figure 18.16 is the classification report for KNN algorithm.

Confusion Matrix of KNN:

	0	1	2	3	4
0	14371	71	55	17	19
1	111	315	4	0	0
2	65	3	1029	14	8
3	21	0	16	105	0
4	33	0	6	0	1248

Classification Report of KNN:

	Precison	Recall	F1-Score
0.0	0.9842	0.9889	0.9865
1.0	0.8098	0.7326	0.7692
2.0	0.9270	0.9196	0.9233
3.0	0.7721	0.7394	0.7554
4.0	0.9788	0.9697	0.9742
Accuracy	0.9747	0.9747	0.9747
Macro Avg	0.8944	0.8700	0.8817
Weighted Avg	0.9742	0.9747	0.9744

FIGURE 18.16   Classification report of KNN from dashboard.

18.3.5 METRICS FROM THE MODEL

Metrics are factors used to judge the progress of a machine-learning model. The metrics which are displayed in the dashboard are precision, recall, and F1-score

- Precision is the ratio between the true positives and all the positives. For our problem statement, that would be the measure of patients that we correctly identified as having an irregular heartbeat or arrhythmia out of all the patients actually having it. Mathematically, we can see in Equation 18.1. Precision also gives us a measure of the relevant data points. It is important that we don't start treating a patient who doesn't have a heart ailment, but our model predicted as having one.

$$P = \frac{TP}{TP + FP} \tag{18.1}$$

- The recall is the measure of our model correctly identifying true positives. Thus, for all the patients who actually have heart disease, recall tells us how many we correctly identified as having a heart disease. Mathematically, we can see in Equation 18.2.

$$R = \frac{TP}{TP + FN} \tag{18.2}$$

- F1-score metric uses a combination of precision and recall. In fact, the F1 **score** is the harmonic mean of the two as mentioned in Equation 18.3.

$$F1 = \frac{2}{\frac{1}{precision} + \frac{1}{recall}} \tag{18.3}$$

Equation 18.3: F1-Score (Figure 18.17).

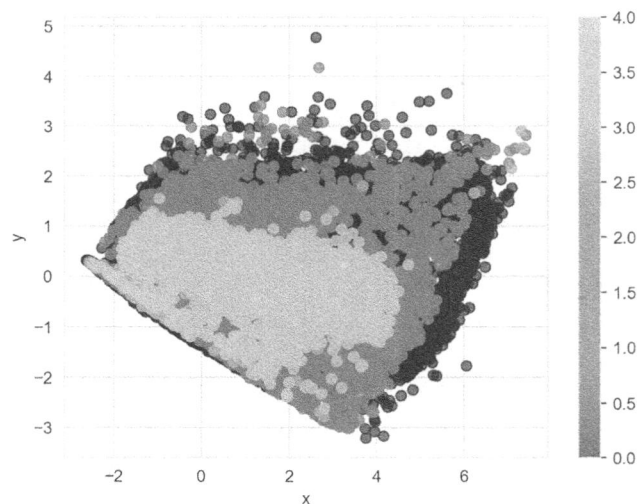

FIGURE 18.17 Heat map for MIT-BIH + PTBDB dataset.

18.3.6 MENU BAR

The menu bar is a well-designed horizontal slide-up window that allows the user to navigate and control through the dashboard and consists of five sections, as seen in Figure 18.18.

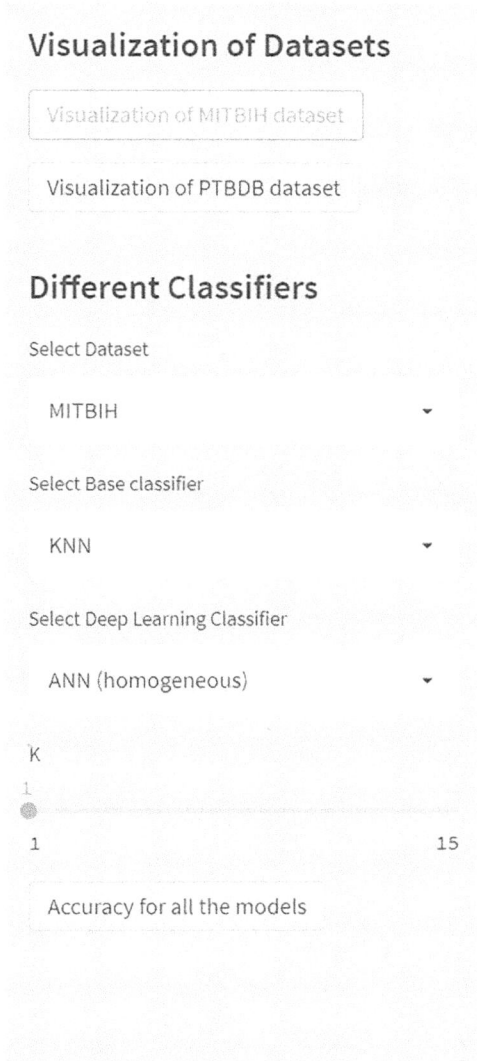

Visualization of Datasets

Visualization of MITBIH dataset

Visualization of PTBDB dataset

Different Classifiers

Select Dataset

MITBIH   ▾

Select Base classifier

KNN   ▾

Select Deep Learning Classifier

ANN (homogeneous)   ▾

K

1

1   15

Accuracy for all the models

FIGURE 18.18   Index bar for the dashboard.

18.3.7   SECTION – 1: VISUALIZATION OF DATASETS

In Figure 18.19, the dashboard allows the user to enter into different windows of the dataset visualization.

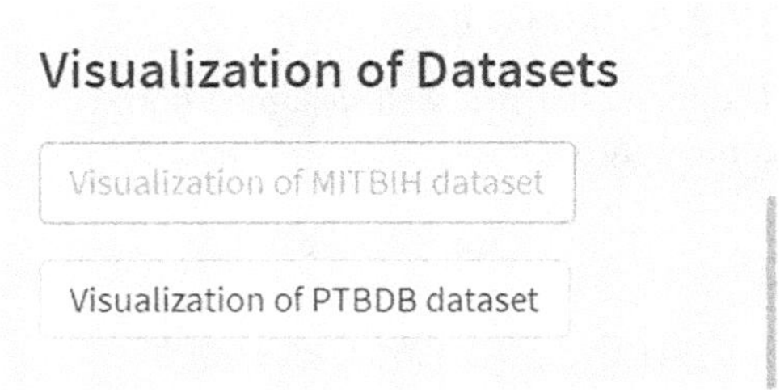

Visualization of Datasets

Visualization of MITBIH dataset

Visualization of PTBDB dataset

FIGURE 18.19   Buttons to select a dataset for exploratory data analysis.

18.3.8   SECTION −2: SELECTING DATASET

As seen in the window in Figure 18.20, the user can select the datasets to be used.

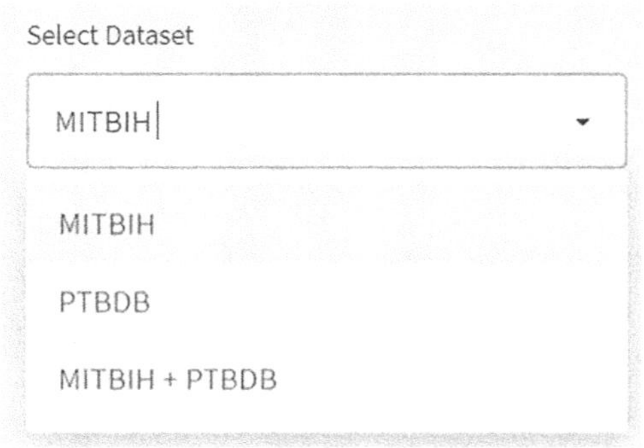

Select Dataset

MITBIH| ▾

MITBIH

PTBDB

MITBIH + PTBDB

FIGURE 18.20   Selecting dataset.

18.3.9   SECTION − 3: SELECTING BASE CLASSIFIER

As Figure 18.21 shows, the user can select the base classifier for the model.

Select Base classifier

KNN| ▾

KNN

SVM

Random Forest

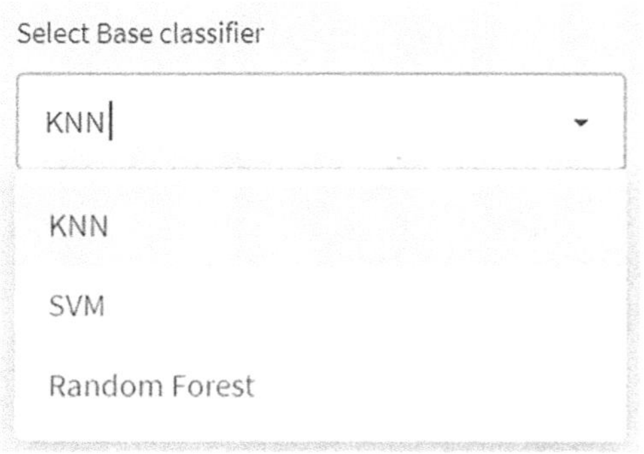

FIGURE 18.21   Selecting a base classifier.

18.3.10   SECTION − 4: SELECTING DEEP LEARNING CLASSIFIER

The user can also select a deep-learning classifier for the model, as seen in Figure 18.22.

Select Deep Learning Classifier

ANN (homogeneous)| ▾

ANN (homogeneous)

CNN

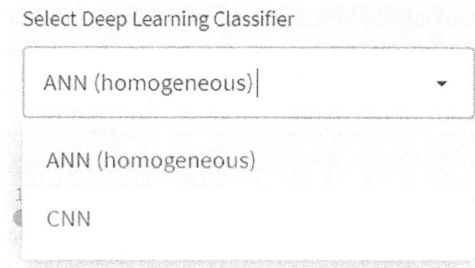

FIGURE 18.22 Selecting a deep-learning classifier.

18.3.11 SECTION – 5: PARAMETERS

Gives the user option to control the parameters of the classifiers, as seen in Figure 18.23.

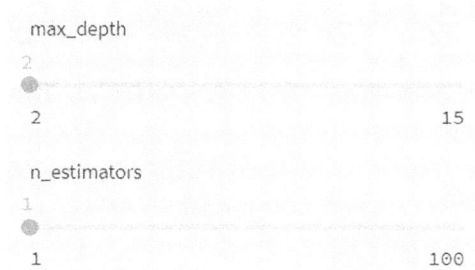

max_depth

2

2   15

n_estimators

1

1   100

FIGURE 18.23 Selecting parameters for Random Forest.

18.4 CONCLUSION

This chapter aims to investigage various machine-learning and deep-learning models and its applications in the analysis of cardiac dynamics. A combination of different models resulted in high accuracy. Three machine-learning models, SVM, k-NN, and Random Forest, reported average accuracy of 85.77%, 86.61%, 94.01% considering the MIT-BIH, PTB-DB, and combined datasets, respectively. Similarly, the average accuracy of three ensemble models viz., Xgboost, Adaboost, and Voting Classifier, reported accuracy of 97.42%, 66.34%, and 91.78%. The mean accuracy of two deep-learning models, ANN and CNN, is 87.95% and 98.92%, respectively, and neural net ensemble models, model averaging and stack ensemble, are 76.8% and 81.2%, respectively. In this investigation, all the models of CNN gave the highest accuracy for all the samples from the datasets. However, detection of anomalous ECG signals that are identifying the type of arrhythmias is left to work in future.

REFERENCES

Alfaras, M., Soriano, M. C., & Ortín, S., "A Fast Machine Learning Model for ECG-Based Heartbeat Classification and Arrhythmia Detection", *Frontiers in Physics*, 7, 2019.

Aziz, S., Ahmed, S., & Alouini, M. S. "ECG-based machine-learning algorithms for heartbeat classification", *Scientific Reports*, 11, 18738, 2021. 10.1038/s41598-021-97118-5

Brownlee, J., "Imbalanced Classification with Python_ Better Metrics, Balance Skewed Classes, Cost-Sensitive Learning", *Machine Learning Mastery*, 2020a.

Brownlee, J., "Deep Learning for Time Series Forecasting Predict the Future with MLPs, CNNs and LSTMs in Python", 2020b.

Brownlee, J., "Data Preparation for Machine Learning - Data Cleaning, Feature Selection, and Data", Machine learning mastery", 2020c.

Celin, S., & Vasanth, K., "ECG Signal Classification Using Various Machine Learning Techniques", *Journal of Medical Systems*, 42, 241, 2018. 10.1007/s10916-018-1083-6

Clifford, G. D. "ECG Statistics, Noise, Artifacts, and Missing Data", 2006. Dataset: https://physionet.org/content/mitdb/1.0.0/

Elgendi, M., "TERMA Framework for Biomedical Signal Analysis: An Economic-Inspired Approach", *Biosensors*, 6(4), 55, 2016. 10.3390/bios6040055

Elgendi, M., Meo, M., & Abbott, D., "A Proof-of-Concept Study: Simple and Effective Detection of P and T Waves in Arrhythmic ECG Signals", *Bioengineering*, 3(4), 26, 2016.

Fandango, A., "Mastering TensorFlow 1.x_ Advanced machine learning and deep learning concepts using TensorFlow 1.x and Keras", Packet Publishing, 2018

Moody, G. B., & Mark, R. G., "The impact of the MIT-BIH Arrhythmia Database", *in IEEE Engineering in Medicine and Biology Magazine*, 20(3), 45–50, May-June 2001, 10.1109/51.932724

Maciejewski, M., & Dzida, G., "ECG parameter extraction and classification in noisy signals," 2017 Signal Processing: Algorithms, Architectures, Arrangements, and Applications (SPA), 243–248, 2017, 10.23919/SPA.2017.8166872

Padmavathi, S., & Ramanujam, E., "Naïve Bayes Classifier for ECG Abnormalities Using Multivariate Maximal Time Series Motif", *Procedia Computer Science*, 47, 222–228, 2015, ISSN 1877-0509.

Rajesh, Kandala N. V. P. S., & Dhuli, R., "Classification of imbalanced ECG beats using re-sampling techniques and AdaBoost ensemble classifier", *Biomedical Signal Processing and Control*, 41, 242–254, 2018, ISSN 1746-8094.

Weimann, K., & Conrad, T. O. F. "Transfer learning for ECG classification", *Science Report*, 11, 5251, 2021. 10.1038/s41598-021-84374-8

Index

For Product Safety Concerns and Information please contact our EU
representative GPSR@taylorandfrancis.com
Taylor & Francis Verlag GmbH, Kaufingerstraße 24, 80331 München, Germany